Complete Physical Education Plans for Grades 7–12

Isobel Kleinman, MSEd

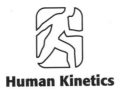

Human Kinetics

Library of Congress Cataloging-in-Publication Data

Kleinman, Isobel, 1946-
 Complete physical education plans for grades 7-12 / Isobel Kleinman.
   p. cm.
  ISBN 0-7360-3248-7
  1. Physical education and training--Study and teaching (Secondary) 2. Lesson plans. I.
Title.

 GV362 .K54 2001
 613.7'071'073--dc21

                                                        00-059787

 ISBN-10: 0-7360–3248-7
 ISBN-13: 978-0-7360–3248-3

Copyright © 2001 by Isobel Kleinman

Acquisitions Editor: Scott Wikgren; **Developmental Editor:** Katy M. Patterson; **Assistant Editor:** Amanda S. Ewing; **Copyeditor:** Jennifer Merrill Thompson; **Proofreader:** Joanna Hatzopoulos; **Permission Manager:** Courtney Astle; **Graphic Designer:** Robert Reuther; **Graphic Artist:** Dawn Sills; **Cover Designer:** Jack W. Davis; **Photographer (cover):** Tom Roberts; **Art Manager:** Craig Newsom; **Illustrators:** Tim Offenstein and Sharon Smith; **Printer:** Versa Press

Printed in the United States of America   10   9   8   7

Human Kinetics
Web site: www.HumanKinetics.com

United States: Human Kinetics, P.O. Box 5076, Champaign, IL 61825-5076
800-747-4457
e-mail: humank@hkusa.com

Canada: Human Kinetics, 475 Devonshire Road, Unit 100, Windsor, ON N8Y 2L5
800-465-7301 (in Canada only)
e-mail: info@hkcanada.com

Europe: Human Kinetics, 107 Bradford Road, Stanningley
Leeds LS28 6AT, United Kingdom
+44 (0) 113 255 5665
e-mail: hk@hkeurope.com

Australia: Human Kinetics, 57A Price Avenue, Lower Mitcham, South Australia 5062
08 8372 0999
e-mail: info@hkaustralia.com

New Zealand: Human Kinetics, Division of Sports Distributors NZ Ltd.
P.O. Box 300 226 Albany, North Shore City, Auckland
0064 9 448 1207
e-mail: info@humankinetics.co.nz

In memory of Rachel Liberman, whose smile on learning that this publication was a possibility will always be a happy memory.

Contents

PART IV   Team Sports Unit Plans 317

Please note that lesson plans for wrestling can be found on the CD-ROM accompanying this lesson plan book.

Acknowledgments

I do not suppose this book would have come to pass if not for several people whose ideals, teachings, and support inspired the process that has brought me to this point.

First, it all began with my parents. My mother, Hermina Kleinman, wanted the best for my sister and me and taught us to do our best, whatever the task and however it came about. My father, Dr. Sol Kleinman, supported my career choice and taught that a career is more than a way to make a living and that passion, competence, and professionalism are always more important than reward.

Then, I must thank the people who have shaped me as a teacher. First, my teacher, role model, and friend, Valerie Drake, for whom action and thought have always been part of the whole. For years and from far away places she has encouraged my growth as a teacher and convinced me to have this book published. Second, I must thank my students, especially those who have become friends, for it is they to whom I attribute my life-long love of teaching. Their effort, humor, and growing success kept me learning alongside them, gave me the confidence to write the book, and motivated my putting our lessons in print.

Finally, my thanks goes out to the people at Human Kinetics, particularly Scott Wikgren, Katy Patterson, and Amanda Ewing, whose input has improved the quality of this book.

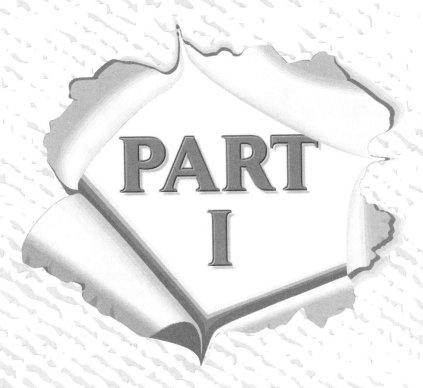

PART I

Introduction

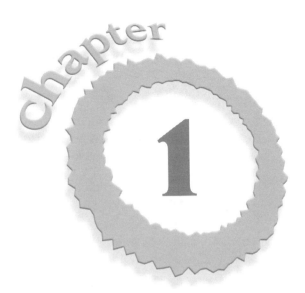

Teaching the Units

Well-thought-out units and lesson plans are as vital to quality education programs as a good road map is to a well-organized vacation. In either situation, without clear direction, you could end up getting lost. Maps help people plan a direct route. And this is what *Complete Physical Education Plans for Grades 7–12* sets out to do—give teachers a direct route to quality physical education. But even the best maps cannot avoid the detours along the way and the inevitable need to adapt to unanticipated conditions. Similarly, well-planned lessons cannot account for *all* variables. With this in mind, I do not detail each drill and demonstration. I do not expect you to follow the lessons exactly as described. In 31 years of teaching secondary physical education, I have yet to plan a unit or lesson that did not require some adjustment, and I suspect the same will be true for you. Sometimes I was lucky and had the time to plan the changes. More often, the need for change was triggered by a "think-on-your-feet" situation that occurred at the last minute.

So, fully aware of the need to make changes, and the national call for accountability in education, I have aimed to give you a comprehensive road map to quality secondary physical education as well as a tool for efficiently altering the map to suit your needs.

Flexibility

This text has been written to provide a solid foundation of highly developed skills progressions that integrate relevant cognitive concepts and comply with national standards, without prescribing all the how-tos. It is not that I'm shy. There are suggestions in this text. But I believe classes thrive when a teacher's creativity and individuality can flourish. Besides, detailed plans cannot be written

Detours on a Teacher's Map

Veteran physical educators know the many things that happen to cause a change in the best of lesson plans. For instance, here are some scenarios:

→ *The weather just won't cooperate.* Physical educators must consider the weather and be ready to adjust plans as necessary. Lessons written for large outdoor spaces must be modified when it rains or is too cold and teachers are forced indoors. The methods for teaching in large outdoor spaces are not practical for smaller ones.

→ *They cut my class time.* Class time is reduced even further when schools shorten classes to accommodate open school night, assembly programs, in-school field trips, fire drills, and pep rallies.

→ *My principal asked me to drop physical education for a few days and teach the state-mandated bus drill and AIDS lecture.* You had planned to end the unit on the 10th lesson—then your administrator tells you to drop physical education to do something else for a few days. Now you'll have to figure out how to finish up the unit and also change the intervening lessons.

→ *I planned a test, but only 10 kids showed up.* Your class suddenly shrinks, but not before you planned to introduce something new, run a tournament, or have a quiz. You're all ready, but only half the class shows up. The other half is on a field trip.

→ *I got to the gym and couldn't use it.* You arrive to meet your class and find you have no place to work because the custodian has decided to change the light bulbs in the middle of the gym floor during your class. Or the grounds crew has decided to mark the field for an interscholastic game. Or a group took over the gym for a blood drive or to decorate for the junior prom. Whatever the reason, the space you had planned for is not available.

→ *My eighth-period class is three lessons behind.* Your classes at the same grade level are like night and day. In one period they are highly mature and skilled; another class later in the day is difficult to keep on task and has much weaker skills.

No lesson plan can cover all these contingencies. All you can do is plan the ideal lesson and then be ready to switch gears.

without knowledge of class size, length of teaching period, kind of facilities and equipment available, level of student experience, and class climate.

The lessons in this text are terrific teaching tools. They give physical educators a clear starting point, encourage the educational use of every minute of the teaching period, and draw that map to quality physical education that everyone hopes to follow.

The CD-ROM in this book allows you to use your own style, pace lessons to meet your classes' needs, use drills that work the best for your students, and end up with customized lesson plans you can print out. With technology, customizing and storing lessons become easy. You can pull up lessons on the screen and then modify and save them for later use. Even the quizzes, handouts, checklists, tournament charts, and skill assessment rubrics are on CD-ROM. Everything is there for you to customize to your needs. Since the chapters are modular and the units are written by experience level, their menu format allows you to pick and choose the right units and lessons for your situation. If you have students who are new to an activity, use the beginner unit. If your students have some experience, move up to the next level in the chapter. Any of the units can easily be added into your existing curriculum or used as building blocks for developing a new curriculum.

Meeting National Standards

While the units and lessons in this book are meant to be flexible, they have a clear direction—to meet the national physical education standards developed by the National Association for Sport and Physical Education (NASPE). Chapter 2 outlines the standards for you and shows how units, lessons, and assessment tools are designed for compliance. If you would like a copy of *Appropriate Instructional Practice—Appropriate Practices for Middle School (or High School) Physical Education*, the document is available from the American Alliance for Health, Physical Education, Recreation and Dance (AAHPERD) at P.O. Box 17040, Baltimore, MD 21298. Their Web address is **www.aahperd.org**.

The Unit Plan Format

Each activity chapter follows a unit plan strategy. Unit introductory material for each activity includes a unit overview listing what will be covered. The unit introductory material also contains teaching tips, facility setup, safety issues, a timeline, assessment tips, and additional resources specific to each activity. Lessons for a range of experience levels and a student portfolio checklist follow this introductory material. After the lessons, quizzes and answer sheets appear. Each unit follows the same format, providing an easy template from which to work.

Unit Overview. The overview outlines the skills, rules, and strategies planned within the lessons from the beginner's level to advanced.

Handout. The second page of many chapters consists of a handout that can be copied from the book or customized on the CD-ROM and printed out. These handouts can be shared with students and parents. Each unit handout includes a brief history, fun facts, benefits of the activity, and Web sites to visit. (The Web site addresses were correct at the time of printing.) Use these fun handouts to stimulate students' interest and to enrich their knowledge.

Unit Extension Project. According to *Appropriate Practices for Middle School (or High School) Physical Education*, appropriate homework consists of learning experiences that occur outside of class and reinforce skills and knowledge acquired within. The third page of most chapters consists of a homework sheet that instructs students to explore each activity. These Unit Extension Projects are designed to help students apply what they learn in class to their real lives out in the community after they graduate. Exploring each sport beyond what is taught in class will help students select a sport or activity as a lifetime activity. I suggest that these projects be assigned early in the units with due dates set toward the end of each unit.

Teaching Tips. This section contains suggestions for implementing the lessons successfully. Included are special considerations that should be anticipated and addressed before beginning the unit as well as unique suggestions that enable medically excused students to be involved in class.

Unit Setup. This section lists specific equipment needs for the unit and spells out how the gym, fields, and outdoor facilities need to be modified to conduct the unit.

Unit Safety. Some units contain specific safety information that generally applies throughout the lessons in the unit. Other units include safety information specific to particular lessons within the lesson plans themselves.

Unit Timeline. This section covers the number of lessons contained in each level and summarizes the main focus of the lessons.

Unit Assessment. This section guides teachers in assessing students and explains which tools to use to assess the students for each unit.

Additional Resources. Each unit contains a list of additional resources, which are among the best available in helping teachers understand the skills to be taught and supplying supplemental ideas for other drills and drill variations.

Student Portfolio Checklist. Student portfolio checklists are included in the unit introductory material as a kind of assessment tool for students' assessment of themselves. These provide a summary of the skills that should be learned for each unit. Students can check what they learned and keep a cumulative record. The checklist identifies broad categories of skills, rules, activity responsibilities, and strategies, grouping them in no particular sequence or priority. The checklist is not a teacher's tool but a personal student record of learning experience.

Performance Assessment Rubrics. You'll find performance rubrics at the end of each unit. Rubrics identify the most important skills for an age level and then break them down into parts to make it easier for you to evaluate progression of accomplishment. Rubrics can be used for self-assessment, peer assessment, or teacher assessment.

Quizzes. Short quizzes located at the end of each chapter are included for each activity at each experience level. Recalling my first attempts at test writing and grading, I have tried to save you from the nightmare of writing tests that take all night to grade. Imagine grading one test at a time from a stack of 400 plus and needing to have grades in the next day. Bad idea. Good teachers need sleep. With that in mind, I've written quizzes that should take no longer than 10 minutes for students to complete and that can be graded by a scanner.

Testing in Class

There are inherent problems in giving tests in a gym. First, anticipate that students will forget they are taking a test and come with no pen or pencil. Or they'll put their pencils down when the games get underway, and the pencils get lost. It's best to keep the pencils yourself, distribute them at quiz time, and collect them with the quizzes. Second, you will have students with special needs. The kind of individual planning for testing students with special needs is spelled out in a student's Individualized Education Program (IEP). The IEP should let you know the kind of testing situation that works best for the student. He might need extended time, a reader, a writer, or a keyboard. Decide with the student (along with his special education teacher) how you will deal with his or her needs. It might be impossible for you to coordinate all the students' needs and still manage the class. If this is the case, plan to let the students take the test with everyone else, but then deliver it, complete or not, to their resource room teacher for completion. Be aware that students frequently do not admit to needing such service, especially in front of peers. When they do not tell you their special needs, it's up to you to determine what is needed.

Scope of the Lessons

Lessons are progressive and grouped by experience level. For a progression to be meaningful, the lessons should be followed in sequence. But since grade levels are combined, you need not cover all *new* material in one grade. However, when dividing a unit's lessons to continue them at the next grade level, I recommend limiting the number of introductory skills planned in the earlier lessons and saving them for the next year so as not to compromise game time. It is important that skills be used in a game situation as early as possible so that they become relevant and so that improvement occurs in the context in which the skills will be used. Also, student motivation is a great deal higher when students are involved in playing rather than just practicing drills.

The Lesson Plan Format

The following paragraphs provide an overview of the lesson plan format, which includes nine sections: Lesson Setup, Performance Goals, Cognitive Goals, Lesson Safety, Warm-Ups, Motivation, Lesson Sequence, Review, and Assessment.

Lesson Setup

This section describes how to arrange facilities and equipment for the lesson. Once a lesson's setup and equipment needs are clear, this section will vanish from the lesson plan until a new arrangement or additional equipment is needed.

Performance Goals

These are the specific activity goals of the lesson. Fitness is the general, unspecified goal of every lesson. Lessons are designed to keep students active in an attempt to develop and maintain physical fitness. Fitness is a major goal and expected by-product of every lesson. That is why the lessons are designed to increase students' knowledge without compromising their active time.

Cognitive Goals

These are the knowledge goals of the unit. They can include concepts, facts, or understandings that enrich the learning experience and encourage critical thinking. They can be specifics of the sport—such as rules and strategies—or scientific physical principles that affect the degree of success in that sport. They may also involve psychosocial factors such as students learning to be responsible citizens, to be realistic about their selves and their teammates, to take initiative, and to assume leadership roles.

Cognitive material should take no more than a few minutes at a time to teach. Sometimes, for convenience, you'll read in one place all the material that you'll share with the class for the lesson. This does not mean that you should deliver all the information to students at once. Restrict cognitive material to a few relevant bites at a time. Explanation should not replace participation.

Along the same lines, while using teachable moments to enhance students' understanding, avoid stopping the whole class to share what happened. Instead, seize the moment, coach the individual, and if the issue is important enough for the whole class, share it later during the review or during introductory remarks in the next lesson.

Lesson Safety

The old adage that an ounce of prevention is worth a pound of cure holds true in physical education. This section will help you prevent accidents before they happen and alert you to factors that may affect the emotional environment of the class. As all physical education teachers know, even the best-planned lesson can leave room for unhealthy social dynamics. The safety tips provided should help you recognize and remedy problems before they get out of hand.

Warm-Ups

Warm-ups in this text serve two purposes. First, they increase the heart rate to get blood flowing, and they prepare the body for activity. Second, warm-ups begin the student's learning process through the use of mimetic exercises. The use of mimetics, which consist of mimicking motions, is a great way to begin teaching new skills and reinforcing movement memory. Essentially, mimetics is the re-hearsal of skills used in a game outside of their usual context and in the absence of a ball. (They can be done using rackets.) By practicing mimetics, students develop the proper kinesthetic feel of complex movements after a step-by-step introduction to the total movement pattern. Mimetics will be thoroughly explained later in this chapter.

Motivation

This section suggests ways to help students see how the lesson is relevant to them and encourages them to be involved at their best level. Used correctly, motivation widens students' perspectives and stimulates their excitement. Your motivational remarks may come from current events, sports records, game strategies, scientific principles, class standings, or personal stories. I've shared some of my stories throughout the book, but try to include stories of your own. The personal touch is usually more successful and warming to students.

Power of Motivation

The ability to motivate can change everything, as it did for me when introducing a dance unit to a class filled with macho eighth-grade boys who did *not* want to dance. One day, when our class time was reduced and too short to get geared up for activity, I showed a video of the major dance scenes from the film *White Knights*. As the video played, I saw how dazzled everyone was at a point in the story when Mikhail Baryshnikov performed 10 pirouettes, challenging his tap-dancing security supervisor to do the same. I replayed the scene. Students loved it. I played the segment again and then asked my class how many pirouettes they could do. From that moment on, teaching dance to that group of students became easier. The boys began to see dance as an athletic endeavor, difficult and worthy of their attention.

Lesson Sequence

This section lists a successful progression for teaching new skills and introducing cognitive concepts in such a way that the class keeps moving. The sequence incorporates awareness of rules, strategies, laws of motion, and socialization in small bits that are relevant to the action of the day and easy for students to learn without causing too much activity downtime.

Review

Here I include suggestions for things to talk about at the end of the lesson. It's best to ask students questions that emphasize important aspects of the lesson. This will get them thinking and let you know how well they understood the lesson.

Assessment

Each lesson requires assessment so you can evaluate student accomplishment and get the information you need to refine lesson plans. Evaluation helps you learn the precise needs of your students so you can adjust your lessons to meet their needs. This requires close observation. You must evaluate if students are reaching your goals for them and decide what to do next. This is particularly necessary during early lessons. Students who are not acquiring the basic fundamentals will need more time. If the class moves on too quickly, many students will become frustrated and stop trying. Wait until most students (90 percent) get it. When necessary, set new, more realistic goals before moving ahead. When the class is ready and just a few students need help, start the next lesson and provide more individualized attention to the few who need it.

Assessment also provides a basis for grading. While some teachers like to get a head start, teach a skill, and grade it a few days later, I like to keep in mind that learning paces differ. I recommend delaying performance assessment until the end of the unit. Students who experience early difficulty in picking up skills can become extraordinary with a little patience and practice.

This Text's Unique Approach

This text does not include specific methodologies, but it does have teaching biases that make it unique. Each bias is a result of my educational philosophy and my many years of experience teaching adolescent boys and girls.

I believe in the Greek ideal—a balanced body and mind. And I believe a physical educator's primary responsibility is to help students learn to be active; therefore maintaining constant class activity is a high priority in my lessons. But since action without thought is not a good idea, this text's lessons integrate thinking and skill while emphasizing movement. This is done by imparting information in small bits so that the student's physical activity does not stop for more than a few minutes at a time. In this way, lessons are weighted to action, not talking, and students have a chance to assimilate the meaning in relevant bits. Needless to say, in writing this text, I have incorporated a teaching style consistent with my desire for lots of activity. First, I always plan for free play (instant activity), an important aspect of my classes. Then I incorporate mimetics in my warm-up.

Instant Activity

Equipment should be out, and the teacher on the gym floor while students are dressing. This enables the students who dress more quickly to practice or play short games with friends before the formal start of class. It also encourages the others to hurry up, since the sitting-and-waiting factor common to so many physical education classes is eliminated. Many colleagues might fear the free atmosphere, believing that discipline problems will increase and that they could not control their classes. But, they are wrong to worry. Allowing free play (instant activity time) motivates students to change quickly and to take advantage of time to play. Plus, free play is educationally productive.

Students are more relaxed when practicing with friends in informal settings. They can learn and improve without worrying about where they rank in comparison to others. They also have easier access to personal attention from their teacher. Also, the free-play period provides an excellent opportunity for teachers to work with individuals who are having difficulty without making them feel singled out. If everyone else is busy playing with friends, the person you're helping does not feel that he is drawing negative attention to himself. His classmates are too involved with their own activity to notice.

Though I often call the instant activity time "free play," there are certain rules. Students are responsible for picking up equipment and using it properly. It generally takes very little encouragement to get students running in, taking some equipment, and practicing or playing. A rack of basketballs disappears in no time. Students come onto the floor, ready to practice with the equipment of the day, be it volleyballs, pickleballs, shuttlecocks, soccer balls, or softball gloves and balls. For dance, just leave "The Electric Slide" on and see how fast the students "slide" in the door to music and begin their warm-up.

In 31 years of teaching, I have found that if there's enough equipment for everyone, both time and equipment are meaningfully used during free play. Rarely have I encountered discipline problems. However, some students fool around inappropriately. If they do, I find correcting their behavior immediately and giving them a chance to do the right thing will move them in the right direction. They become cognizant of their actions and learn to become better class citizens. Experience has taught me that with a patient but firm hand, even the most difficult student appreciates the latitude of free play and learns to be a responsible member of class.

Mimetics

Using mimetics for the warm-up phase of a physical education lesson has been used here to accomplish several things. The idea came to me some years ago when, frustrated with the brevity of class time and motivated to get the most out of every learning opportunity, I started teaching movement patterns before the game, before giving out equipment, before I even knew what to call what I was doing. It was a reaction born out of observation. Students were having a tough time developing a correct bump pass in volleyball. Drills that had been successful in other classes simply did not work with them. They needed something more fundamental. And that is how I started using mimetics.

Mimetics are exercises that mimic skills. During mimetic exercises, students mime game-playing skills, without words and without the ball. Mimetics can begin and fortify the learning process while they increase blood flow and warm up muscles. When mimetics are used as part of the warm-up, the time spent is both educationally profitable and physically beneficial. What makes me such an advocate of them is that since their incorporation in my class routine, students have had real performance gains in half the time. The best part is seeing the pleasure students get from being able to do something they did not think they knew how to do. Because mimetics are so easy to perform, complex movement patterns quickly become natural and flowing. They can be used to build correct movement patterns for many skills: the football throw, chest pass, overhead throw, lay-up shot, bump pass, set, spike, block, rebounding, tennis serve, in fact, any action that requires timing and coordination. When repeated correctly, mimetics make movement patterns routine, comfortable actions, easily transferable from completing a simple exercise to using the ball and playing the game.

All told, the results have motivated my continued use of mimetics whenever possible. What follows is an example of how I would use mime in a basketball lesson when the performance goal is rebounding.

First, I do *not* explain the purpose of my instructions; I just get them moving correctly from the start. Once the whole pattern is put together, I give it a name. This takes no time from the physical activity. I start out by simply asking the class to follow me while I guide the activity, giving them movement cues and voice calls that keep them moving while I continue to increase the complexity of what they are doing, a little at a time. This is done by pacing commands like a square-dance call. As they finish one, I introduce the next. Each should be done two to five times:

"Jump as high as you can. Let's do it together. Ready, jump."
"Jump, but this time reach your hands up as high as possible when you're in the air."
"While you're up there, make sure the palms of your hands face each other—now jump."
"This time *stretch* those arms as high as you can. Imagine them grabbing a ball out of the air."
"Land with spread feet, so they take up lots of space."
"Bring your arms down with the imaginary ball in your hands."
"Come down from your jump with spread feet and elbows out."

When I finish, I ask, "Who can tell me what we are practicing?" Students are now warmed up and can be taken directly into the motivation aspects of the lesson.

The next time class meets, all you need to say is, "Let's do 10 jumps to rebound." The students can follow you or a student leader while either of you lead the exercise, everyone following in unison. When students are ready for more complexity, ask them to "move in to rebound." With verbal cues, guide them a few steps forward, telling them to take steps to get to that "imaginary position" in front of the rim and inside the basketball key. (Have them each pick a spot on the ground a few feet in front of them as their imaginary spot.) The class can be instructed to run to their spot, jump straight up, and, when they come down, look at the spot they jumped from. Did they land in the same place they took off from? Expect to hear "no." Try again and ask them again. "No." Ask them to try running to the spot, jumping, and coming straight down so this time they are landing where they left the ground. Again, do a spot check to see if they landed in the same place they took off from. The exercise and the checking provide feedback about their bodies' momentum. When the exercise is done, you have warmed up the class, taught them a new skill, enhanced their basketball technique and knowledge, taught biofeedback, introduced a lesson in avoiding loose-ball fouls when rebounding, and taught it all without specific explanation, which will follow during the motivation or the procedural part of the lesson.

Of course, this one example is not meant to represent a full warm-up. Warm-ups should include other mimetics, too. For instance, during basketball alone, mimetics can contribute to success in skills such as pivoting, shooting, stopping, guarding, making jump shots, doing lay-ups, and turning to shoot. The warm-up should also target exercises for the abdominals and for stretching. Students should stretch after they have raised their heart rate. For efficiency, students can stretch (once they learn the proper form) while you do the motivation part of the lesson.

Drilling for Skill Acquisition

For the most part, lessons here aim to introduce one new thing at a time and allow students to feel comfortable before going on. However, to keep interest up, muscle-fatigue down, and the learning curve rising, several fundamental skills can be combined and practiced, even in early lessons. For instance, if kicking a ball is the objective, the exercise must also include trapping the ball. The receiving partner needs to stop the ball so she can kick it back. If the lesson is throwing, catching needs to be included as well. Also, since it's unwise to repeat the same motion an entire period, you might add another skill, such as base running, without taking up a lot of time to reorganize the class. Most students at the secondary level have experience throwing, catching, dribbling, and kicking, so combining several fundamental skills in a first lesson is not the leap it might appear to be. That said, the idea of focusing on one skill or concept during each lesson remains the guiding force behind this text's lessons.

The drills you run in class are important. Running drills never seemed much of a challenge to me until the early 1970s, when I gave a student teacher complete responsibility for teaching an eighth-grade class. This particularly memorable day, she was set to teach basketball dribbling. She wrote a complete lesson plan, then, prepared and confident, she set out to teach it. She took attendance, led the warm-ups, explained the lesson, and lined the students up for the drill. The students were motivated. They listened and were cooperative, but they simply could not understand what she wanted them to do. The first result was chaos. She stopped them when she saw the drill was not working, and she repeated her instructions. As I listened, it was hard, even for me, to visualize what she wanted. But in good spirit, the students tried again. Their renewed efforts were still a mess. She stopped them again and repeated her instructions a third time. The plan, her great drill, was not coming out the way she'd hoped, but she kept trying and so did they. I watched, realizing that repeating her explanation was an exercise in futility, that the drill was too complicated for the best basketball players in the junior high school, and that an ordinary class of eighth graders would simply not be able to master it. I knew she would be better off changing her plan so no one got more frustrated, but I did not interfere. Ten minutes into the lesson she stopped addressing the class, turned to me, handed me her grade book, and said, "Take the class. This is not working and I don't know what to do anymore." Then she fled the gym.

There are two points here. The first is that it's important to think on your feet. It's not always possible to gauge how a group will respond to your plan. Be ready to make changes. Second, when it comes to setting up drills, follow the KISS principle: **K**eep **I**t **S**hort and **S**imple. Students do not need to be razzle-dazzled with complex drills. They just want to learn, have time to practice, and feel successful. Make your drills interesting and relevant, efficient and safe. Drills should provide lots of repetition and should be accompanied by feedback.

The organizational formations I suggest in the lessons are intentionally simple. They are designed to allow students to practice safely and have the most repetitions possible so they can refine their skills in the shortest amount of time, all while permitting you a clear line of vision of the entire group. As students progress, simple variations can facilitate goal changes, refine targets, and make practice more sophisticated, while not overwhelming students with information overload. For instance, when you first teach the soccer dribble, allow students their own ball with an uninterrupted area in which to dribble. As they get more competent (or more tired), you might want to give them a breather by having several of them share a ball as they would in a simple relay or a shuttle drill. You might add to their dribbling skill by having them run alongside one another and pass on a slant. Or you can use one student as an obstacle or a receiver. You might tell them at halfway to the original goal to pass to a target or to a student waiting for the ball. In each case, you are incrementally adding to their use of the dribble by combining it with other skills and formations.

Keeping Competition Educational and Enjoyable

Competition can be a negative experience for students if the only ones who feel like winners are those with the best scores. While some competitive events eliminate "losers" until only the best players remain, your goal should be to encourage maximum participation against a variety of opponents in an equal field where everyone is included in every game, every day.

Competition has too many benefits to avoid it because of its possible negative factors. Competition is a great motivator and, in the right environment, can be a useful educational tool. It encourages improvement and greater physical effort, and it makes games more exciting for students. To ensure a healthy competitive experience, teachers must set meaningful goals, maintain a positive learning environment, provide students with an even field in which to play, and teach them to feel like winners no matter the score.

Here's a story showing how a teacher can improve self-concept before and during a competitive situation. I began teaching senior high school students after teaching junior high for 18 years. I came to the high school unconsciously programmed to believe that the older students I would now be working with wouldn't need as much skills work or encouragement as my former younger students needed. Boy, was I surprised. During the basketball unit, many high school students—boys mostly—hung their heads during games, avoiding the ball, afraid to make a mistake. Many seemed generally intimidated because their skills compared poorly to their classmates' skills. That first year I tried convincing them that they should shoot when open and reasonably near the backboard. I told them the worst-case scenario would be that they would miss, and their teammates would try to rebound and put the ball back up again. It took almost the whole unit to convince these students to try. When they finally did try, they got so much pleasure from their efforts. I felt sad that they had been so humbled for most of the unit. There had to be a better way.

There is a better way, but I did not discover it until we were fortunate enough to have both sides of the gym and the use of all eight backboards. With eight backboards and more space, I could line up my large class in eight small groups. They grouped with friends, perfectly legitimate since we were just practicing, so the groups were not of equal ability. We began that day by combining the performance goals of two earlier lessons: dribbling and shooting. We dribbled across the gym to shoot at assigned baskets before dribbling back. After everyone had a few turns, I told students to stay at the basket once they got down there and keep shooting until their shot dropped in. Then they were to dribble back to their lines. After a few turns for everyone, I changed the instructions, telling them that if they shot and missed, they should dribble to another basket and shoot again. If the shot did not drop in, they should go to the next basket and shoot again, continuing on to different baskets until they sank a shot, before dribbling back. The class did this for several minutes. One by one, everyone eventually saw the ball drop in.

Then I suggested keeping score and finding out which group, given an equal amount of time, could accumulate the most points. We did the simple drill first—dribble down, shoot until it goes in, and dribble back. It was easy to explain. From the time I would say "go" until they heard "stop," they would score two points each time a member dribbled to the basket, sank a shot, and dribbled back. The instant opinion was that the practice group with the best athletes in the class would outscore everyone else by a mile. Interestingly, it did not work out that way. When three minutes were up, a group with lesser-ability athletes scored one basket more than the team everyone thought would win. We did it again. The high score was 28, the next 26, the next 22, most others had 16 to 18 points, and the caboose scored 12. Were they excited? You bet. Why? Everyone was able to score and make a contribution to the group of friends they were playing with.

Variety being the spice of life, I mixed the drill up a little. Sometimes the players had only one shot and had to come back, sink it or not. Sometimes I told them to stay until it dropped in. Sometimes I asked them to dribble to the zone where they practiced their outside shot, shoot from there, and if they scored then come back immediately, but if not, get the rebound and try a lay-up shot. If that dropped in, they scored two points for their group, and whether or not they scored, they had to come back and let the next person in the group go. No matter the rules, the objective of scoring and the success in doing it proved to everyone that they could score. Meanwhile, they learned a lot. Those drills enhanced their self-confidence, as well as their awareness that more than the best athletes could score and that they all were capable of shooting and scoring when no one was interfering with their view of the basket. You can appreciate the merits of this shooting experience if you have seen players get the ball when they are completely open and within range of the basket, then spend precious seconds hesitating until they decide what to do and end up passing it to someone else.

My classes did not have a reluctant shooter thereafter, and the tenor of each class changed. Games and tournaments no longer depended on heroes but on whole teams. All the students felt free to shoot and were convinced that they could make both an offensive and a defensive contribution because they knew they could score. Once they were part of a team effort, class cooperation was high, teams played like teams, and the goals I set for them were met. In such an atmosphere, everyone won no matter who had the best score.

Understanding the Importance of Game Play

As your students move toward graduation, their goals may change from acquiring skills to using them in real games. Game play, if approached and supervised appropriately, is wonderful and should not be avoided, even at younger levels. Sometimes it brings out the best in people. I have watched the most disengaged students become excited, rush to get to class, and be out there practicing during free play just so they can play better for their teams. I recall a particularly reticent girl who had been extremely timid during basketball drills but who wanted to do her part for her basketball team. By the tournament's end, she played so hard that she came back to the locker room all sweaty. "Wow," she said to me. "I never knew sweating could be so much fun." Isn't that what it's all about?

If students leave us without enjoying what we teach, without enjoying activities that will keep them vigorous, they run the risk of becoming sedentary adults. Physical educators are responsible for preparing students for a *lifetime* of activity. To meet that responsibility, what we teach, and what students master, should be fun. For this reason, while this text emphasizes lessons that help students refine their skills, it also puts those skills into use as soon as possible. The end product is designed to meet physical educators' ultimate goals for their students: enhancing their fitness, stimulating their interest, encouraging their effort, generating good class relationships, and, win or lose, finishing with good feelings.

Enjoying the Game Experience

I firmly believe that success is vital to enjoyment, and that achieving success requires mastering skills that only come with confidence and motivation. So, helping students achieve skills is very important, but it is also essential to have them use those skills in a real game.

Many people while studying the learning process studied the "games for understanding" or "tactical games" approach and how it helps students reach success. They advocate that students play the game before learning the skills, believing that it's best to understand the context in which skills are used before learning how to do them properly. As a teacher who began her career teaching only girls, I would say it took working with boys for me to realize how useful the tactical games approach can be.

Experience has taught me that there are gender differences in preferred learning style. Of course my findings aren't universal, but this is what I generally found to be true.

→ Boys generally want to play first. They really don't think about needing to learn how. Once they play the game and realize how difficult it can be, they stop fighting efforts to teach them how to do it better.

→ Girls generally want to know what and how to do what they are supposed to do before doing it. They are much more patient about learning skills and repeating them. The prospect of the game does not excite them until they feel they know how to play it.

I learned more about the benefits of the tactical games approach when I was observing several eighth-grade football lessons at a new school. The boys and girls got out on the field, lined up, and each day practiced some kind of passing or defensive drill. Whenever I watched, they were always drilling. I never saw them play a game. Later, I noted when taking out my 9th- and 10th-grade classes that the average student had a pretty impressive success rate when it came to passing drills. Both genders were accurate when throwing to a person on the run if they were up to 10 yards away. They could run square out, square in, button hooks, and posts. They could also hang on to the ball when they caught it. They really looked ready for a game. Then the belts and flags came out for flag football. Surprise! They needed to learn how to use them. After learning flag use and the kickoff rules, students were sent out to play. They sauntered to their playing field, obviously in no rush. After five minutes, half the group was on the field, ready for the game. The rest had to be rounded up and cajoled. Finally, the game began. The quarterback made a good throw. The receiver caught the ball, ran a few steps, and threw the ball to someone else. That person caught the ball and ran a few steps. Then she too threw the ball to someone else. In shock, I stopped the action to correct it and learned that these students, who had had two to three years of football lessons, had learned only to throw and catch in all that time. They never were taught to play the game. That explained everything—their lack of overall enthusiasm, their sauntering to the field, their inability to use belts and flags, and their not having the foggiest idea how to use the skills they had learned.

Playing the game without the skills can be frustrating; however, learning skills without ever playing the game is also frustrating. It's like learning to read words but never getting the opportunity to read a book. No one would approve of that. Why approve of the other?

Planning Successful Tournaments

An essential and fun part of almost every unit is tournament time. Once students have begun to master games skills, they will want to apply these skills in competitive settings such as matches and tournaments. I have found tournaments to be rewarding and enjoyable, but making them successful requires planning and supervision. In the next few passages I'll offer some ideas for creating and running a successful tournament.

Making Up Teams

If you have two to six teams in a class, make sure each is equally skilled. To do this, you must know each member's skill level. Then, after you account for all factors that you can think of in a particular sport, such as height, speed, throwing accuracy, jumping ability, and prior experience, create teams whose combination of players is equal to the others. This gives every team an even chance to win.

If you want to teach students to work together, make new friends, and learn to respect individual differences, it's best to split up cliques and have a strategy for preventing domination by just a few players on a team. Such players will try to control the ball between themselves and avoid the rest of their teammates. I've dealt with this situation in several ways. In basketball, I had students play their first practice games without a dribble. This way, the ball had to be passed before the ball carrier could move. Doing that for 15 minutes was amazingly effective. It forced the domineering player who would have dribbled to the basket and done all the shooting to pass to his teammate in order to get in better court position. In volleyball, rather than allowing teammates to run in the way of someone else and smack the ball over the net, I praised those who could hit a bump pass that went to the center of their own side of the court. I also made a big thing of good sets sent to the dominant net person, which of course encouraged the net person to be there to receive them. In football, when all else failed, I coached the other team, forcing the quarterback to eventually come around. The quarterback could not stand the constant interceptions that came with having his opponents double- and triple-team his receiver, which happened when the opponents anticipated who the likely receiver would be. Pretty soon, the negative situation got the quarterback to look at other members of his team so he could find an open receiver. At that point, no more needed to be said—no receivers were ignored and teams had to play like teams.

When the competitive field is large, as it would be when doing individual and dual sports (a class of 24 would have 12 doubles teams or 24 singles teams), you can run class tournaments in separate divisions, each with a different skill level. By creating divisions, games can be played within each student's skill level—the best athletes play each other in one division, the average in another, and the least skilled in another. This makes it more fun for everyone.

Most decisions about forming tournaments will depend heavily on the nature of the class. One constant should be your expectation that students use a good work ethic and that their competition leaves no one feeling intimidated.

Teaching During Tournaments

While tournaments are going on, don't stop teaching. Tournaments provide a great opportunity for you to teach students to apply the skills you've taught them in an authentic situation. Some tips include the following:

- As you observe, use the teachable moment, offering advice, corrections, and positive reinforcement during the action. Take advantage of the fact that some students learn more out of necessity than when just drilling.
- Make sure everyone plays by the same rules and code of ethics.
- Get around to all the groups, complimenting individuals on their accomplishments.
- Cheer out loud for accomplishments most students don't recognize. For example, you might cheer what seemed an unsuccessful effort to come up with the ball if the effort forced an opponent's error.
- Cheer for assists, good defense, or using the right strategy, even if the effort did not succeed.

- Encourage leadership, an understanding of the dynamics of the game, teamwork, and initiative.
- Encourage anticipation so that teammates are backed up, and not overrun.
- Teach students to be realistic, to appreciate the progress and effort of each team member, and to understand that students can only do what they can do.
- Set up progressive goals that students can measure up to despite the score.

Creating a Feeling of Success

Create a tournament atmosphere in which all students feel successful. Unfortunately, unless you're a magician, you cannot create success. That requires students' efforts. If students refuse, teachers must find a way to get them involved. Finding the right words and doing the right thing to get a disinterested student moving is almost an art. Resistant students need to trust you and the environment before they'll risk anything that might lead to failure. Most can be won over if the class atmosphere is consistently active, emotionally reinforcing, socially healthy, and cognizant and appreciative of individual growth.

In our culture, which emphasizes winning, students must learn that participation is far more important than the final outcome. Take action that praises and rewards effort over outcome. By recognizing good sporting behavior, good hustle, fabulous team play, good effort on defense, most improved performance, and so on, students can think more about values and less about winning.

The Goal: Physically Educated Students

This text has something for everyone. Students who are sports enthusiasts will be prepared for playing in an adult world of leagues, tournaments, and pickup games. Others can simply enjoy playing the game for its own sake, as well as the camaraderie of working as a team. Others who love moving just for the fun of it will find pleasure in many weeks of noncompetitive activities. Among them are units on fitness (including aerobic dance), weight training, exercise machines, self-testing activities, and social dance. The social dance unit includes folk, ballroom, disco, Latin, Cajun, country, square, and line dancing. Students who experience the entire package will be physically educated. They will be aware of the need to stay active, mindful of how good it feels to really move, and confident enough in their learning skills to keep searching for that special activity that turns them on, an activity that might never have been taught in class—cycling, scuba diving, climbing, skiing, or kayaking.

The 14 units in this book (plus the extra unit on the CD-ROM) do not cover all physical activities, but they cover enough to guarantee a well-rounded approach, with experiences in many types of sports and lifetime activities. The units are based on limitations I've experienced in the Northeast, where gym space is at a premium and winter brings us indoors much of the year. Some units are longer than others. The units that afford the highest level of participation in small spaces, such as volleyball, dance, aerobics, and fitness training—activities that can accommodate everyone without forcing students to sit out—are given the most attention.

Some activities reappear every year (volleyball, fitness, football, basketball, dance); others do not (golf, badminton, pickleball, tennis). Some chapters have just one unit, written for beginners; others are for beginners and intermediate; and others are for all three experience levels (beginner, intermediate, and advanced). The activities that reoccur from level to level provide fresh content and build on past experience, so you can be assured that students will not be doing the same thing every year.

My approach is holistic, in hopes of educating the whole person, body and mind. But just as English teachers can't cover every worthwhile book in one course, physical educators can't cover all activities. Our job is to set a tone for participation. An educated person doesn't know it all, but does know how and why to learn more.

Facilities

You will need adequate facilities for your units and lessons. If facilities are inadequate, you need to ask and answer several questions before making major decisions:

Should I go ahead with the activity? Many bend over backward to teach an activity they love, never thinking of more appropriate alternatives. Would you teach swimming without a pool? I doubt it. To allow for full participation among students, you need to adjust to the facilities available. Once I had 50 students, three tennis courts, and no wall close by for hitting balls against. The equipment situation was fine, but I had no space. Students would have had too little activity, too little experience with the equipment, and too little time to practice the fundamental skills. In this atmosphere, introducing tennis would have been a lesson in frustration. Could I have taught the students tennis with so many students waiting to play?

Can I keep the students active most of the period? If the answer to the question is "No," perhaps you should not teach the activity. Curriculum decisions should not be automatic. If a tradition does not make sense given current circumstances, start a new tradition.

What can I do to enhance participation when facilities are not optimal? Here are some ideas:

- Create additional learning stations that require less equipment and space, and divide the class into smaller groups so everyone rotates to each station.
- Modify the games to increase participation. You could
    change the number of players on a side,
    shorten the length of the game, or
    rotate players between games and practice stations.

For instance, say you want to teach a class of 20 to play tennis, and you have three tennis courts. Playing doubles accommodates only 12 players. How can you modify your lesson, engage all 20 students, and limit the educational compromises?

- Devote one court to drilling skills with a teacher, a highly skilled student, or a ball machine feeding balls and plan a systematic rotation from the drill court to the doubles courts.
- Divide regulation courts into minicourts, changing the focus from practice and games on full courts to practice and games for small-court control.

19

- Create a schedule so students get equal court time. Have 12 students play doubles on the three regulation courts and have the remaining 8 students work at stations outside the courts. Send them to work on the control or volley drills you taught at the beginning of the unit. Or have them practice serving through a hanging hoop or a target on a wall. Or have them practice hitting against a wall. After a specific amount of time, assign them to doubles play and the others to practice.

What do you do if you have 30 students and just three courts?

- If you must maintain class in one place—on the tennis courts—stick to skills, assign 10 students on each of the three courts, and have a student leader, teacher, athlete, or ball machine feed balls to each of the lines.
- Divide the class into three equally able groups and assign two groups to neighboring fields to play a team sport they already have learned while the other group has tennis lessons (assuming appropriate supervision is possible). Rotate the groups so everyone has the same number of tennis lessons before the unit ends.

If you have 50 students and just three courts, it might not be worth it to teach tennis.

Tennis can be one of the more challenging activities to teach efficiently, since most schools do not have enough courts to accommodate all students at once. The United States Tennis Association (USTA) has publications designed to help teachers deal with less than ideal conditions. For information, contact the USTA at 800-990-8782 or at 70 West Red Oak Lane, White Plains, NY 10604. The USTA Web address is **www.usta.com.**

Suggestions for Curriculum Development

Teaching a sport during its normal season makes it easier to motivate students. Those trying out for the school team, watching friends play, seeing the game on TV or in the stadium, or reading about it in the papers have had their interest aroused already. You have the further benefit of using current examples of rules and strategies by citing something that happened in a real game. All this adds greater insight to your lessons. For instance, if you're teaching the importance of protecting the ball, the value of the lesson is heightened when it takes place soon after a game is won or lost as a result of someone having the ball stolen away.

Unfortunately, it's not always possible to take advantage of sport seasons. Many parts of the country have about three months in the fall and spring when the weather is good enough to play outdoors. Most of the year is spent indoors in crowded facilities. If your school is like mine, the gym is used all year; it is crowded and in constant demand. Given the limitations of facilities and the size of staff and classes, it's a challenge to provide a program that includes individual sports. Sometimes you'll need to tiptoe around each other and be willing to compromise.

Knowing how varied each teaching situation is, and realizing that several activities—movement education, swimming, modern dance, gymnastics, track and field, lacrosse, field hockey, project adventure, and table tennis—are not in this book's table of contents, I cannot prescribe an entire curriculum. But I can tell you that the sample I've presented here really works. Given a school year similar to ours—with 38 weeks of classes, 40 weeks of school, classes on alternate days, and 45 minutes bell to bell—this curriculum has an excellent selection of activities and gives you a useful example of how to organize and arrange the units.

Seventh Grade

Have long units, and emphasize fundamental skills and team cooperation.

Locker room use, the use of combination locks, and getting dressed quickly and in public (one day)
Fitness testing for a fitness index baseline (two to three days)
Soccer (seven weeks)
Football throwing and catching skills (one week)
Volleyball (seven weeks)
Aerobic-dance physical fitness (five weeks)
Basketball (five weeks)
Physical fitness reassessment (two to three days)
Track and field (four weeks)
Softball skills and modified game using fielding concepts (remainder of the spring)
Locker cleanup and completion of student portfolios or cumulative records (one day)

Eighth Grade

Expect more consistency in fundamental skills, begin encouraging strategic control, and seek more team involvement.

Football (six weeks)
Soccer (two weeks)
Dance, or a movement education approach to gymnastics (three weeks)
Volleyball (six weeks)
Aerobic-dance physical fitness (five weeks)
Fitness testing (one week)
Basketball (five weeks)
Pickleball or paddleball (five weeks)
Softball (six weeks)

Ninth Grade

Increase the skills vocabulary, promote strategies when repeating activities, and introduce more individual and dual activities.

Badminton (five weeks)
Football (three weeks)
Soccer (three weeks)
Dance—folk, square, and country-western (three weeks)
Volleyball (six weeks)
Fitness—weight training (four weeks)
Basketball (five weeks)
Fitness testing (two days)
Tennis or pickleball (four weeks)
Softball (four weeks)

Tenth Grade

Expect greater control of the skills learned in ninth grade and more strategy and team-work. Introduce more individual activities.

A racket sport, preferably tennis (four weeks)
Football (three weeks)
Soccer (three weeks)
Dance—square, line, and folk (three weeks)
Volleyball (six weeks)
Fitness (five weeks)
Basketball (five weeks)
Fitness testing (one week)
Badminton, pickleball, or paddleball (four weeks)
Softball (four weeks)

Eleventh Grade

Provide new athletic opportunities and leisure-time activities; promote social skills, leader-ship opportunities, group strategy, and the creation of an athletic advantage.

Team handball (five weeks)
Golf (five weeks)
Football or soccer (three weeks)
Social dance (four weeks)
Volleyball (six weeks)
Fitness—circuit training in the weight room or aerobic training (four weeks)
Basketball (four weeks)
Handball or paddleball (four weeks)
Softball or tennis (four weeks)

Twelfth Grade

Provide some new team sports and more lifetime activities.

Team handball or tennis (four weeks)
Football (two weeks)
Soccer (two weeks)
Badminton, handball, or pickleball (four weeks)
Volleyball (seven weeks)
Social dancing—ballroom, country-western, and Cajun (four weeks)
Basketball (four weeks)
Golf, wrestling, or modern dance (six weeks)
Softball or tennis (four weeks)

Meeting the National Standards for Physical Education

The National Content Standards, published by the National Association for Sport and Physical Education (NASPE) in *Moving Into the Future: National Standards for Physical Education* (1995), are consensus statements that express what students should know and be able to do once they have completed a quality physical education program. NASPE also provides guidelines for appropriate practices meant to facilitate the creation of physical education programs that result in physically educated individuals. These guidelines help teachers educate students so they graduate with the skills, knowledge, and motivation to engage in a life of physical activity and other healthy lifetime practices. The appropriate practices do not outline a curriculum plan for physical educators but provide a framework that educators can use to create a quality program.

The national standards recognize that to achieve a quality physical education program, developing physical skill is not enough. In *quality* physical education, cognitive, social, and emotional skills are developed as well. What follows is a general overview of how this text can help you design a physical education program that meets the national standards.

An Overview

The lessons in this text are well balanced, complying with a main tenet of the national standards. Lessons introduce and allow refinement of motor skills, promote a level of participation that improves physical fitness, and develop related cognitive, social, and emotional understandings. Here are some ways the text can help you develop a quality physical education program that complies with the national standards:

- The lessons contain both performance goals and cognitive goals.
- The practice of having instant activity (free play) and developed warm-ups helps ensure a high level of participation from the onset. The warm-ups also help students acquire sport skills and reach fitness goals.
- The students develop social and emotional skills.
- Teams are selected by the teacher, not the students.
- Class instruction and individual coaching hints during game play aim to teach students how to work together.
- The older grades' lessons focus more on socialization, responsibility, initiative, cooperative learning, and ethics than on skills acquisition.

Satisfying another tenet of the national standards, this text offers a broad range of activities. There are 14 diversified units in this text. Note that this book's table of contents is not the definitive list of activities a secondary school should offer its students. Curricula can appropriately vary with regional differences and still meet NASPE's recommendations. For example, I teach handball, a popular game in my metropolitan area and an excellent lifetime activity. It's inexpensive, it can be played against almost any wall that has a concrete foreground, it has great fitness benefits, and it's a great social outlet. However, though handball is an excellent addition to my physical education program, I know that what's popular in New York at the beginning of the 21st century might not be so popular where you live. The lessons in this text should be used as examples. You should modify lessons as you see fit.

The West Coast might favor in-line skating; the country's northern states, downhill skiing; the farm belt, cross-country skiing; and areas near lakes and beaches, beach volleyball. Regions that offer other popular lifetime sports are not wrong to do so. Nor is it wrong for this text to omit them. It's impossible for this book to cover every activity that might interest students. Still, my job and yours is to provide students with a solid foundation of skills, knowledge, and motivation that can apply across many activities, including ones that haven't been invented yet, so that students are willing, able, and interested in seeking a lifetime of activity.

Another goal of physical education addressed in the appropriate practices guidelines is that programs use a variety of approaches when promoting fitness, developing knowledge, and increasing emotional and social skills. To meet this goal, each lesson in this text is designed to maximize activity while encouraging students to think. I do this in a variety of ways. Sometimes skills are taught outright, and sometimes they are developed in response to a task (game situation). But activities always begin at the bell, giving students opportunity to practice and refine their skills. Afterward, we talk about ideas and concepts that have been woven into each demonstration, each drill, and each competition so students can benefit cognitively as well as physically.

Critical thinking, elicited in each lesson, helps students learn skills, improve their game plan, and answer questions during the review at the end of the lesson. The knowledge and understanding integrated in each lesson are later assessed through written quizzes. While beginners' lessons emphasize skills more than subsequent units do, they still include guidelines for teaching students appropriate social and emotional behavior. Students must learn to adjust to classroom work ethics, teacher-designated teams, responsibilities during a tournament, winning, losing, and team game strategy. The units have clear and realistic performance goals. Performance rubrics, included at the end of each ability level, are suitable for self-assessment, peer assessment, or teacher assessment.

Appropriate Practices

The sections that follow take a broad look at how this text addresses the appropriate practices outlined by NASPE in its guidelines for physical educators.

Curriculum Guidelines

A physical education curriculum should be designed to educate students appropriately about physical education so that they become physically educated individuals, as defined by NASPE. A teacher can design an effective program by using the suggestions in the appropriate practices document.

Program Choices.   This text provides goals and objectives within each lesson that guide students in their achievement.

Refinement of Skills.   Skill refinement, an essential goal of any physical education class, occurs over many lessons. In this text, many lessons begin with mimetics. These mimicking actions are a great way for students to practice while warming up. Without taking time from the activity of the day, through mimetics students practice how they should move during games. Lessons progress from completing movement patterns in isolation to completing them with equipment; they also progress by increasing goals for speed, distance, and accuracy. A skill's rationale, its practicality, and its real game purpose are identified early on and, when possible, practiced as they would be used in a game. The practice first occurs with no defense in the way (i.e., dribble to a goal and shoot, or set to a player who spikes). Then, after several days, defenders are added to the equation. At this point, most students are ready to try to play the game. The few students who aren't ready will have time to catch up on basic skills, with the help of the teacher, during subsequent free-play periods and with the help of their teammates during team warm-up.

As an example of how mimetics can help refine the skills process for volleyball's bump pass, I'd begin with students learning to hold their arms properly and practicing quick arm alignment. Then they would learn and practice positioning the body. I'd ask them to get to an imaginary ball while readying their arms. Then they would learn to squat in the proper stance, under the imaginary ball. That's when they'd practice a forward split stride with bent knees. Then the focus would turn to the follow-through, where I'd ask them to practice using their arms to guide the ball up.

You'll need to judge how far to go the first day, but soon you can add the footwork that gets students down and under the imaginary ball. Varying footwork patterns comes next. Ask students to run back, meet a ball that is passing them on their side, and get their arms behind the ball, ready to follow through so their bump gets the ball to the center of the court.

After students practice these mimetics during the warm-up, distribute balls and begin the next phase in the skills progression. Students now learn to relate to the ball and coordinate their movement patterns toward meeting a moving object. This aspect of the lesson has students learning to bump the ball straight up and rebump it when it comes down (self-bump practice). They do that for several seconds, taking turns if necessary, and are given several trials. Then they learn to bump forward to a wall. When the wall sends the ball back, students move under it and redirect it back to the wall. They repeat this until their turn is over or they have lost control of the ball. Do this for several seconds and several trials. Then someone tosses the ball gently and low so that it can be redirected up and back to the tosser. Repeat this for several tosses and several trials. At this point, students are ready to react to the random variety that occurs in a game. Students get into groups of six, make a circle, and practice bumping so that the height of the ball goes toward the center of the circle (circle volley drill). Students on the circumference learn to react, get under the ball, and bump it up to others in the group. As competence improves, you can turn the circle volley drill into a game: "Let's see which group can legally keep the ball alive and hit the most bump passes before the ball gets out of control."

With a good amount of repetition, students have a moderate degree of success and, after learning the serve, the basic tools to begin a game. Games make clear the need for more control. Students learn that controlling the bump pass when using it to block a serve is harder than bumping a ball from a soft toss or high pass. The reality of the game often inspires a desire for more practice and control. In this scenario, the next lesson would set aside time to practice receiving serves with bump passes and would help students improve both those skills for the game.

Physical Fitness Activities. This text plans for physical activity to be enjoyable while increasing awareness and improving fitness. Fun is a great motivator and thus a key prerequisite for any good physical education program. If students learn that participating is fun, they'll be more likely to have a lifetime filled with physical activity. But enjoyment is often not experienced until students have real success and feel like they are in some control. To achieve these goals, sport-specific skills, strength, and stamina (fitness) are necessary. Admittedly, for many, the process of learning does not start out to be fun, and some students can be resistant. I am very familiar with students' lack of enthusiasm and have tried to develop lessons they'll find enjoyable.

Besides each lesson's aim for fitness, this text has a fitness unit for each school year that focuses exclusively on fitness acquisition, health knowledge, and health safety. Though it's an annual unit, fitness activities vary from year to year, as do the skills, safety, and concepts that students learn. Lessons promote continuous feedback from such activities as monitoring heart rates, measuring recovery rates, charting daily circuit training progress, and recognizing biofeedback. For instance, when new muscle groups are called into action, some students are left stiff and sore—their body is telling them something. They are taught to listen. When activity is strenuous and leaves some students dragging, they learn why and how to recognize their progress when their endurance and muscle strength improve.

Chapter 3, the fitness testing chapter, explains how to administer the New York State Fitness Test, which I started using because I teach in New York. Other states may also have similar information that you can make available so students can individually compare their performance to that of their peers. The fitness unit (chapter 4) makes extensive use of the test's standardized norms and teaches you how to use them as learning tools that give students another way of picturing themselves. As a bonus, using this test helps students understand statistics, such as the concepts of mean, median, and mode.

The New York state norms allow comparative analysis so that students can measure themselves against a large population (the state of New York) instead of just against their classmates. They can compare their raw scores to the scores of others the same age, gender, and grade level to find out where they rank in the skill being tested. The lessons go beyond testing fitness and giving grades. They plan to have the normal bell curve, standard deviation, scaled scores, and percentile ranks explained. Everything that will help that explanation is here in this text: the fitness forms, the normal bell curve diagrammed with scaled scores below it, and all the charts broken down by age group, grade level, and gender.

The results of two days of testing and the information derived are meaningful, as well as motivational, to students. Their interest and reaction over the years have led me to believe that this is important information for them. Knowing where they place among peers is not a turnoff. It motivates them to do their best, especially when so often our students are surrounded by mediocrity. This motivates students because it makes them aware of what the standard for other students like them is. It is important to stress that fitness test scores should be used as a tool for monitoring personal improvement and goals. If a student thinks he is top dog and finds out he isn't, he will make the extra effort next time to prove he is. If a student accepts the notion of being average among her peers and suddenly learns her sense of average is not accurate, she will try harder next time. For some students, being "average" is not good enough because they have aspirations of making athletic teams. These students should be looking at fitness levels of athletes. On the other hand, students with low fitness levels should not be concerned about the fitness levels of other students, but rather on improving their own fitness so they can achieve at least a basic level of fitness needed to maintain health. If the standardized population performed better than they did, then all their teacher's prodding and pushing is more meaningful, and students will react more favorably to future lessons.

The standardized norms used in the New York State Fitness Test do not provide health criteria, so you'll want to explore other tests that do provide criteria-referenced standards to give your students an idea of what their scores mean in relation to good health. Consider using FITNESSGRAM since it provides "Healthy Fitness Zones" developed through extensive research. FITNESSGRAM is also endorsed by Physical Best, a top-quality fitness education program developed by the American Alliance for Health, Physical Education, Recreation and Dance

(AAHPERD). The Physical Best program is an excellent choice for expanding the health-related fitness education component of your physical education program.

Knowledge.   Cognitive goals, a basic tenet of the national standards, are written right into the lesson plans. Take, for example, the teaching of the dribble in basketball. Along with learning to dribble, students learn the reasons for dribbling, the rules surrounding dribbling, the strategy involved in dribbling, and the choices dribblers have. They'll learn some of the strategy up front, such as the reasons for not looking at the ball. They'll learn the physical laws affecting the ball's return from the floor and the feel of equal and opposite reactions.

Student understanding is stimulated by learning about events, people, times, and places they are unfamiliar with. This new information, included in the lesson's Motivation section, sparks interest and encourages participation. Experience has taught me how valuable outside information can be in helping kids get past the attitudinal and emotional barriers they sometimes set up to prevent learning. For instance, when I introduced the dance unit the first years I taught coed classes, the boys reacted badly, not wanting to have anything to do with dancing. Thank goodness for Lynn Swan, a professional wide receiver who attributed ballet training to his miraculous midair receptions and the ability to land on his feet, ready to move on the football field. Hearing this, many boys began to put more into their dancing. When children can relate to the information you give them, you can help them alter their perceptions and attitudes.

Positive Social Behavior.   The National Content Standards call for the development of positive social behavior. Ethics, leadership, and citizenship are incorporated into the lessons in this text, as are the values of teamwork, personal responsibility, and appreciation of individual differences. Some units are social in nature (such as dance), and there are phases within other units where socially oriented activities are encouraged. Behavioral skills are important aspects of each unit, though they are not assessed until training and maturity have a chance to take effect. Behavioral standards are part of the assessment system in the intermediate and advanced performance rubrics. The shaping of positive social behavior is left primarily to teachable moments. These moments occur when teachers take the time to set up a sound learning environment, group teams so they are equal, and work to have everyone follow the same set of rules and conditions.

What leads to a behavior teachable moment can be hard to predict. It might be that interest in the activity being offered is preferred or dominated by one gender, or that some poor behavior must be addressed. This is particularly true of immature groups. I recall an incident that occurred during a coed eighth-grade football unit. I made up the teams as I always do and saw many of the boys, whose vision of football excellence was running 40-yard post patterns on every play, looking downcast when they saw only one or two males on their team. Their reaction: "Who am I going to throw the ball to?" Some refused to play. Others passed only to other boys.

I understood that the situation offered a potential teachable moment. First, I set about teaching students how to plan, making use of the skills they had and accepting and working around their weaknesses. The understanding of themselves went hand in hand with encouraging defensive matchups that made sense (equal height, speed, or knowledge). This stifled some of the bad behavior, but not all. When one boy continued to construct plays that used only boys, I pointed out that play after play, the girls were not covered, so it made sense to throw them the ball. Still the boy threw to the tightly covered boys, believing that somehow they would come up with the ball. At this point, I encouraged the other team to send their defense after the boy they knew would get the ball, double- and sometimes triple-teaming him. Eventually I made my point and the boy started throwing to the girls. After a girl caught a pass and ran for a winning touchdown, the boy's attitude toward throwing to girls flip-flopped quickly.

Bad language and attitudes are harmful to an emotionally healthy learning environment—don't tolerate them. What I usually do is temporarily remove the student from activity, explain that such behavior hurts feelings and—once the student recognizes that the class and teacher were hurt—ask him or her to apologize. With an apology to the class, the offending student gets immediate reentrance to the game. Most often students learn to apologize. It takes a few minutes of cooling down before it happens, but once it does, there's rarely a reoccurrence. Meanwhile, the point is made and the situation resolved quickly without anyone feeling victimized.

This text addresses the necessity of manipulating the environment so that there is a place for everyone and the learning atmosphere is healthy. It reminds teachers of their homework—making up equal teams. It is expected that teachers will not let students talk their way off of teams and that, like the Girl Scouts' motto, students will be encouraged to "make new friends and keep the old—one is silver and the other gold." Lesson plans encourage a realistic acceptance of individual differences and discuss ways to identify strengths and weaknesses and how to use them appropriately. But in the final analysis, it is you, the teacher, who must maintain the atmosphere that promotes working together, accepting each other's limitations, living by the same rules, and eliminating egregious behavior.

Variety. Another recommendation in the appropriate practices document is variety. To meet that goal, this text includes 14 different activity units—two on fitness, six on lifetime sports, and six on team sports (plus the wrestling unit, which only appears on the CD-ROM). There are approximately 400 different lessons, each teaching something new, be it a skill, an idea, a strategy, a principle, or a formation. Even a sport or activity repeated from year to year (i.e., volleyball, basketball, fitness, and dance) is not repetitious in learning. Every lesson contains something new, and better performance and increased knowledge are expected at every rising grade level.

Sports activities are taught in a variety of ways that students should enjoy. The emphasis of skills is placed on how they can be used in real play, real life, and real environments. Every lesson is designed for action. When relevant knowledge is imparted, it is done so in short segments so it does not detract from activity and so it can be assimilated easily.

Dance is a chapter unto itself. Numerous folk, square, country, social, and ballroom dances are suggested in three different units and done so to ease learning and produce a lot of different experiences. Variety ensures that some aspect of each lesson will appeal to different tastes and be fun to do. Dance skills have an immeasurable lifetime social benefit. Dancing skills are tapped during the aerobic fitness unit, a seventh- and eighth-grade unit, and also may turn into the chosen option that juniors and seniors take when developing their personal fitness program.

Instruction

The national standards challenge physical educators to use instructional practices associated with the following:

Success. In this text, activities are designed to increase basic skills incrementally so that within a lesson or two, students are comfortable with the skills being taught. Lessons are designed in such a way that students can reach 100 percent success during the skills acquisitions phase of the unit. This is accomplished through the setup of the class practice and drills. For example, when teaching throwing and catching, start the students at a close distance and with little pace. As you become satisfied with the students' progress, back them up. If what is being taught is more complex, such as batting in softball or net recovery in volleyball, and the practice sessions require rotations, make sure the class doesn't rotate until the person up has had three successes.

If a student has problems with timing and is preventing the group from rotating, draw the student aside and work with him individually. This can be done during the class period, during free play the next class period, at the end of the period, during lunch, or after school.

Learning time. This is adapted to the class's needs. Goals are realistic. Although it's likely that most students will meet the goals by the end of each lesson, this text suggests abandoning the idea of moving ahead until 90 percent of the class is successful. Lessons are on the CD-ROM to enhance a teacher's ability to make such adjustments.

Learning environment. This text gives tips about how to deal with the frustrations that might come up during the learning process and addresses some successful strategies for avoiding them. It also identifies activities and the progression so clearly that intermediate goals are apparent, thus allowing teachers and students alike to honestly cheer for accomplishments that might have seemed trivial to the uneducated eye.

Feedback. This can be a wonderful teaching and motivational tool. A social environment such as a gym is never absent of feedback, although sometimes it can be the wrong kind. Teacher feedback is necessary to undo the harm of demeaning and disrespectful comments from classmates. This requires constant feedback, a sense of the mood of each student—those berated and attacked frequently are unwilling to come forward and ask for help—and a willingness to involve oneself in the social drama of the group setting.

Teachers can be a great source of positive feedback. They should be ready to compliment students on all kinds of intermediate successes, because students frequently do not recognize the value of their actions or others, especially when their performance does not result in a score or a win. Games frequently have an unrecognized hero—or two or three. It is up to teachers to recognize the unrecognized—your words are inspiring and a great learning tool if used in a meaningful way. Unfortunately, if positive reinforcement is the only goal, it becomes meaningless if inaccurate. I remember a well-respected physical education teacher-coach asking an untenured teacher whether he was being observed that day because she heard him make so many positive comments during class. As it turned out, he was. Positive feedback should not wait for a teacher's day of observation. It should be ongoing.

I worked with someone who was so positive, he could make everyone feel better about themselves. He never tired of trying. One day he asked someone to demonstrate her bump pass and then, though it was totally out of control, told the student and the class it was great. Feedback stops serving a good purpose when it is too general and when it is untrue. It also undermines the veracity of the person giving it and, unfortunately, does not teach students to improve on what they have. Teachers can be truthful and still say nice things about a poor performance, but they must be selective. In this example, there were positive details the teacher could have addressed and been accurate. The student got up and had the courage to demonstrate in front of her peers. She reacted to the ball well, got under it, had her arms prepared properly, and had her knees bent. Those aspects were excellent and worthy of having a class remember. But it was clear to the demonstrator and to the class that something had gone wrong. The ball sailed wildly out of control. It was up to the teacher to point out why, without being so general. In this case, the student's follow-through was incorrect and the ball went flying behind her. Teachers who want to make kids feel good about themselves can do so by highlighting the good aspects and going on to explore for improvement. Students appreciate honesty. In this case, "great job" did not do it.

Feedback should not be dependent on the teacher. Other forms should be available, too. Feedback should be available in self-testing situations, from scores and statistics, and from classmates.

Inclusion. This is an issue addressed in the national standards under "Instruction Practices," which speaks to including "experiences and instructional strategies for all students regardless of level of ability, gender, race, or ethnicity." In this text, every student on the register is included in planning. That includes those with medical problems or disabilities. There are some suggestions for including all students in the "Teaching Tips" section of each unit; however, the topic of including students with disabilities is too broad to cover thoroughly in a lesson-plan book. At the end of this chapter, I've included a list of sources that covers inclusion in greater detail. There are a lot of sources out there on this topic, so I recommend teachers do a little research of their own.

Practice. Practice makes perfect (when practice is done correctly), and in this text, there are many opportunities for more. A short free-play period is set aside at the beginning of each lesson during the first half of every unit so that students can practice individually and teachers can work with those who are having difficulties, without taking up class time or making learning problems obvious to classmates. Warm-ups that include *mimetics* provide daily practice of correct movement patterns. Drills are uncomplicated and allow a lot of repetition. Every effort is made to provide enough practice that students become proficient within their own age group and experience level.

Group formation. Groups are arranged in a variety of ways. During practice, students are organized by attendance rows or some other nondiscriminatory arrangement. Occasionally students assemble with friends. Tournament teams are always prearranged by the teacher.

Teaching styles. Styles vary according to the goals of the lesson. Sometimes groups are addressed as a whole and perform in unison. Other times, the problem to be solved is given to everyone but developed individually. Other times, lessons are specific to need and student. For example, an eighth-grade football captain complained that his team dropped his passes and that not a soul on his team could hold onto the ball. He was frustrated because he used the pass exclusively and because, without catching his passes, his team could never score. He was tired of losing. For him, it was just a discourse that got him learning what to do. We talked on the way to the football field. I asked him a number of questions: "Does your team practice throwing and catching before the game starts?" It does. "Could they catch during practice?" Yes, they never had problems at close ranges. "What other ways are there to advance the ball?" He could run it, but he had never tried. By answering leading questions, he realized he could control the ball with short passes or with the run, get a few yards each play, use the clock, and avoid incompletes and interceptions by just going for the downs markers and taking all three plays to get there. He got so excited, this young man who had been so patient and had worked so hard, that it did not matter that he had lost all the previous games, that it was the end of the tournament, that he and his team could never win it. He could not wait to try his new strategy. When we got to the field, he ran off to start the game. He was beaming on the return. I guess you can imagine how excited everyone on his team was when they used their strengths, avoided their weaknesses, and came up winners.

Learning styles.   Teachers should plan learning experiences with students' learning styles in mind. Various teaching methods include demonstration, sound cues, blackboard diagrams and charts, kinesthetic feedback, biofeedback, repetition, and, when possible, technology.

Warm-ups.   These vary. They are planned and are guided in a safe, focused, and productive way.

Assessment

This text addresses the assessment practices covered in the NASPE guidelines:

Role of assessment.   Assessment plays an important role in the national standards, one that this text meets. Assessment is ongoing. Daily observation serves to help decide the best approach for subsequent lessons and appropriate ways to divide the class in teams and tournaments.

Achievement.   This is based on defined goals, which are specified for each experience level and can be found in performance rubrics. It also is based on short quizzes that conclude each unit.

Physical fitness testing.   This is a form of assessment that allows students to compare prior performance to new performance, as well as compare themselves to others within the same age group, gender, and grade level.

Classroom atmosphere.   Assessment is reality based. It occurs during activity, when students do what they do and are not concerned about being graded.

Techniques available for assessment.   These come in many forms in the text: the student portfolio checklists, biofeedback (checking heart rates and output), a recognition of one's own performance among peers, a measure against statistical norms, and objective assessment based on performance rubrics and quizzes.

Outside assignments.   These are varied and will lead to learning enrichment and parent feedback. The fitness unit asks students to inventory the lifestyles of their families and encourages sharing the information received at school with those at home.

Interpretation to the public.   The text includes a letter to parents explaining the reason for fitness and identifying the fitness ranking of their child as well as a sheet for every unit that explains the value of the activity and the benefit to the youngster playing it.

Class attire. This is a school policy and is not addressed in this text with the exception of the dance unit, when students are asked to wear street clothes and sneakers and are told that social dancing usually is done in street clothes and not in a special gym uniform.

Inclusion Sources

Please refer to the following resources for ideas for adapting your physical education program to include students with disabilities.

Auxter, David, Jean Pyfer, & Carol Huetting. 1993. *Principles and Methods of Adapted Physical Education and Recreation* (7th ed.). St. Louis, MO: Mosby.

Block, Martin E. 1994. *A Teacher's Guide to Including Students With Disabilities in Regular Physical Education.* Baltimore, MD: Paul H. Brookes.

Moon, M. Sherrill, ed. 1994. *Making School and Community Recreation Fun for Everyone.* Baltimore, MD: Paul H. Brookes.

Seaman, Janet A, ed. 1995. *Physical Best and Individuals With Disabilities: A Handbook for Inclusion in Fitness Programs.* Reston, VA: American Alliance for Health, Physical Education, Recreation and Dance.

Sherrill, Claudine. 1997. *Adapted Physical Activity, Recreation, and Sport: Cross Disciplinary and Life Span.* Boston: WCB/McGraw-Hill.

Sport Science Review. Adapted Physical Activity 5 (1996): 1–88.

Winnick, Joseph P, ed. 2000. *Adapted Physical Education and Sport* (3rd ed.). Champaign, IL: Human Kinetics.

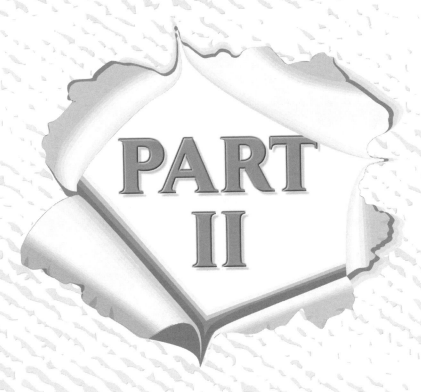

PART II

Fitness Unit Plans

Chapter 3

Fitness Testing

Unit Overview

1. Teach what is being measured and why:

- The ability to change direction, a helpful skill in sports such as basketball, tennis, and soccer
- Abdominal strength, a health issue that prevents back pain and improves posture
- Speed, an essential skill for track sports, as well as sports like football and soccer
- Endurance, a benefit that reflects a healthy heart
- The best performance on a given day in four statistically measured subtests

2. Teach the general benefits of measuring fitness:

- It represents an opportunity to measure self-improvement over time.
- It enables students to compare themselves to the performance of other students the same age, gender, and grade level as students from New York state.
- It helps motivate improved performance if scores fall in the 16th percentile or lower.
- It teaches responsibility in following the rules of the test and scoring accurately.
- It helps students relate to statistical mathematical concepts based on real activity.

3. Teach what it means: Scores are statistical comparisons of learned skills to other students of their own age, gender, and grade.

4. Teach them to compute and record their fitness level index.

Fitness Testing Teaching Tips

The following steps detail how to implement the New York State Physical Fitness Test.

1. Identify students with difficulty in following instruction and pair each of them with a helper.
2. Do a "reality" check for scores that appear unreasonably high or low.
3. There is a learned element to doing these tests, but to have them done correctly, you could organize a partial practice run to review procedure and scoring. Most students have more trouble scoring accurately than they do in taking the test, though some come up with variations that need immediate correction.
4. Have students fill out their cards before taking the test to eliminate time problems. Have a supply of pencils and pens handy.
5. To test efficiently, do the following:
   * Have half the class perform the agility test at a time, then switch. When students are not doing the test, they should score and record for their partners. Do the same with the sit-ups.
   * For the shuttle run divide the class in equal lines, put each line behind a cone, which is 10 feet away from the cones on either side and 45 feet from a far cone, and run one person from each line at the same time.
6. Have students complete the mile walk/run in one period, using a marker system to help, and then track how many laps they have completed.
7. Provide all students with their achievement-level score. This score is a ranked score from 0-10, with a score of 4-6 being average. This score indicates where on the performance scale an individual's score falls. These statistics are provided in conversion tables found in appendix C.
8. Using a multidisciplinary approach to making scores meaningful, provide students with an explanation of the statistics:
   * Explain how they were gathered and made into a normal frequency distribution.
   * Explain how the score distribution turned into a normal bell curve.
   * Tell then what a percentile rank is and how it is based on a frequency distribution.
   * Describe how the achievement-level scores are scaled scores, which are based on the total range of scores, lowest to highest. For instance, a broad population took the 10-second agility test. Their scores were collected and sorted. The lowest score was assigned a 0 and the highest score a 10. In the 7th grade, the lowest scores, which only 1 percent of the population reported, were 0-6 sidesteps in 10 seconds. This score got an achievement score of zero. The highest scores, also reported by only 1 percent of the population, were 23+ sidesteps for girls and 25+ sidesteps for boys. These scores were assigned an achievement score of 10. The median score, which was reported the most, was assigned an achievement level score of 5. This range of scores fell into the 50th percentile, meaning that 50 percent of the reported scores were higher and 50 percent of the reported scores were lower.
   * Assure them that fitness scores will not affect students' grades.

Unit Setup

Facility

Clean gym floor

Pre-measured and marked gym areas can allow the teacher a lot of flexibility and ease with testing transitions. Once the space is measured and marked, there would be no need to measure it again. A suggested layout to accommodate all indoor test items safely is shown in figure 3.1.

Track free of obstructions

Equipment

Physical fitness cards for each student; fall/spring sides available for entries

Pens or pencils for every two students in the class

A stopwatch

Blackboard and chalk or marker board with markers

Enlargement of the statistical norms for each age group and for each grade level so it is visible to students 20 feet away. Have them locate their own scaled scores (achievement-level scores) at the conclusion of the test and enter the ranked scores on their fitness cards.

Hand-held markers

Unit Timeline

Seventh grade—four full days in the fall:

Day 1: Teach, demonstrate, and have students practice scoring each of the first three subtests.

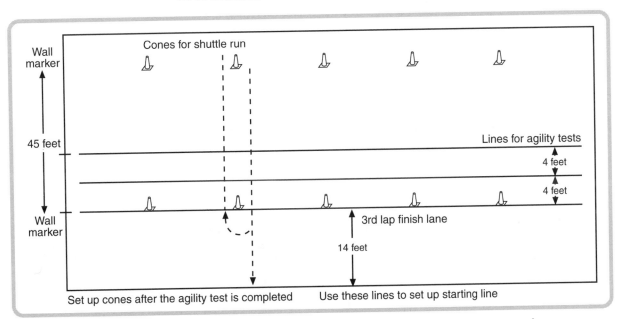

Figure 3.1—Fitness testing gym layout.

New York State Physical Fitness Test, reprinted, by permission, from NYS Education Department. (Albany, NY: NYS Education Department)

Day 2: Test and record the scores of the agility, strength, and speed items of the fitness test.

Day 3: Test and record the mile walk/run.

Day 4: Find the achievement-level scores, explain their significance, and complete the fitness card, finding the total level of fitness.

Eighth to twelfth grades—a maximum of three full days of testing each time the test is repeated:

Day 1: Review agility, sit-ups, shuttle run, and scoring as they come up, test, and record the scores. Provide immediate feedback via the achievement-level scores if possible.

Day 2: Give and complete the mile walk/run, record the scores, and locate the achievement-level score.

Day 3: Complete the physical fitness cards, include reminders about what the achievement-level scores mean, and teach students to calculate their total fitness level.

Unit Assessment

All students should be held accountable for completing all four items of the physical fitness test prior to the conclusion of the marking period in which it is given:

The school should report the fitness test scores to parents.

Students whose achievement level falls in the 16th percentile and below should consider improvement, because 84 percent of other similar students perform better. This can be done with
- a general class discussion about average performance,
- a private discussion with the student, or
- a letter sent home communicating the school's concerns and addressing lifestyle changes that might improve the health and performance of the student in the future.

A student portfolio checklist is provided here for student use (table 3.1). Encourage students to track their progress as they master new skills.

Additional Resource

Heyward, Vivian H. 1998. *Advanced Fitness Assessment and Exercise Prescription*. (3rd ed.). Champaign, IL: Human Kinetics.

Physical Fitness Testing Lesson 1 — Beginner level

Lesson 1 is for first-year students only. It is not recommended for classes that have already taken the fitness test once. For grade levels with experience, skip to the next lesson.

Table 3.1　Fitness Testing Student Portfolio Checklist

STUDENT NAME _____

- ☐ Has completed the 10-second agility test
- ☐ Has completed the sit-up strength tests for one minute
- ☐ Has completed the shuttle run by running three times around cones separated by 45 feet
- ☐ Has completed the one-mile walk/run
- ☐ Understands what achievement-level scores mean
- ☐ Knows own achievement-level score for agility
- ☐ Knows own achievement-level score for abdominal strength
- ☐ Knows own achievement-level score for the speed dash
- ☐ Knows own achievement-level score for the mile walk/run
- ☐ Knows, statistically, if in the range of performance that is considered average fitness, below average, or above average
- ☐ Is considered to be performing at least in the average fitness range
- ☐ Is improving performance on the fitness test, though not yet in the average range
- ☐ Is using best effort when being tested
- ☐ Is self-motivated to pursue fitness on own

From *Complete Physical Education Plans for Grades 7–12* by Isobel Kleinman, 2001, Champaign, IL: Human Kinetics.

Lesson Setup

Facility

Place tape, a minimum of 14 feet from the long wall, for the length of the gym.

Put down two more lines, four feet from either side of the previous one, so there are three lines separated by four feet that run the length of the gym.

For the shuttle run, place a permanent marker 45 feet from the starting line of the agility test so that the agility line can be used as the starting line for the shuttle run. If the marker is made on a wall, it will be a lasting reminder of where to place cones for the 45-foot shuttle running lanes:

- Make certain that the running lanes for the shuttle run are 10 feet apart.
- Make certain that the finish line is 14 feet from a wall.

Performance Goals

Students will

follow instructions as given,
score accurately and within the rules, and
complete a heading on the physical fitness cards.

Cognitive Goals

Students will

understand the reason for being tested,
learn what is being measured by the test,
learn to follow group instructions, and
learn the rules and procedures of each subtest.

Lesson Safety

You should set up lanes and running areas so there is adequate space between each and students are in no danger of running into the walls or into each other.

Warm-Up

Students will

1. Jog around the work space for one to two minutes
2. Stretch the quadriceps, hamstrings, gastrocnemius, and lower back

Motivation

Tell your students that they are going to learn to take a four-part fitness test. A good thing about this fitness test is that it is like the Olympics of fitness. When everyone is finished, students can find out the best scores reported by students of the same age, gender, and grade level of all students who have taken these tests, not just the best or most common scores in the class. When the test is taken again later in the year and in subsequent years, students can see how they've improved, as well as if they've scored higher within their age and gender group as they've gotten older.

By comparing scores, students can tell whether they've improved or not and set goals for themselves based on that information. The most valuable aspect of taking this test is the opportunity for self-evaluation and self-improvement.

Lesson Sequence

1. Distribute physical fitness score cards (table 3.2) and pencils and have students fill out headings only.
2. Point out the four subtests and explain that the class will learn the first three today.
3. Collect the cards.
4. Demonstrate the agility test performance and teach how it is scored (figure 3.2).
5. Have students count the lines that the demonstrator passes. Have them count out loud and in unison during a slow demonstration.
6. Allow half the students in class to try the side-stepping test, scoring for themselves first and then a friend. When they are scorers, they are to stand

TABLE 3.2 New York State Physical Fitness Scorecard

NAME _____ GRADE _____

TEACHER _____ AGE _____

PERIOD _____

	RAW SCORES (ACTUAL SCORE FROM THE TEST)	ACHIEVEMENT-LEVEL SCORE (BASED ON NEW YORK STATE NORMS FOR AGE OR GRADE)	PERCENTILE RANK (COMPARISON SCORE OF SAME AGE GROUP ACROSS NEW YORK STATE)
Agility Ten-second side-stepping test (passing over three lines separated by four feet)			
Strength One-minute sit-up test			
Speed Shuttle-run test (three times around 45-foot spaced-out cones)			
Endurance One-mile walk/run			
Total fitness-level scores rankings			

New York State Physical Fitness Test, reprinted, by permission, from NYS Education Department. (Albany, NY: NYS Education Department)

off to the side. Practice this several times until there is no scoring confusion and you're certain each line passed over is counted in the score.

7. Demonstrate a proper sit-up (elbows to knees with ankles held stationary by a partner).
8. Allow students a limited time period to try sit-ups themselves, correcting incorrect form and instructing partners to correct or not count any sit-ups done improperly.
9. Demonstrate the shuttle run (figure 3.3), with the timer calling out the time on the stopwatch once the first person turns around the far cone and begins the last lap back to the starting line (i.e., "19, 20, 21, 22, 23, 24, 25, 26").
10. Have students do a trial run.

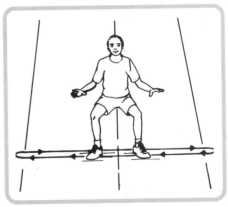

Figure 3.2—Straddling the line to begin the agility test

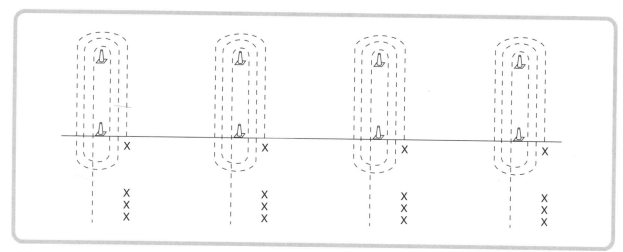

Figure 3.3—Organizing the class for the shuttle run test.

Review

Tell students that the next class will be the real test. All tests should be a measure of their best work, so tell them to get "psyched," sleep well, have a good breakfast in the morning, and remember to bring a change of clothes to the gym.

Assessment

Observe the students' ability to respond to instruction.

Physical Fitness Testing

Lesson 2 Beginner level
Lesson 1 Intermediate/
Advanced level

Lesson Setup

Facility

Refer to the setup in lesson 1 of the Beginner level.

Performance Goals

Students will complete and record their raw scores for the 10-second agility test, the 1-minute sit-up test, and the shuttle run test.

Cognitive Goals

Students will learn their day's personal best for the specific items.

Lesson Safety

Do not allow students to perform any task with cards or writing implements in their hands.

Have students who are waiting to do the shuttle run sit well behind the starting line.

Warm-Up

Students will

1. Jog around the work space for one to two minutes
2. Stretch the quadriceps, hamstrings, gastrocnemius, and lower back

Motivation

Tell students that they should try to do their very best. After they get their raw scores, they can find out if what they did was average, above average, or below average.

Lesson Sequence

1. Distribute fitness cards and pencils to students and their partners.
2. Begin the agility test after answering any questions and reminding students to count each line that the person being tested passes over during the 10-second test. Remind them that the scoring is the hardest part of the test. They want to go as fast as they can and still make sure their foot passes the outside line. Remind scorers to count all lines, including the center line, but count only the lines the foot passes:
   - The performer straddles the line and slides in either direction on the "go."
   - The partner counts the lines passed and records the score when hearing "stop."
   - The entire class should be done in two shifts, while you check for clear mistakes, incorrect scoring, and unrealistic numbers. Use a third trial for corrections only.
3. Begin the strength test with sit-ups. Have half of the class line up facing the same direction. Emphasize the rules: the student must curl to a seat, arms must be folded in front of the chest, elbows must touch the thighs coming up, and midback must touch the ground when down. Remind the scorer to be accurate. Emphasize that if students are tired, it is all right to slow down. Ask them to try to do as many as possible. Call out "go," one minute later "stop," and have the partner mark the score in the second raw-score box. Do two shifts.
4. Begin the shuttle run:
   - Line up students in equal lines behind each running lane.
   - Remind them that they must be behind a cone until the "go" signal, then they should complete three laps and run past the cone on the final lap at their top speed. It helps students to let them know how much time is left.

45

- Remind the scorer to give scores to the closest half-second once the runner passes the cone for the last time. Tell the class that the scorer will only know the score if she can hear the timer calling out the time. If students get too excited and start cheering (which they usually do), the times will go unheard and it will be impossible to record the scores.
- Run the first person at each station at a time, making sure that the scorer records the score on the runner's fitness card.

5. If time allows, give students the achievement-level scores and have them record them in the achievement-level column.
6. Collect the cards and pens or pencils.

Review

Doing one's best, even in a short time, is tiring but rewarding. Congratulate everyone whose scores reflect their personal best. Now it is time to get mentally prepared for the next class. Tell students that they are going to do four laps around the track—the mile walk/run. Remind them to sleep well, have a good breakfast, and bring a change of clothing.

Assessment

Check that the collected fitness cards have raw scores for tests one through three.

Physical Fitness Testing — Lesson 3 Beginner level / Lesson 2 Intermediate/Advanced level

Lesson Setup

Facility

Quarter-mile track free of obstructions

Equipment

Semicomplete physical fitness cards
Enough "markers" to provide three to each runner at a time (examples of things easily available and light for a runner to hold: Q-Tips, ice-cream sticks, tongue depressors, straws)

Performance Goals

Students will

complete four laps around the track (one mile) prior to the end of class, and convert their raw score for a mile to an achievement-level score.

46

Cognitive Goals

Students will

understand a mile's length and the time required to complete it,
learn what is being measured by completing a mile—endurance,
learn a strategy for completing the mile:
- Pacing oneself
- Using it as a test of self-improvement, trying to complete it in less time than before

understand that tests generally reflect the best one can do that day, and
understand the rules;
- No cutting across the track
- Student must have three markers and complete four laps to get a score

Lesson Safety

Be alert to any health problems: falls, wheezing, fainting, seizures. It might call for a simple rest, require the attention of the nurse's office, or require suspending the testing for that student.

Warm-Up

Students will

1. Complete jumping jacks, sit-ups, and push-ups to elevate their heart rate and warm their muscles
2. Stretch the quadriceps, hamstrings, gastrocnemius, and lower back

Motivation

Announce that the mile is the last item of the physical fitness test. Tell students that as soon as they are done, they will take their raw scores and convert them to achievement-level scores. Then they'll be able to compare their scores each year and aim for improvement.

Tell students that the mile will test their aerobic endurance, that is, if they can get past the "pleasure" principle. They should try to get their best performance even though they are feeling tired. Inform them that most people walk three miles per hour, or 20 minutes a mile. But they shouldn't: This is supposed to measure their best physical output, not serve as a casual walk. Tell them to do their best!

Lesson Sequence

1. Explain the purpose of the marker, how it will be given out (one for each lap completed), and how the score (time for the mile) will be given once the runner completes the fourth lap, three unbroken markers in hand. See figure 3.4 for a general picture of what a whole class running the

mile would look like during the period, and how to space out the teacher and the person handing out markers.

2. Remind students that any run longer than a typical dash requires pacing, but if they cannot sustain the same pace, it is perfectly all right to slow down. They should continue moving forward or run the risk of not completing the distance within the class time.

3. Teach that the inside of the track is the shortest distance and, when possible, runners should stay on the inside.

4. After a mile is completed, have students locate their fitness card and record their raw scores.

5. If time remains, have students research their achievement-

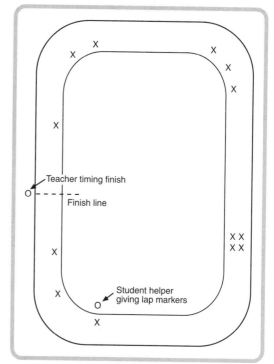

Figure 3.4—Suggested stations for timing the class doing the mile run.

level results and record that as well. This can be done with the assistance of someone who has been taught to read the "norms," an unprepared or medically excused student who is available, or the first few runners who have run ahead of the class.

6. Collect the fitness cards.

Review

Ask students if this is the first time they've completed a mile. Congratulate them!

Discuss whether they did better than the previous year, when they were younger.

Ask if their scores meet the health criteria.

Review where their scores fall in the statistics.

Find out who did best in the class, which boy had the best time, and which girl had the best time.

Ask students what the best time in the school was.

Advise them to take a warm shower, get a good night's rest, and remember their gym clothing for the next class.

Assessment

Make a comparison with statistics and with previous performance.

Physical Fitness Testing

Lesson Setup

Facility

A quiet space in which to communicate
A flat, firm, clean floor on which to sit and write or chairs for each student

Performance Goals

Students will complete their physical fitness cards:

Each raw score will be converted to an achievement-level score.
Achievement-level scores will be tallied.
The total of achievement-level scores will be converted to the total achievement-level score and percentile rank.

Students will begin their next unit when the paperwork is done.

Cognitive Goals

Students will learn what a comparative score is:

Percentile ranks
Scaled scores
Where their performance stands when compared to their own gender, grade, and age

Students will draw conclusions about fitness, achievement, and personal results.

Warm-Up

Students will complete a long warm-up since the majority of time in this lesson will be academic:

1. Slide side to side, jog backward and forward, and complete sit-ups, push-ups, and jumping jacks
2. Stretch the quadriceps, hamstrings, gastrocnemius, and lower back

Motivation

Now that the raw scores are entered, have the students see where they stand. Ask if anyone has taken this test before. Can they tell whether their raw scores improved? Ask if they did more sit-ups this year than last, had a better mile, did more side steps, or ran the shuttle faster. Discuss whether their better scores reflect a notch up in their peer group or that they all are older and better.

Lesson Sequence

1. Draw a normal distribution curve on the blackboard, including standard deviations, means, the range of each scaled score as a baseline, and the percentile rank (figure 3.5).
2. Explain the normal distribution curve, the meaning of average range in terms of the scaled scores (achievement-level scores), and how students can find out their own achievement-level scores by reading the posted charts.
3. Explain what a percentile rank means and how students can find out their own.
4. Return all physical fitness cards, distribute pens or pencils, and have students enter their achievement-level scores.
5. Point out that some students do much better in some test items (the practice effect, natural speed) than others but that now it's time to look at the whole picture.
6. Teach students to calculate their total level of fitness.
7. When all entries on the cards are complete, collect them.
8. Seek out students who could only reach the 16th percentile and privately discuss the findings with suggestions for future growth.

Review

Discuss the significance of where students stand now and where they should stand in terms of their physical fitness. Suggest they share this information with their parents.

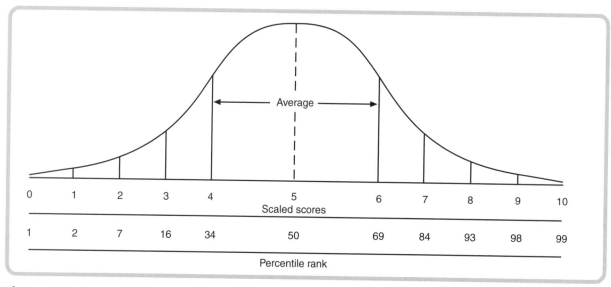

Figure 3.5—Normal bell curve with scaled scores and percentile ranks below.

Assessment

Compare student raw scores with statistics available from New York state. See appendix C for appropriate grade levels. Students whose fitness levels do not approach the average range should be encouraged to improve their effort in class and be more active at home. Enlisting the help of the students' parents is advised. Refer to the sample letter that follows.

A Sample Letter to Parents/Guardians

Dear _____ ,

We have just completed a physical fitness program designed to promote _____'s health, fitness, and understanding of the importance of an active lifestyle. In concluding our unit, all students in class took the New York State Physical Fitness Test and measured their performance against others in the same grade, of the same age, and of the same gender with scores that New York state had gathered and statistically analyzed. The results of the comparisons have left some concerns. After a concerted effort of conditioning in class aimed at improving everyone's physical fitness, _____ was not able to perform in the average range for his/her level.

He/She achieved a total percentile score of_____ , meaning that_____ percent of the students the same age, grade, and gender performed better. While this score is not necessarily reflective of _____'s state of health, it did lend comparison of his/her performance in agility, abdominal strength, speed, and endurance to many in a rather large sample. I am writing at this time to ask you to help me and _____ improve his/her chances for a long and healthy life full of activity.

Would you help me and help _____ by stressing a lifestyle that sets aside more time for and interest in gross motor activities? Activities of an aerobic nature are very helpful. Walking, jogging, dancing, "jazzercise," kickboxing, bike riding, swimming—activities that raise _____'s heart rate, activities that can be sustained continuously for 20 minutes—are wonderful for cardiovascular improvement and fitness. Aerobic effort as well as stretching and strengthening activities will help elevate _____'s quality of life now and in the future.

Since none of us can trade in our bodies for a new one when we feel they let us down or we are tired of them, it is prudent to teach our youngsters how to take care of theirs now. Thank you for your time and effort.

Please feel free to contact me. I can be reached at [school phone number and hours accessible].

Sincerely yours,
[Your name]

Introduction to Fitness

Unit Overview

1. Each lesson should focus on one key health-related fitness concept, include a minimum of 20 minutes of physical activity, and include a warm-up and cool-down. Explain the relevance of health-related fitness in everyone's lives and how your students can improve their fitness:

   - The short- and long-term benefits of fitness: looking and feeling better, being able to do more, better health, a longer life, avoiding major diseases, having a better quality of life
   - How different activities have a different intensity and how intensity affects the burning of calories
   - How cardiovascular health improves through regular activity and why that is important to good health
   - Basic concepts in understanding the cardiovascular system and its functions:

     The resting pulse and how to measure it
     Finding one's maximum heart-rate (MHR)
     Finding a beginner's target heart rate (THR)
     Finding the THR of someone who is regularly active
     Why working in the target zone improves cardiovascular fitness
     The significance of a recovery pulse

     How long it takes for one's healthy heart to return to rest after vigorous activity
   - The definition of fitness as it relates to good health:

     The role of flexibility and how to correctly and safely improve it
     The role of muscular strength and how to correctly and safely improve it
     The specific benefit of abdominal strength
   - How aerobic and anaerobic activity differ
   - The role of endurance and appropriate methods for developing endurance
   - The roles of warm-ups and cool-downs during vigorous activity and appropriate methods for warming up and cooling down
   - Body composition—muscle bulk versus body fat—and its relationship to good health
   - Safety concerns during workouts
   - The types of activities that would most enhance cardiovascular fitness

2. Students will develop a personal program of fitness that includes activities to address muscular strength and endurance, aerobic fitness, flexibility, and body composition.

Fitness Teaching Tips

1. The fitness unit lends itself to using an interdisciplinary approach in several ways. Multiculturalism and physics are two disciplines that can be covered during a fitness unit.
   - Dance provides opportunities to enhance the learning experience while getting fit. Students can learn multicultural facts when doing dances from around the world.
   - Weight training provides the opportunity to teach the laws of physics (i.e., how gravity affects concentric and eccentric muscle contraction; how pulleys increase the burden on muscles, as opposed to lifting free weights; and how fulcrums can be changed, which in turn changes what muscles are exercised).
   - Teach how physiological principles apply to all the variables of fitness, from resistance training for improving strength to muscle extension for improving range of motion.
   - Teach how, historically, people needed strength for their jobs. Now most people don't need strength and fitness for their work, so physical fitness has become an extracurricular activity.
   - Discuss why a physician might "prescribe" physical activity.
2. Students are more motivated to work hard to achieve fitness if the program you offer is fun and challenging and if you join in. Too often, teachers sit on the side and turn on a TV, allowing a commercial fitness video to do the job for them, when the most effective teacher, the true role model, is someone who practices what she preaches. It is not always possible to swing into action, participating the whole period with every class, but students do need a sense that you believe what you teach and will follow your own prescription. I have found that the use of videos is a poor substitute for an active teacher, particularly in large classes where only those close to the TV can hear and see what is going on. Television simply cannot be amplified sufficiently to be heard in a gym, especially when students are moving. Besides, nothing quite compares to a live role model, responding to silliness with a smile, encouraging and enthusiastic, right there in front of class demonstrating. If you feel there is no choice, that you simply cannot do the routine with your class and need to resort to video, make sure the best students are nearer the TV so everyone can emulate them, and try to find an amplifier to increase the volume of the TV sound so that everyone can hear the music. Without the music, you have lost an important motivational factor.
3. If you choose an aerobic dance physical fitness unit, you can use the dances in the dance unit. In addition, I have found that choosing popular music and choreographing four 16-beat passages that are repeated over and over works very well to keep the students' interest. Of course that means you have to take more time to create them, but it is worth it. A collaboratory effort with students, colleagues, your kids, or friends makes the effort fun. In the meantime, the following available dances can serve the purpose of filling in the gaps. Once you have planned and taught all your dances, tape the music together so that the movements from warm-up to final stretching are continuous. If you have students who flatly refuse to dance, have them jog the outside of the gym in time to the music. This ensures that they are

exercising at the same activity level as everyone else. When the class stops for abdominal work and stretching they should rejoin the class. Here are some dances to use in your aerobic dance routine:

- For warm-up and cool-down—the Electric Slide, Macarena, Saturday Night Fever Walk, Stepping Out, Pata Pata, Virginia Reel, Oh Johnny Oh, Bingo, and Miserlou
- For moderate activity—the Seljanica Kola, Mayim, Hot Lips, To Ting, Ve' David, Teton Mountain Stomp, and any square dance that has everyone moving at once
- For the highly energetic—the Salty Dog Rag, Hora, Jessie Polka, Nebesko Kolo, Sevila Sebela Loza, and Sicilian Tarantella
- A good five-minute song for an abdominal exercise routine—"Man in a Mirror" by Michael Jackson or "Nikita" by Elton John
- A great way to end is by doing a stretching routine to "Imagine" by John Lennon

4. Students who perform the same activity have different cardiovascular responses. Those who are overweight or typically inactive will find that activities that are easy for others are too taxing on them. They are likely to raise their heart rates so they exceed their target zones. To avoid drawing attention to them, teach everyone in the class how to reduce the stress placed on their heart by reducing the level of energy required for what they do without stopping. Such adaptations can be made by reducing the range of movement—for instance, not jumping when everyone else is—reducing the repetitions, or using less arm motion.

5. Have students understand that mild discomfort is a necessary part of improving fitness levels but that the old adage "no pain, no gain" is not true. Take care not to push too hard. It is better to make small gains so that everyone can keep participating than to wear students out. They may become fatigued and get a charley horse and want to stop. Teach the students how to calculate their target zones and set appropriate goals. Then encourage them to stick to it.

6. Create a learning environment that encourages students to work at their own rate and level.

7. A complete aerobic program has been designed for the seventh- and eighth-graders in this book. Its fundamentals can be used at any age. If you are introducing this age group to the weight room, emphasize correct technique and safety first and foremost. Have students use their own body weight, resistance bands, or light weights, but emphasize repetition for improving strength and endurance. Avoid maximal and overhead lifts completely.

Unit Setup

A large work space that is clear and completely clean, especially since students will be lying on the floor on mats during part of the period.

The weight room should be a designated area. All equipment should be checked for safety. Students who are so small that the major pieces of equipment cannot be adjusted to their bodies should not be allowed to use that kind of equipment. Most Nautilus and Cybex machines used in health clubs are designed for a wide range of adult sizes, but they may not be appropriate for small seventh graders. Be sure to check that the machines can safely accommodate your students, and that after all possible adjustments, their joints are properly aligned with the weights.

Equipment

Free weights
Health-related fitness profile forms (table 4.1)
Pencils
A stopwatch or wristwatch with a second hand
Blackboard and chalk or marker board with markers

TABLE 4.1   Health-Related Fitness Profile

NAME _____

CLASS _____ DATE_____

Body Weight _____   Height _____   Age _____   Gender _____

FITNESS COMPONENT	TEST ITEM	HEALTH STANDARD	TEST 1 SCORES	TEST 2 SCORES
Flexibility	Sit and reach	25 cm		
Cardiovascular endurance	Mile walk/run	10 minutes, 30 seconds		
Abdominal strength	Sit-ups	34		
Upper-body strength	Pull-ups			
Body composition	Skin fold—triceps			
Weight	Skin fold—calf muscle			

Health Standards for Mile

Age (years)	Gender	Health standard
13	Female	11 minutes
	Male	8 minutes 30 seconds
14+	Female	10 minutes 30 seconds
	Male	8 minutes 15 seconds

A student personal chart on which to mark classroom work on a daily basis

A cassette deck, compact disc player, or a sound amplifier that plays sound over the noise of the students as they work out

Selected music, videos, or both

A heart-rate monitor

A skin-fold calibrator

A weight scale

Recreational supplies such as jump ropes, basketballs, and so on

Unit Timeline

There are three units in this chapter, each including the following:

Six lessons are required to introduce the cognitive approach in segments. Each lesson should have a minimum of 20 minutes of physical activity.

Six lessons should be set aside in which 95 percent of the lesson time is student physical activity.

Two lessons are for

- assessing student performance, taking care to base grades on improvement and correct technique;
- culminating the activity; and
- getting a written measure of the students' cognitive understanding (a quiz).

Unit Assessment

Students in a circuit/weight-training program will make daily entries on a workout chart. By the conclusion of this unit, students enrolled in an aerobic program will be able to

move *continuously* without pausing for rest periods,

complete a five-minute choreographed warm-up,

complete 20 minutes of activity in the target heart-rate zone,

have a five-minute cool-down, and

have attained mastery of the following:

- seventh and eighth grades—concentrating on an aerobic workout
- 9th and 10th grades—using weight-efficient workouts
- 11th and 12th grades—independent study, with students making many of their own choices and designing their own programs around your master plan

A student portfolio checklist is provided for student use (table 4.2). Encourage students to track their progress as they master new skills.

Additional Resources

AAHPERD. 1999. *Physical Best Activity Guide: Secondary Level.* Champaign, IL: Human Kinetics.

AAHPERD. 1999. *Physical Education for Lifelong Fitness: The Physical Best Teacher's Guide.* Champaign, IL: Human Kinetics.

Andes, Karen, ed. 1999. *The Complete Book of Fitness: Mind, Body, Spirit*. New York: Three Rivers Press.

Power, Scott K., and Stephen L. Dodd. 1996. *Essentials of Total Fitness: Exercise, Nutrition and Wellness*. Boston: Allyn and Bacon.

Strand, Bradford N., Ed Scantling, and Martin Johnson. 1996. *Fitness Education: Teaching Concept-Based Fitness in Schools*. Scottsdale, AZ: Gorsuch Scarisbrick Publishers.

TABLE 4.2   Student Portfolio Checklist

STUDENT NAME _____

- [ ] Understands how, what and why of cardiovascular fitness
- [ ] Understands how, what and why of agility
- [ ] Understands how, what and why of muscle strength
- [ ] Understands how, what and why of having physical endurance
- [ ] Understands the measure of body composition and how to change it
- [ ] Understands how body weight is affected by physical activity
- [ ] Understands that fitness is related to personal health and happiness
- [ ] Acknowledges whether personal fitness level meets the established health standard
- [ ] Has followed a school plan to reach or sustain the health fitness standard
- [ ] Has knowledge of safety factors involved in any physical improvement program
- [ ] Is aware of impact of activity on fitness, weight control, appearances and stress
- [ ] Is developing interests and skills in lifetime activities
- [ ] Has developed a lifetime plan to maintain and improve physical fitness

From *Complete Physical Education Plans for Grades 7–12* by Isobel Kleinman, 2001, Champaign, IL: Human Kinetics

Physical Fitness Lesson 1   Beginner level

Lesson Setup

Facility

An area large enough for the class to safely move in

Equipment

Popular and peppy music
  For doing a line dance—the Macarena, Electric Slide, or Saturday Night Fever Walk
  A videotape of an aerobic dance routine

Performance Goals

Students will perform

  a rhythmical, low-impact aerobic warm-up; and
  the appropriate method of stretching all muscle groups.

Cognitive Goals

Students will learn

to associate health with fitness;

a short history of the national health crisis;

that *aerobic* is activity that increases respiration and heart rate without making one lose one's breath;

that by not being out of breath, one is allowed continuous aerobic movement for 20 minutes or more; and

why flexibility is important and how to maintain it by stretching.

Lesson Safety

The class will need appropriate space, large enough to allow everyone to move safely. The cleanliness of the floor is extremely important to reduce the possibility of infection when students lay down.

Warm-Up

Students will

1. Complete a rhythmical use of all large body groups
2. Jog for three to five-minutes with music
3. Dance using choreographed movements to music for three to five minutes, such as a popular line dance—the Macarena, Electric Slide, Achy Breaky Heart, or Saturday Night Fever Walk

Motivation

Announce to students that they can learn a healthy and socially enjoyable way to warm up their bodies for an aerobic fitness unit (figure 4.1).

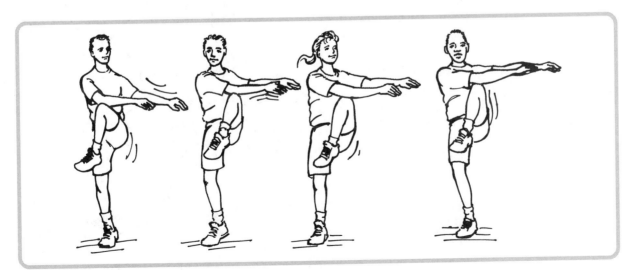

Figure 4.1—An aerobic dance class.

Lesson Sequence

1. Give a short explanation of the national health crisis of the 1960s that heralded the fitness movement and describe the current state of our population—dangerously overweight and inactive. In 1960, President John F. Kennedy was the first national leader to make national fitness a priority during peacetime. He encouraged the first national 25-mile walk, set up a youth council on fitness, and became a role model for living a vigorous lifestyle. Since then, with research and education, we have learned more about the nature of fitness, the benefits of activity, and the importance of both to a long and happy life.

2. Discuss briefly how fitness and health are interrelated: the heart, bones, cancer, aging, attitude, social life, and stress.

3. Demonstrate and teach, in segments, the warm-up chosen for the aerobic unit: it can be a line dance as in figure 4.1, which is a generalized warming of the large muscle groups, or it can be special exercises to focus attention to each large muscle group.

4. Teach a segment, and have the students duplicate. Allow for repetition.

5. Put the segments together, practice as a whole, and perform to music without stopping.

6. Teach students to stretch the following: the quadriceps, hamstrings (figure 4.2), gastrocnemius, lower back, shoulder joint, and neck.

7. Count and encourage a static stretch, 16 seconds for each stretch. Let students know that for stretching to be most effective they should
   • hold the position, reaching further only as they loosen up; and
   • know that physical therapists recommend holding a position for one minute.

Review

Discuss whether it is possible to be healthy if a person is not fit.

Review that students have started an aerobic dance unit designed to promote their physical fitness and that they have learned one aspect of fitness—stretching for flexibility.

Tell them that they have begun a unit of healthy movement that will improve their cardiovascular fitness.

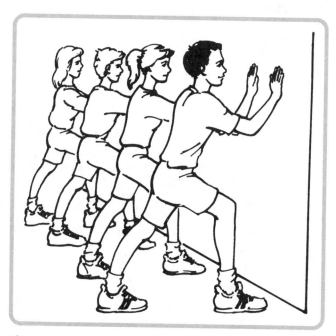

Figure 4.2—Group of students stretching their gastrocnemius muscles.

Ask students to take home a health index (see the index on page 97). Ask them to read it over with the family, complete it, and bring it back.

Physical Education Lesson 2   Beginner level

Lesson Setup

Equipment

Music passages three to five minutes long for two moderate aerobic activities or an appropriate video passage for a moderate routine
Music for an abdominal/thighs exercise routine or an appropriate video passage

Performance Goals

Students will

warm up,
measure their resting heart rate, and
learn a moderate activity:
- Aerobic dance—a square dance, folk dance, or novelty dance that includes walking, some skipping, and a little jumping
- Aerobic videotape—find a moderate section, break it down, teach it in parts, and then perform the whole thing through
- An abdominal routine
- Stretching

Cognitive Goal

Students will learn

the importance of *flexibility*:
- It enables them to move through a full range of motion.
- It prevents joint and muscle injury.
what a resting heart rate represents

Motivation

Tell students that they will increase the work their heart has to do by asking it to do more.

Lesson Sequence

1. Discuss flexibility.
2. Provide an explanation of the heart rate and how it translates as a pulse.
3. Explain that the heart works even when it doesn't seem to (involuntary muscles).

4. Teach students to feel their pulse on the wrist below the thumb or on the right side of the neck, as in figure 4.3.
5. Count pulse beats for a timed interval while students are at rest.
6. Begin the more active part of the lesson, teaching simple routines that include walking, limited jogging, jumping, or skipping. Break it down into parts before performing it as a whole. Play the entire music once each part is learned separately. Choose something that has no more than three simple parts and is self-repeating (e.g., Mayim,

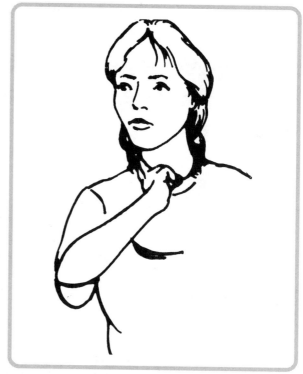

Figure 4.3—Finding the heart rate.

Bingo, Ve' David, or Seljancica if using folk dance).
7. Teach a routine for strengthening the abdominals and lower back muscles.
8. Conclude with the stretches learned in the first lesson, performing them as part of a routine to music, making sure each stretch is held for one musical phrase (16 beats).

Review

Ask students what they can do to avoid tearing muscles and dislocating joints.
Ask for someone to explain whether the heart is an involuntary muscle or a voluntary muscle.
Discuss whether it works even when they are resting.
Ask if students can remember their resting pulse.

Physical Fitness Lesson 3   Beginner level

Lesson Setup

Equipment

Highly energetic music such as Salty Dog Rag, Nebesko Kolo, Hora, or Jessie Polka, or something choreographed to popular music—Beat It, Gloria, or Tell Me What the Papers Say

Performance Goals

Students will increase their heart rate so it is within their target heart-rate zone and sustain it for at least 10 minutes. (Since students are still in the process of learning, they might not reach their target zones during this lesson. Future lessons will strive for continuous activity that is in the target zone for a minimum of 20 minutes.)

Cognitive Goals

Students will

understand what the cardiovascular system is and its importance to health and fitness;

learn to find their own theoretical maximum heart rate (220 beats − one's age = the maximum heart rate); and

learn the expression, "If you don't use it, you lose it," and what that means in fitness.

Motivation

Tell students that today they will learn what to expect from their heart rate if they work longer, faster, and harder.

Lesson Sequence

1. Discuss how frequency, intensity, and time (number of body parts, amount of work against gravity, and duration) can change the output requirement on one's heart.
2. Start activity with a designated warm-up.
3. Introduce and teach activity that is more vigorous—more jumps, runs, and arm movements and perhaps a little faster (use the Hora, Doubleska Polka, Jessie Polka, Kerry Reel, or novelty dances to popular music that have jumps and arm swings):
   • Teach the activity in segments.
   • Combine all parts, having students sustain the activity until the music is over.
   • Have someone in front of the class performing properly so students can see a role model.
4. Conclude the active part of the lesson with the moderate routine learned in the previous lesson, followed by the abdominal routine (if time), concluding with stretching.

Review

Review how students can make activity more demanding.
Discuss how they can make activity less demanding when it is too vigorous.
Ask what they can expect their hearts to do.

Physical Fitness Lesson 4 — Beginner level

Lesson Setup

Equipment

Heart rate monitor
Watch with a second hand

Performance Goals

Students will

measure their heart rates after they speed up;

perform an aerobic dance routine that includes a warm-up, moderate activity, vigorous activity, an abdominal strength item, and stretching; and

move continuously without stopping other than to count their pulse rates after the warm-up and after the most vigorous part of the routine.

Cognitive Goals

Students will understand, via demonstration,

how the cardiovascular system is affected by activity,

what happens to their pulse rates when doing a different activity, and

how high their heart rates go when doing the most rigorous part of a routine.

Motivation

Talk about how many times students' hearts beat during rest, during warm-up, and during vigorous activity.

Lesson Sequence

1. Have the class find and count the pulse rate before beginning the warm-up. Technology can help, as in figure 4.4,

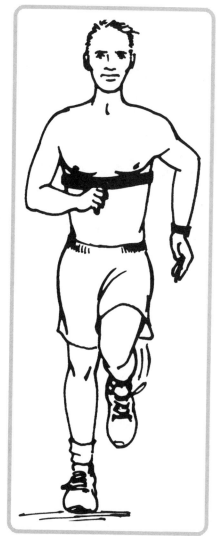

Figure 4.4—Using a heart rate monitor.

where a student is shown wearing a heart-rate monitor. Students should do the following:

- Learn to locate and feel their pulse rates
- Count for 15 seconds and multiply what they count by 4

2. Have the class do the warm-up. When it is over, instruct students to find their pulse, beginning to count on your signal.
3. Have them follow the same instructions for vigorous activity; after it is over, they should find their pulses and count on the signal.
4. Instruct the class to cool down with the moderate routine, followed by the abdominal routine, and then take a pulse rate again.

Review

Review, via questions and answers, what happened to students' heart rates as the work got harder and then what happened when it got easier again.

Ask anyone who has a heart-rate monitor at home to bring it in for the next few weeks.

Physical Fitness Lesson 5   Beginner level

Performance Goals

Students will

perform the aerobic routine;
calculate their own target zones: heart-rate range 60 to 75 percent of their maximum heart rate (220 beats – their age); and
work in their target zone during the lesson.

Cognitive Goals

Students will

understand the components of the target heart rate—time, heart rate, and air;
be brought up to date on current research that recommends the most effective route to cardiovascular fitness (frequency, intensity, time, and type—as of 1997, the suggested minimum is 30 minutes or more of activity every other day with a minimum of 15 minutes in the target heart-rate zone);
learn what is meant by *target heart rate*; and
understand what makes each person's zone different and what it takes to reach it.

Motivation

Students will find out today if this routine gets them into their target zones and for how long and what to do if it makes them work harder than they should.

Lesson Sequence

1. First, discuss and then compute the heart-rate zone mentally. Assist students by figuring their ages and doing the arithmetic orally: 220 − age (.60 or .75) = the zone.
2. Start the warm-up, move directly to moderate activity and then vigorous activity without pausing:
   - Have students check their heart rates at the highest activity point.
   - If there is someone with a heart-rate monitor on, have him read the monitor to the class at each point in the routine that he thinks they have entered into vigorous activity.
3. Lead the class in performing a moderate cool-down activity—an abdominal routine and stretching routine.

Review

Discuss having too high a heart rate and losing breath.
Ask students how they can reduce the effect doing the same activity.
Discuss having too low a heart rate.
Review how they can increase the effort doing the same activity.

Physical Fitness Lesson 6 — Beginner level

Lesson Setup

Equipment

Two more vigorous musical selections

Performance Goals

Students will

learn a second vigorous, highly energetic dance routine or activity,
perform a routine that reaches the maximum target zone for at least 15 minutes of the routine, and
be able to complete the activity already learned with no pauses.

Cognitive Goal

Students will review the minimal requirement to get and keep cardiovascular fitness.

Lesson Safety

Remind students that if they are experiencing more than the usual discomfort, to reduce their energy levels and alert you.

Motivation

Tell students that it's time to add to the routine developed so far so they are in the target zone for the recommended length of time.

Lesson Sequence

1. First discuss the minimum recommendation of time sustained in the target zone for enhancing cardiovascular fitness.
2. Teach one to two more vigorous routines so that the total time used to perform vigorously is at least 15 minutes. Activities chosen should have more running, jumping, skipping, hopping, and arm movements or be done with more speed.
3. Repeat as much of the intended routine as there is time for, while leaving time for a full cool-down, which can be a moderate dance activity, such as the Pata Pata, Stepping Out, or Virginia Reel, or abdominal exercises or the stretching routine you already taught.

Review

Ask if students had too high of a heart rate and were losing their breath.
Ask students how they can reduce the effect doing the same activity.
Ask whose heart rate never reached the target zone. Discuss having too low a heart rate.
Review how they can increase the effort doing the same activity

Teacher Homework

Once all the routines have been taught for the warm-up, a moderate increasing activity, a high-energy activity, an abdominal routine, more moderate activity, a cool-down, and stretching, and class time is used up when doing the routines continuously, tape the music together so that the sequence just rolls and students can just keep dancing.

Physical Fitness Lessons 7-12   Beginner level

Lesson Setup

Equipment

The seventh/eighth grade aerobic routine with all the music compiled

Performance Goals

Students will perform the class-developed aerobic routine that provides for *continuous* movement the entire period starting with a warm-up, progressing through activity levels until reaching the target heart rate, then bringing down the heart rate and finishing with a cool-down.

Cognitive Goals

Students will learn what it feels like to move continuously for 28 to 32 minutes.

Motivation

Students can get fit! Ask them if they know that when adults join health clubs, many take fitness classes for *an hour*. This class only has a certain number of minutes (mention the number). Explain that fitness can be improved with small amounts of activity that add up through the course of a day. However, tell students that the class is aiming for the optimum level for fitness and that the best way to reach that level is to work at the target heart rate zone for 15 to 20 minutes every day.

Lesson Sequence

Put the music on as soon as the five-minute dressing time is up. Students should enter the room and, without pause, begin their routines. You should do relevant class organization without interfering with the movement of the class activity. The full routine ends with a stretching segment for the cool-down. Pictured in figure 4.5 is a group of students, in varying degrees of tightness, stretching their hamstrings.

Review

Ask students if the routine is getting easier for them to complete.
Discuss if they are accomplishing their goal of being able to maintain constant energetic activity without needing a rest while they are in their target zone.

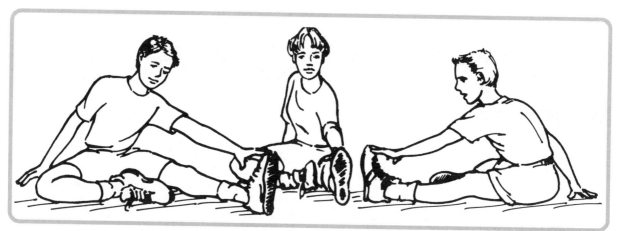

Figure 4.5—Part of a cool-down and stretch routine.

Ask if they are making gains, and if they think they're improving their fitness. If they keep this up, and stay exactly the way they are now, ask if they think they are fit.

Physical Fitness Lessons 13-14   Beginner level

Lesson Setup

Equipment

Posted grading standards

Performance Goals

Students will

perform their routines, and
assess their recovery rates.

Cognitive Goals

Students will learn how the body assesses its fitness—the *recovery rate*:

What the recovery rate is
How to measure theirs

Motivation

Mention to the students that they have been doing this for themselves for a while now and they know if it is getting easier or not. They probably can safely guess that as it is becoming easier to get through the whole routine, they also are getting fitter. Tell them it's now time for you to evaluate how accomplished they are and grade the variables they've been working on. Announce that there's another measure of their fitness, so they do not have to just guess it. To try to read their own body's reaction more scientifically, they can measure how long it takes their heart rate to slow down and get back to resting once they stop their activity and just rest. Inform students that it is believed that the faster one's heart rate returns to resting, the fitter one is. Suggest they see how long theirs take.

Lesson Sequence

1. First discuss the recovery rate and that the students' pulses will be taken at the conclusion of stretching.
2. Have them do the entire routine from start to finish.
3. Instruct them to take a recovery pulse at the end of the routine's stretching and cool-down sequence.

Review

Review the fact that stretching requires effort, too.

Ask students how many of them had heart rates that decreased during the stretching routine.

Ask how many had heart rates that got down to 100 beats per minute toward the last few minutes of their stretching routine. Tell them the fact that it's going down is great.

Five minutes after the completion of an activity a good health standard to watch for is that their heart rate has returned to its resting pulse.

Discuss whether students have learned enough to share with their parents and help them stay healthy.

Assessment

Assessment should be based on cognitive and performance gains. A written quiz (page 98) and performance rubric (table 4.3) can be used for this assessment. Also advisable is concluding with a measure of physical fitness for the sole purpose of student self-awareness.

Chapter 3 introduces and has lesson plans for a fitness test devised, used, and statistically analyzed in New York state. Though many tests are available—newer and better ones for measuring physical fitness—the book includes this performance-based test because it is short and has separate statistical norms for each gender, grade level, and age. For those seeking comparative scores, this might be advantageous. But comparative scores do not necessarily reflect fitness, and being average or above does not necessarily reflect one's state of health. Also, the items measured—agility, speed, abdominal strength, and endurance—are not complete measures of fitness.

If you are looking for the best way to assess fitness, you might want to seek out a criteria-based test. Scores from such a test allow students to learn the relationship between fitness and health, whereas statistical norms, as those used in the New York state test, only provide information on where a student ranks in comparison to others. Such a measure occasionally can be a good motivational tool, particularly when groups feel that they are doing enough because it is better than the student next to them.

Physical Fitness Lesson 1 — Intermediate level

Lesson Setup

Facility

An area large enough for the class to be able to safely move in

Universal and/or Nautilus machines that have been certified as safe

Free weights if nothing else is available

Equipment and/or floor space for aerobic activity that can accommodate the whole class at the same time while they
- jog in place and
- use aerobic equipment such as bikes, treadmills, Stairmasters, or rowing machines

Enough space to accommodate the whole class stretching at the same time

TABLE 4.3 Beginner Fitness Performance Assessment Rubric

NAME _____ DATE _____

TEACHER _____ CLASS PERIOD _____

	0	1	2	3	4	5
Flexibility While sitting can reach	Must bend the knees to reach with hand	Can reach knees	Can reach calves	Can reach ankle	Can grab sole of foot	Nose to knees
Aerobic fitness Mile walk/run	Cannot complete	Takes the full period to complete	Completes between 13 and 16 minutes	Completes between 11.9 and 12.9 minutes	Completes between 10 and 10.9 minutes	Completes in less than 10 minutes
Abdominal strength Sit-ups for a minute	Less than 9	Between 10 and 19	Between 20 and 24	Between 25 and 29	Between 30 and 39	40 or more
Upper-body strength Push-ups or pull-ups	Girls: 2 or less Boys: 3 or less	Girls: 3-4 Boys: 4-6	Girls: 5-6 Boys: 7-9	Girls: 7-9 Boys: 10	Girls: 10 Boys: 11-13	Girls: 11 or more Boys: 14 or more
Agility Stepping in 10 seconds	Girls: 0-6 Boys: 0-8	Girls: 7-8 Boys: 9-12	Girls: 9-10 Boys: 13-15	Girls: 11-13 Boys: 16-18	Girls: 14-17 Boys: 19-20	Girls: 18 or more Boys: 21 or more
Speed Shuttle run (in seconds)	Girls: 29+ Boys: 27+	Girls: 27.9-28.9 Boys: 25.5-26.9	Girls: 25-27 Boys: 23-25.4	Girls: 23.5-24.9 Boys: 22-22.9	Girls 22-23.4 Boys: 20-21.9	Girls: Less than 22 Boys: Less than 20
Balance Standing on one leg (in seconds)	0-2	3-4	5-8	9-12	12-18	19+

Equipment

Music for the aerobic warm-up and stretching
Audio/video equipment with good sound amplification

Performance Goals

Students will

take their resting pulse, and
begin working on a circuit training program using the weight room:
- Performing a warm-up routine to be done daily
- Beginning work on upper-body strength
- Performing a good stretching routine to be done daily

Cognitive Goals

Students will

review a history of fitness and why it is relevant to them and needed by all:
- The lack of exercise in daily lives leads to a natural state of poor fitness.
- Personal health is enhanced by fitness.

receive a quick summary of current research on the effects of fitness;

reflect on personal fitness strengths and weaknesses;

learn what circuit training is and how it improves fitness;

learn what every good circuit should include—warm-ups, aerobic exercise, and specific exercises for improving strength, flexibility, and agility;

learn what machines provide the aerobic aspect—the rowing machine, stationary bike, treadmill, steps machine; and

identify machines or weights for exercises dedicated to strengthening the upper body.

Lesson Safety

The facility must have appropriate space to allow the entire class to move safely.

It must be clean so students can be comfortable and be without risk of infection while lying on the floor.

The equipment must be certified for safety.

Students must be monitored for the following:
- To use safe amounts of weight (this is a fitness program, not a body-building program or a program to see how much a student can lift at one time; approaches and safety precautions differ for each individual)
- To breathe properly
- To go through the entire range of motion
- To stay away from machines that do not adjust to their sizes
- To behave appropriately:
  No throwing free weights
  No overloading the bar
  No using free bars without spotting

Warm-Up

The warm-up should be a rhythmical activity that uses all or most large body groups and is done everyday. It can be

a three-to-five-minute jog to music,

choreographed movement to music,

a review of a warm-up from seventh and eighth grade or something completely new and dance related, or

the use of aerobic equipment available in the room:
- bikes
- steps machines
- treadmills
- rowing machines

Motivation

Mention to the class that many people choose to work out in a weight room: A lot of people use the weights to get stronger and develop more bulky muscles. Others use weights for getting firm in hopes of sculpting their bodies. Tell students that they will begin to learn how to work out so they get all the benefits they want without causing any injuries to themselves.

Lesson Sequence

1. Give a short explanation of
   - the national health crisis of the 1960s and of the 1990s;
   - how fitness and health are interrelated—the heart, bones, cancer, stress, aging, attitude, social life, and stress;
   - the concept of working a circuit for total body fitness; and
   - the ingredients of fitness:
       Aerobic fitness
       Strength
       Flexibility
       Agility
2. Conduct a general aerobic warm-up of three to five minutes—jogging (could be in place), using any machine that induces cardiovascular fitness (the steps machine, treadmill, bicycle, or rowing machine), or doing a dancing warm-up learned during the seventh-and-eighth-grade unit.
3. Introduce exercises for the deltoids:
   - Have a student demonstrate at the appropriate machine or Universal station or with the correct hand-held equipment, making sure to emphasize proper alignment.
   - Have the class practice, with or without weight.
   - Have students do a set of 10, teaching them to breathe properly.
4. Do the same procedure at the appropriate stations for the biceps, triceps, latissimus dorsi, pectorals, and neck. You or one student should use the machine,
   - demonstrating the proper seat alignment,
   - teaching the class to find a weight that allows 10 repetitions of the exercise,
   - having students mimic the exercise, as seen in figure 4.6, without weight, and
   - Reminding everyone to breathe properly.
5. Conclude with a stretching routine (e.g., the routine from the seventh- and eighth-grade aerobic dance program).

Review

Discuss how the class has started a unit designed to safely improve physical fitness while using weights. Tell students that this kind of training, also called resistance training, has positive benefits, but only if they do it right. Some students have weights at home, some are on football or other sports teams and have been in a program to bolster their fitness, but most have done many of these exercises without ever having used weights before. Discuss your hopes that their workouts

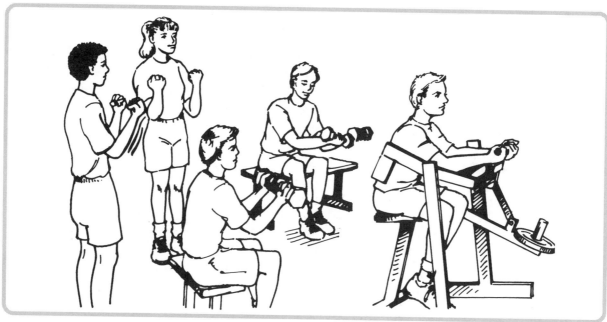

Figure 4.6—Using mimicry to get a point across.

are healthy ones: If weight training speeds up the process of firming up, getting one more fit and strong, it also can speed up the process of getting injured.

Ask the class why people work out with weights if they can hurt themselves: because it requires fewer repetitions to exert the same effort and get the same health benefit. Have the students guess the number of repetitions it would take to duplicate the energy used to do 10 contractions while bearing 40 pounds. Assure them that it would take a lot of repetitions and lots of time. That is why exercise regimens use weights. Someone on a tight schedule can complete a good workout in less time.

Physical Fitness Lesson 2 — Intermediate level

Performance Goals

Students will

perform warm-ups,
complete the introduction to upper-body muscle groups that were missed in the previous lesson,
perform exercises for the legs, and
cool down while stretching.

Cognitive Goals

Students will

learn the danger of using supplements to enhance performance;
understand the value of a warm-up (to prevent injuries);

understand the value of stretching (to maintain and improve flexibility to prevent injuries);

learn the "leg curl" and injury-prevention aspects of strengthening the hamstrings (most people develop the quadriceps for power and ignore the hamstrings, endangering the stability of the knee joint, which can overextend and tear ligaments);

identify exercises and machines for the gastrocnemius and quadriceps muscle groups; and

identify exercises for the ankles and hip-joint muscle groups and actions.

Warm-Up

Students will perform a rhythmical use of all large body groups in an established routine to be done every day in this unit.

1. Jog five minutes to music
2. Complete a choreographed movement to music
3. Perform exercises on rowing machines, bikes, steps machines or treadmills
4. Complete a specific dance routine

Motivation

Tell students that sometimes the power they teach their body to generate makes for better athletic performance. This brings to mind Mark McGuire and Sammy Sosa and their strenuous weight training, as well as their use of supplements. Mention the use of supplements since some students may have reached the age where they want to bulk up and get a lot stronger as quickly as possible. Ask if the issue of natural supplements has come up in health class. Find out if anyone is using natural supplements. First, they should learn how to use the equipment to build lower-body strength, then the class can talk about supplements later.

Lesson Sequence

1. Discuss the following:
   • The widespread use of supplements and how it has changed over time:
     The historic dangers of supplements
     The monetary enticement to get more power
   • Why warm-ups and stretching are important to a trained athlete or someone working out with weights:
     Warmth makes muscles more elastic; without elasticity, muscles can tear.
     Stretching reminds muscles to return to their longest state after they have been working so hard to shorten themselves by contracting.
     Rigorous training programs inadvertently promote shrinkage of muscles.
2. Introduce whatever upper-body muscle groups have not been taught and practiced previously:
   • Use a student to demonstrate:
     How to align the machine correctly to one's size
     How the exercise is performed on the machine

- Have students all do the exercise with or without the weight for today.
- Emphasize and make sure that everyone breathes properly while doing the exercise.

3. Demonstrate the "leg curl" and the proper alignment for the hamstrings:
   - Explain the necessity of building up hamstrings to 75 percent of the strength of the quad, to avoid hyperextension and possible tearing of crucial knee ligaments.
   - Have students duplicate the exercise even if they're not at a machine.
   - Show all the machines that use the curl for hamstrings.

4. Demonstrate extension and proper alignment for the quadriceps:
   - Have students duplicate the exercise even if they're not at a machine.
   - Show all the machines and the proper alignment for the upper quads as well as lower quads.

5. Repeat the process for the gastrocnemius muscle and for all ankle flexors.

6. Leave time to complete a stretching routine.

Review

Tell students that the more advanced an athlete is, or older, or stronger, the more important warm-ups and stretching are. Review that the class now has learned the machines for the upper body and the lower body. Ask if anyone remembers why the leg curl is so important to do every time one strengthens the quads.

Physical Fitness Lesson 3 — Intermediate level

Performance Goals

Students will

warm up;

perform the remainder of the exercises for the lower body that are yet un-learned;

perform, with safety (proper alignment and breathing), a routine for each exercise;

perform proper exercises for the abdominal muscles, back, and neck;

cool-down while stretching.

Cognitive Goals

Students will

learn the value of working out the abdominal muscles:
- The back is structurally vulnerable and many people complain of back pain.
- The abdominal muscles help avoid the structural weakness of being human and standing on our feet.

learn how to properly perform the remaining exercises for the lower-body muscle groups;

identify and learn to align and safely use the machines for the remaining muscle groups—the abdominals and back;

understand the differences among upper-body, lower-body, and torso categorized exercises; and

understand and establish a safe routine for using the weight room and working out with weights.

Warm-Up

Students should perform the rhythmical use of all large body groups in a routine done every day in the unit.

Motivation

Tell students that after this lesson, they will have been introduced to every machine for every muscle group. Then they can begin working out with a partner at their own pace.

Lesson Sequence

1. Complete whatever exercises have not already been introduced for the lower body, using the procedure already indicated.
2. Discuss the following:
   - General body alignment and why the back is prone to difficulties
   - Why abdominals are so important to strengthen
3. Introduce any machine or exercise that students are to use daily for strengthening a muscle group: have everyone perform with or without weight resistance.
4. Discuss the importance and method of making sure to work the body safely. Students should develop their muscle groups equally; if there isn't time to do it all in one period, they should alternate among upper, lower, and torso exercises.
5. Allow students to begin their own workout after warm-ups are completed.
6. Leave time to complete a stretching routine.

Review

Tell students that you now have introduced all the exercises. They might have forgotten the exercise names or how to move the machines so they align properly with their body, but you will be there to answer all questions in the days to come. They shouldn't fail to ask questions when they have them.

Ask if anyone remembers why so much attention is given to developing one's abdominal muscles.

Review whether it's necessary to have a special machine or setup to do it.

Physical Fitness Lesson 4 — Intermediate level

Performance Goals

Students will

learn what is meant by *muscle fatigue*,
pick a partner to work with,
follow the established routine, and
work out on their own.

Cognitive Goals

Students will understand

that breathing is important:
- Working with weights can be done aerobically.
- Weights themselves will not enhance cardiovascular fitness.
- Blowing the air out of one's lungs on the thrust is important.
- Counting out loud helps guarantee that one breathes.
- Holding one's breath is dangerous!

that one increases endurance by increasing, gradually, the following:
- The length of time (minutes, hours, weeks, months of working out)
- The frequency one works out (number of days a week)
- The intensity of the exercise (more weight, greater speed, or more repetition)

that many people find weight training more successful if they have one day on and one day off, with the off day dedicated to aerobic fitness.

Lesson Safety

Students must be monitored to use a safe weight and move through the entire range of motions.

Make sure that students count out loud or breathe in when lowering the weight and exhale when lifting the weight.

Warm-Up

Students should perform the rhythmical use of all large body groups in a routine done every day in the unit.

Motivation

Tell students that they are now almost completely ready to take the information they have and begin marking their own progress. In the next class, they will receive a chart to record their progress. For now, they should use as much of the equipment as they have time for and ask whatever questions they have. Tell them that you'll be moving around to see that their equipment is properly set up, that they are breathing correctly, and that they are trying to move through the whole range of motion instead of just part of it.

Lesson Sequence

1. Discuss breathing:
   - Aerobic breathing allows participants to complete more repetitions, which improves cardiovascular fitness
   - Compare it to the limitations of the weight-training approach, which is an anaerobic activity (starts and stops) that doesn't allow for continuous motion. Ask students to train on weights with as few starts and stops as possible.
   - The importance of good breathing technique while working on equipment
2. Discuss the meaning of endurance and how to improve it:
   - The length of practice
   - The frequency of practice
   - The intensity of practice
3. Have students warm up and then proceed with their own workouts.
4. Have everyone pair up so that while one is about to work, the other can set the alignment, put the pin in at the proper weight, and be the "cheerleader" encouraging the other student to complete the set of repetitions (reps). Then, of course, the roles reverse.
5. Make sure students move off the machines after one set, use the full range of motion, breathe properly, and use weights that do not make them reach muscle burnout before 10 reps. Explain that muscle burnout is another term that means muscle fatigue, which occurs when a muscle reaches the point where another repetition is not possible.
6. Leave time to complete the stretching routine.

Review

Discuss whether students have begun to build their endurance and how.
Have them do an inventory of what they've accomplished working through most of the period:
- Ask how many have exercised their abdominals.
- Ask how many did as many sets of exercise for their lower bodies as they did for their upper bodies.
- Ask how many were able to complete a full set of 10 reps without their partners having to change the weight.

Physical Fitness Lesson 5   Intermediate level

Lesson Setup

Equipment

Pens or pencils
Weight room chart for each student

Performance Goals

Students will

complete a daily circuit while training for fitness in the weight room,
record the weight they use at each piece of equipment they go to and the
number of reps they do, and
perform safely.

Cognitive Goals

Students will

understand that muscles are strengthened by repetition of exercises up to the
point of muscle fatigue, resting the muscles, and gradually increasing resistance;
understand that pushing the muscles beyond muscle fatigue damages the muscles;
learn how to increase strength by increasing frequency, intensity, time, and
type (a specific type influences which muscles are receiving a workout):
• The length of time (minutes, hours, weeks, or months of working out)
• The frequency one works out (number of days a week)
• The intensity of the exercise (more weight, greater speed, or more repetition)
learn to identify and follow all instructions on their individual weight-room chart; and
learn how to work efficiently with a partner.

Lesson Safety

Students must be monitored for the following:

Using proper alignment
Using a safe weight
Moving through the entire range of motion
Breathing properly

Warm-Up

Students should perform the rhythmical use of all large body groups in a daily
routine to be done every day in the unit.

Motivation

Announce that in this lesson and each one that follows, students will pick up
their own workout charts (table 4.4). The charts are for them to see the progress
they make as well as to remember what weights they should start with or that it
is time to increase the weights. Tell them to make an entry every day on everything they work on. Advise them not to overlook the entries about the amount
of weight used and the number of repetitions. If they have used weights that
were too easy and they did not reach muscle fatigue by the 10th rep, they shouldn't
do the set again. They should wait until the next class to raise the weights. In this
class, ask them to make a notation on their workout chart that tells them to add
weight. There also is a section for how long they did the cardiovascular warm-

TABLE 4.4 Charting Progress—A Workout Chart

NAME _____ CLASS PERIOD _____

DATE OF ENTRY										
Duration of aerobics exercise										
type (row, jog, bike, dance)										
Check if you stretched										
Number of abdominal curls done today										

COMPLETE ONE SET OF EACH OF THE FOLLOWING ACTIVITIES. RECORD THE WEIGHT. ENTER IN DATE COLUMN.

Bench press										
Shoulder press										
Lat pull downs										
Bicep curl/forearm										
Leg extenison										
Leg curls										

OPTIONAL EXERCISES IF TIME REMAINS. ENTER ON DATE DONE ONLY.

Squats										
Toe raises										
Hip and back extension										
Dips										
Chins										
Side lateral raises										
Triceps press down										
Decline press										
Arm cross										
Rowing torso										

From *Complete Physical Education Plans for Grades 7–12* by Isobel Kleinman, 2001, Champaign, IL: Human Kinetics.

ups, stretches, and abdominals; tell students not to forget them, even if they did them as a class. Entries should remain in the column for the date entered.

Lesson Sequence

1. Have the class do a warm-up.
2. Discuss strength, its meaning, and how to improve it:
   - The length of practice
   - The frequency of practice
   - The intensity of practice
3. Discuss muscle fatigue
4. Discuss how to most advantageously work with a partner:
   - Partners should check alignment.
   - They should check for proper weight and move the pin as needed.
   - They should record the last workout weight and the number of reps accomplished.
   - They should be a coach or cheerleader, encouraging the other student to get through the whole set before stopping.
5. Distribute charts and pens or pencils.
6. Allow students to proceed with their own workouts, using the chart shown in table 4.4.
7. Encourage students to ask questions, such as the following:
   - How do I move the seat?
   - Where are the pins?
   - Which exercise machine do we use for rowing?
8. Keep reminding the class as a whole and students individually to move through the full range of motion.
9. Students should be given time to complete their stretching routine.
10. Have students complete their entries on their charts and return pens or pencils and charts.

Review

Ask if the class has any questions.

Review how many students have completed all the required exercises.

Ask if anyone did more than one set at any machine.

Discuss whether anyone had time to do more than the required number of exercises.

Ask students why they think the required exercises only allow one set.

Physical Fitness Lesson 6   Intermediate level

Performance Goals

Students will

work in pairs, and

continue to complete the circuit and record their work on their charts.

Cognitive Goals

Students will understand that differing goals define someone's workout style and results:

Some work out to increase strength and muscle cross sections:
- The greater the cross section of muscle, the stronger the muscle.
- They want to create the image of bulk.

Some work out to become more fit:
- They try to exercise all the components.
- They expect firmness, not bulk.

Students will begin to understand some of the training program safety issues:

Prevention—clothing, water, breathing correctly, using equipment correctly
Recovery—muscle fatigue, muscle injury, joint injury, dehydration
Miracle enhancers for success

Warm-Up

Students should perform the rhythmical use of all large body groups in a daily routine to be done every day in the unit.

Motivation

Present students' charts to them. Ask them to be sure to make an entry every day that they work out. The entries should remain in the column for the date entered. Comment that physical improvement takes time—and it's time to start.

Lesson Sequence

1. Discuss the different training approaches as a review and motivation:
   - Strength
   - Total fitness
   - The class goal: for everyone to get more fit
   - The general use of training enhancers:
       Ask the students if they know of anyone using steroids, creatine, or other drugs.
       Save the lecture for another time—it's better to get kids to let you know how familiar they are with the enhancers, and what, if any, they use. This will create an open learning environment.
2. Tell students that fitness is impossible if the environment and the approach to training are not safe:
   - Prevention of injury—proper clothing, water, proper body mechanics, breathing
   - Recovery—from illness, fatigue, dehydration, injury
3. Distribute charts and pens or pencils.
4. Have students warm up and then proceed with their own workout.
5. Give students time to complete the stretching routine.
6. Have students complete their entries on their charts and return pens or pencils and charts.

Review

Ask if there are any questions.
Discuss if students remember how they can build strength.
Ask how many of them completed all the required exercises.

Physical Fitness Lessons 7-12 — Intermediate level

Performance Goals

Students will

work independently (in partners) on the goal of personal fitness and follow the established routine for developing fitness in the weight room:
- A cardiovascular warm-up of five minutes
- Stretching each muscle group
- Working on the abdominals
- Alternating upper-body with lower-body exercises done in one full set
- Completing a minimum of three sets for the upper body and three sets for the lower body

follow established safety procedures:
- The proper clothing
- Intake of water as needed
- Working with weight that allows muscle fatigue after 10 reps

monitor their own progress via daily entries on their weight-room charts.

Cognitive Goal

Students will become aware of the serious implications and dangers of using drug and natural substance enhancements.

Lesson Safety

Students must be monitored for the following:

Using proper alignment
Using a safe weight
Moving through the entire range of motion
Breathing properly

Warm-Up

Students should perform the rhythmical use of all large body groups in a routine.

Motivation

Present students' charts. Remind them that physical improvement takes time, and they should use their class time wisely.

Lesson Sequence

1. When students enter, distribute their charts and have them begin their workouts promptly. The attendance procedures can be done during the class without intruding on workout time.
2. Coach for the following:
   - Proper breathing
   - Full range of motion
   - Correct alignment while lifting
   - Monitoring, cheering, and recording for one's partner
   - Using class time wisely

Review

Ask students if there are any questions, and if this is becoming easier for them.

Bring up the enhancers that students may have mentioned they've used, and tell them what you've learned about them. It's important to discuss all the positives before discussing the negatives. Be honest about your concerns. Mention that the use of creatine was growing in 1999—major sports figures had great personal success with no life-threatening alterations. Comment that the long-term effects are unknown, and the unknown is scary. Discuss how steroids and Phen Fen got so widely used and the result 5 to 10 years down the line. Alert your students.

Ask anyone who has a heart-rate monitor to wear it for one lesson and see if his work approaches the set targets.

Assessment

Review the charts submitted by each student.

Grades can be based on the following:
- The ability to complete that which is required,
- Increasing the weight over time,
- Increasing the number of additional sets and muscle groups exercises,
- The quality of stretching and warm-up effort,

The performance rubric (table 4.5)

A quiz (see page 99).

Physical Fitness Lesson 1   Advanced level

Lesson Setup

Facility

An area large enough for the class to be able to safely move in

Universal and/or Nautilus machines that have been certified as safe, with pins for each machine being used

TABLE 4.5 Intermediate Fitness Performance Assessment Rubric

NAME _____ DATE _____

TEACHER _____ CLASS PERIOD _____

	0	1	2	3	4	5
Flexibility While sitting can reach	Must bend to reach with hand	Can reach knees	Can reach shins	Can reach ankle	Can grab sole of foot	Nose to knees
Aerobic fitness The mile walk/run (in minutes)	Girls: +15 Boys: +12	Girls: 14.1-15 Boys: 11.1-12	Girls: 12-14 Boys: 10.16-11	Girls: 11-11.9 Boys: 8.46-10.15	Girls: 10-10.9 Boys: 8.15-8.45	Girls: 9.9 or less Boys: 8.14 or less
Abdominal strength Sit-ups for a minute	Less than 15	16-21	21-26	27-34	35-40	41 or more
Upper-body strength Push-ups or pull-ups	Girls: 2 or less Boys: 4 or less	Girls: 3-4 Boys: 5-6	Girls: 5-6 Boys: 7-8	Girls: 7-9 Boys: 9-13	Girls: 10-11 Boys: 14-16	Girls: 12 or more Boys: 17 or more
Agility Stepping in 10 seconds	Less than 8	9-12	13-15	16-18	19-20	21 or more
Speed Shuttle run (in seconds)	Girls: 29+ Boys: 27+	Girls: 27.9-28.9 Boys: 25.5-26.9	Girls: 25-17 Boys: 23-25.4	Girls: 23.5-24.9 Boys: 22-22.9	Girls: 22-23.4 Boys: 20-21.9	Girls: Less than 22 Boys: Less than 20

Equipment

Music for aerobic warm-up and stretching
Appropriate audio or video equipment with good sound amplification

Performance Goals

Students will

take a resting pulse at the conclusion of the discussion;
do a 20-minute, uninterrupted exercise that they have learned before:
- A warm-up—three minutes
- Moderate activity—three minutes
- Vigorous activity—eight minutes
- Moderate activity—three minutes
- Stretching—three minutes

take their pulses before stretching and after stretching; and
take their pulses after the summary.

Cognitive Goals

Students will

discuss the validity of fitness and its value to a good and healthy life,
examine their current health profiles and discuss them,
learn about new relevant research, and
be reminded of the difference between a resting pulse and a working pulse.

Lesson Safety

The class needs appropriate space:

• Large enough to allow the entire class to move safely
• Clean enough for students to comfortably work out while lying on the floor

The equipment must be certified for safety.

Warm-Up

Students will complete the rhythmical routine that uses all of the large-body muscle groups.

Motivation

Tell your students that these are the last high-school years for them to learn, realize, and pattern a healthy lifestyle that will work for them forever. After high school, they won't be able to get that kind of education without paying for it in a college course or at a health club. Instead of learning all of these fitness skills in a health club, which could cost hundreds of dollars, students can maybe save a little money while they get moving in a healthy, fun way. Assure them that the money is not half as important as the health issues. Have them review what they've learned and where they are in the fitness/health profile.

Lesson Sequence

1. When the students enter, have them sit and come to a resting pulse during the review discussion.
2. Take a resting pulse.
3. Begin an activity routine that will go uninterrupted for 20 minutes and include a warm-up, moderate activity, vigorous activity, moderate again, and a stretching activity, in that order. Use previously learned aerobics routines, aerobics videos that can easily be imitated, or circuit training so that activity does not stop.
4. Take a pulse prior to stretching.
5. Take a pulse after stretching and have students note the number of beats that it has come down.
6. Take a pulse after the summary and have them note again whether it has returned to resting.

Review

Review students' recovery rates and their memory of their strengths and weaknesses in fitness. This knowledge is for them. At this point, it needs to guide them, not you, on how they should be vigilant about the best ways to work out and what they need to improve. Some students may not need to improve—maybe maintenance is all they need. In any case, these young adults hopefully will consider making their life as healthy as they want it to be.

In order to do that, tell students they should know whether their health profiles reach a health standard. They should know whether their fitness levels allow them to complete an activity, without undue stress, for 20 to 30 minutes. They should know whether their cardiovascular systems are able to recover after vigorous activity in a reasonable amount of time.

Assessment

Observe the students' abilities to follow instructions, how they join in discussion, and if they keep up with activity demands.

Ask students who have a heart-rate monitor to wear it for one lesson and see if their work approaches the target ranges they should be working in to bring up their cardiovascular fitness levels.

Ask if any students have an exercise video they like or a dance routine they want to follow; suggest they bring it for the next class.

Physical Fitness Lesson 2 — Advanced level

Lesson Setup

Equipment

Music and/or video of student choice either in the teacher library or brought from home

Recreational supplies and equipment that can be safely accommodated in the classroom environment, such as Ping-Pong, jump rope, a pool table, or, if there is a large gym area, basketballs, volleyballs, handball, badminton, or paddleball

Heart-rate monitors—as many as available (it would be great if there were one for each student)

Performance Goal

Students will choose to do either recreational, aerobic exercise, or weight-training activities for fitness improvement.

Cognitive Goals

Students will

analyze if the exercise of their choice yielded the cardiovascular benefit they
were aiming for,

understand the value and necessity of cardiovascular fitness,

understand how to reach cardiovascular fitness:

* The need to elevate the heart rate continuously for 20 minutes
* Cannot be continuous if needing to stop to catch one's breath

know their heart-rate target zone:

* How it varies by age
* The formula (220 – age x 60-75 percent = the average target heart-rate goal)

learn if the physical work of their choice yields performance in the heart-rate zone.

Lesson Safety

There will be many things going on if this lesson is followed in the way it is written; therefore, proper attention must be given to the need for the following:

Appropriate space for each independent activity so that none interferes with the other

A clean room so that students can work out while lying on the floor without risking infection

A weight machine that is certified for safety

Free weights that are used without dropping, throwing, or choosing extremes that might require spotting

Motivation

Tell students that in today's lesson, they will get to guide their own activities. They can choose whatever they want to do among certain things in their environment (you might have to restrict choice to accommodate location and safety). Tell students to try to keep doing whatever they are doing, even when you tell them to find their pulse and count it. They will be measuring to see if their activity of choice elevates their heart rates to a level that is sufficient to maintain cardiovascular fitness. Tell them to see if they can get their heart rates in the target zone that they need to be working in.

Warm-Up

Students will warm up on their own doing exercises they like.

Lesson Sequence

1. Discuss the lesson aim of the day, to see if activities of choice get students into their target zone and facilitate physical fitness.
2. Instruct students to respond to teacher direction to take their pulse:
   * They should anticipate this 15 minutes into the period.
   * They should do it while they are working.
3. Have the class proceed with activities of choice, noting whether students remember to warm up.
4. Observe if all students maintain their activity level throughout the period.
5. Fifteen minutes into the period, ask students, while they continue working, to locate their pulses.

6. When all students appear to have successfully found their pulses, give the signal to begin counting their pulse rates until they are told to stop counting. Try to encourage them not to stop activity while they do their counting.
7. The summary should be question centered to review the findings of this experiment.

Review

Discuss what you've observed of class warm-ups and work ethics.
Have students share what they learned about their heart rate during the activities of choice:
- Did it approach a sustainable target zone?
- Did it require rest that would cause heart-rate fluctuation?
- Do they think the highs and lows averaged into the target zone?

Tell the class that if anyone has a heart-rate monitor, it would be great to wear it. Even if students think they have this all figured out, it would be nice if they had the monitor with them. In fact, they might lend it to a friend so others can get an accurate reading of their heart rate, too.

Physical Fitness Lesson 3   Advanced level

Lesson Setup

Equipment

Music and/or video of student choice either in the teacher library or brought from home
Teacher-directed activities that gradually increase physical effort (you decide what that activity will be so there is the proper equipment to meet your goal)
Forms that outline the method of setting up one's own workout program:
- An aerobic dance/step/jazz routine format
- A circuit-training format
- Weight-training charts

Performance Goal

Students will burn some calories.

Cognitive Goals

Students will

correlate the value of activity with that of weight control;
examine the caloric-burning values of some popular activities;
learn how to increase the burning power of each activity; and
learn that to get the most value from exercise, one cannot get too fatigued to complete a full program.

Lesson Safety

Be vigilant that the high-energy part of the routine you lead is not exceeding anyone's heart rate.

Warm-Up

Students will complete the rhythmical routine that uses of all large-body muscle groups.

Motivation

Tell students that today you will lead them through your choice of activities for getting and maintaining fitness. They should pay attention to the physical effort required, because at the end of the lesson, you will assign them a project in which they complete their own routines or workout program.

Remark that fitness is necessary, but they need to realize that to do the work, they should stick to a routine that makes them do it as frequently as needed. The effort is something that they must enjoy—or else, at the earliest opportunity, they run the risk of giving it up.

Lesson Sequence

1. Discuss the value of food and the implications of using more than we can burn up each day:
   - Where one gets energy
   - How activity burns one's food intake
   - How caloric burn is related to intensity
   - Which activities yield the most burn at a moderate level of intensity:
     The highest value—.078 to .063 calories per pound per minute
     A stationery run at 70 to 80 steps per minute = .078
     Jogging at 13.5 miles per hour, handball, or soccer = .063
     The middle value—.045 to .05 calories per pound per minute
     Weight lifting or biking = .05
     Basketball = .047
     Tennis = .046
     Dancing = .045
     The lowest caloric burn—.036 calories per pound per minute
     Volleyball or walking = .036
   - How weight can be affected by the amount of activity one does
   - Getting a feel for the effort and burn of each activity
2. Announce the warm-up and lead the class in a classic warm-up.
3. Announce the moderate activity, increasing intensity, with students following.
4. Announce the target zone, increase the intensity, and have students follow.
5. Announce the next moderate activity, scale down the requirement, and have students follow.
6. Lead them in a stretch and cool-down.
7. Assign committees:
   - Give them a work sheet that will help organize their creativity.

- Look over the charts that they will be developing and show how you would have filled yours out based on one routine you did for today's class.

Review

Tell students that you are giving them a form to fill out and a responsibility to design, with their committee, part of a class routine that, when put together with the other committees' ideas, will fulfill the requirements of a good workout. The form simply outlines their plan and gives them a guideline for how to approach meeting their plan. Students will have some class time to finish some of the work, but they might need to do a little planning at home, too. Suggest they look the form over, and if they have any questions, they should ask before they leave class. You also can offer to be available after school to provide answers.

Students also should start thinking about what kind of music they like or what they would like to plan if left up to their own devices. Remind them that, whatever they choose to do, the whole class must be able to do it as a group.

Physical Fitness Lesson 4 — Advanced level

Lesson Setup

Equipment

Cassette players for each group
If the class is using a video, try to get a method of duplicating the part of the video that the students choose (if choosing a pretaped commercial tape) or a video camera to record their own movement choreography.

Performance Goals

Students will

work on developing their own warm-up, no-break, aerobic, or stretching routine to fulfill their assignment, and
burn some calories and use exercise to reduce stress.

Cognitive Goals

Students will discuss the following:

What is stress and what are the negative indicators
How to relieve muscle tension

Warm-Up

Students will warm up as the groups plan and practice their routines for presentation to the class.

Motivation

Announce to students that today they are starting to create their own routines (table 4.6). Once their routines are complete, you will tape each group's routine so you have a complete set of all the groups' routines that the class will use for the remainder of the unit. Until the students supply the warm-up, they should stick to yours.

Lesson Sequence

1. Discuss stress, what causes it, the negative indicators, and how to rid one's self of it.
2. Assign groups of no less than two to different aspects of developing the class routine. One group should develop each of the following, if in aerobics:
   - A warm-up routine
   - A moderate routine of three minutes
   - A second moderate routine of three minutes
   - A vigorous routine of three minutes (with the heart rate at the target zone)
   - A second vigorous routine of three minutes
   - A third vigorous routine of three minutes
   - An abdominal and lower-back routine
   - A stretching routine for all large muscle groups

Review

Remark that you hope the class is being creative. Students should find the music that they like moving to and choose movement that they enjoy doing, that they can teach to someone else, and that they can do, with their group, in front of the class. Once you get each group's routine, you can tape the whole thing together and play it through—the entire class has contributed to making an aerobic tape. Tell students that once it is taped together, you will keep the class copy so they don't have to bring their music back and forth anymore. And, when each group's section of music comes on, those students will come to the front of the class and be the leaders, so that everyone can dance along with them. Tell the students that it's going to be fun, and they may even teach you a few new steps.

Physical Fitness Lesson 5   Advanced level

Performance Goals

Students will

complete their group routines and prepare to present them to class; and be active for the full period, without a pause.

Cognitive Goal

Students will assume responsibility for one aspect of the class's road to improving aerobic fitness.

TABLE 4.6 Worksheet for Creating an Aerobic Dance

NAME _____

TEACHER _____ GRADE _____

STUDENTS IN GROUP	RESPONSIBILITY
1	
2	
3	
4	
5	
6	

RESPONSIBILITIES: MUSIC, CHOREOGRAPHER, TEACHER OF GROUP, WILL TEACH CLASS, A DEMONSTRATOR, SECRETARY

Musical selection	Group formation
Duration	Direction of movement
Beats per measure	Energy level
Length of introduction	Target heart rate
Dance attributes	Goal of this routine

GOALS: WARM-UP SPECIFIC MUSCLE GROUPS, STRETCH, HEART RATE IN FAT-BURNING ZONE, RAISE HEART RATE TO MAXIMUM, MAINTAIN CONTINUOUS MOTION, COOL-DOWN

The Choreography Explained:

Four measures

Arms _____

Body _____

Legs _____

Four measures

Arms _____

Body _____

Legs _____

Four measures

Arms _____

Body _____

Legs _____

Four measures

Arms _____

Body _____

Legs _____

Warm-Up

Students will practice and work on their choreography.

Motivation

Tell students that it's time to finish what they started and practice so they can teach and demonstrate their own routine. Instruct them to practice so they all can be in unison and each of them can be part of the leader demonstration when their music comes on. Tell them that in about 10 minutes, they will begin making presentations to the class and setting up their class aerobic routine.

Lesson Sequence

1. Have the groups complete their practice in 10 minutes, writing down the sequence of activity on a form, shown in table 4.6.
2. Have students begin their presentation, teaching their routines:
   • A warm-up routine
   • A moderate routine of three minutes
   • A second moderate routine of three minutes
   • A vigorous routine of three minutes (with the heart rate at the target zone)
   • A second vigorous routine of three minutes
   • A third vigorous routine of three minutes
   • An abdominal and lower-back routine
   • A stretching routine for all large muscle groups

Review

Review what has been finished so far. Announce how many routines the class has left to learn. Tell students you will take their music and make a master tape, and then return their cassettes and CDs to them. Tell them you're looking forward to learning their routines and letting them teach you some new things. Tell students that if they haven't left their music and plan with you already, they should remember to bring it in next class.

Assessment

You are aiming for fitness and joy here, so keep the tone light and enthusiastic.

Teacher Homework

Make sure that all student music is taped on one tape in the proper sequence, so the class can perform each group routine with continuous motion. As routines are taught in the order called for, tape them on one class tape that can run without interruption later on.

Physical Fitness Lessons 6-12 — Advanced level

Lesson Setup

Equipment

Any equipment the groups need for their routine—steps, light free-weights, and so forth

Performance Goal

The class will be active for the full period. Students will come to the front of the class to lead the section of the routine they developed themselves.

Cognitive Goal

Students assume partial responsibility for everyone's fitness and fun.

Motivation

If all the routines have not yet been presented, taught, and taped, tell the class that it's time to finish learning what classmates have so diligently created so that the routine can be done in its entirety after today.

Lesson Sequence

Groups lead the part of the routine that is theirs on the tape by coming to the front of the room during their routine and returning to the group and becoming the class when it is not.

Review

Discuss what is meant by "no pain, no gain."
Ask students if they really have to be in pain to have a gain.

Assessment

Have the class retake the physical fitness test profile and see how it changed. Skills assessment can be based on a variety of performance standards:
- The performance rubric
- Improvement in physical fitness levels
- Effort in assuming responsibility and being self-directed

Assess knowledge through a written quiz (located on page 100).

Physical Fitness Quiz—Intermediate Level

NAME _____ TEACHER _____

DATE _____ CLASS PERIOD _____

True or False: Read each statement below carefully. If the statement is true, put a check under the True box in the column to the left of the statement. If the statement is false, put a check under the False box in the column to the left of the statement. If using a grid sheet, blacken in the appropriate column for each question, making sure to use the correctly numbered line for each question and its answer.

True **False**

☐ ☐ 1. The heart rate increases if one does an activity with increased weight.

2. Reduced flexibility reduces the risk of injury.

☐ ☐
☐ ☐ 3. A working heart rate of 100 beats per minute for someone 16 years of age is too slow to significantly improve cardiovascular fitness.

☐ ☐ 4. Common aerobic activities are tennis, volleyball, and basketball.

☐ ☐ 5. To gain the most positive cardiovascular improvement, activity should not stop for 20 to 35 minutes.

☐ ☐ 6. An ideal "set" in basic weight training is a minimum of 8 to a maximum of 12 repetitions.

☐ ☐ 7. Muscle burnout is a symptom of muscle fatigue.

☐ ☐ 8. Good activities that are done incorrectly are still beneficial.

☐ ☐ 9. It is best to warm up your muscles before you stretch.

☐ ☐ 10. A person can be physically fit without being fast.

Extra Credit: Match the columns.

_____ 1. Pulse   **a.** Moving through the whole range of motion

_____ 2. Flexibility   **b.** Increases the heart rate

_____ 3. Anaerobic activity   **c.** Sixty to 75 percent of one's maximum heart rate

_____ 4. The target zone   **d.** Evidence of a contracting heart muscle

_____ 5. Faster and higher   **e.** Running sprints

From *Complete Physical Education Plans for Grades 7–12* by Isobel Kleinman, 2001, Champaign, IL: Human Kinetics.

Physical Fitness Quiz—Advanced Level

NAME _____ TEACHER _____

DATE _____ CLASS PERIOD _____

True or False: Read each statement below carefully. If the statement is true, put a check under the True box in the column to the left of the statement. If the statement is false, put a check under the False box in the column to the left of the statement. If using a grid sheet, blacken in the appropriate column for each question, making sure to use the correctly numbered line for each question and its answer.

True	False	
☐	☐	1. A 120-pound girl is carrying a backpack with 50 pounds of food and clothing. Her body will have to work as hard as someone who weighs 170 pounds.
☐	☐	2. Stretching teaches your muscles to be shorter, thereby reducing your range of motion.
☐	☐	3. Seventy year olds who elevate their heart rates to 100 beats per minute work near the same cardiovascular efficiency (75%) of an 18 year old with a heart rate of 144.
☐	☐	4. You get more cardiovascular benefits from dancing than from bowling or playing ping pong, billiards, softball, or football.
☐	☐	5. The purpose of working within a target zone is to maintain activity that challenges your cardiovascular system without making you lose your breath.
☐	☐	6. You cannot achieve cardiovascular benefits from activity unless you work in your target zone for 20 minutes.
☐	☐	7. Your resting pulse rate will be lower if you're older or more fit.
☐	☐	8. It is better to stretch before you warm-up since cold muscles are more elastic.
☐	☐	9. Improper alignment while lifting weights can cause serious muscular and structural damage.
☐	☐	10. If the activity you are doing is fun, you cannot be working hard enough to improve your cardiovascular system.
☐	☐	11. Weight lifting burns about the same number of calories as biking.
☐	☐	12. Running in place at 80 steps per minute burns more calories than just about any other activity you can do.
☐	☐	13. There is bound to be some mild discomfort when raising your fitness level.

☐ ☐ 14. You know your fitness is improving when you are too tired to finish the routine.

☐ ☐ 15. A day on followed by a day off suggests giving muscles a chance to rest from lifting weights.

Matching Questions: Read one numbered item at a time. Then look at each of the possible choices in the column on the right. Decide which item in the right-hand column best matches that of the left-hand column and put the corresponding letter on the blank space to the left of the number it best matches.

_____ 1. Recovery rate   **a.** Shortens, thickens, and strengthens muscles.

_____ 2. Adding weight   **b.** Increases the heart rate

_____ 3. Active person's THR   **c.** Time it takes to return to resting pulse

_____ 4. Inactive person's THR   **d.** 60% of their maximum heart rate

_____ 5. Lifting weights   **e.** 75% of their maximum heart rate

From *Complete Physical Education Plans for Grades 7–12* by Isobel Kleinman, 2001, Champaign, IL: Human Kinetics.

Lifestyle Fitness Index Answer Key

Scoring: three points for each A, two points for each B, and one point for each C.

25 to 30 points: Congratulations. You are probably taking good care of yourself.

16 to 24 points: Not bad, but review your exercise program; increase intensity or duration and flexibility.

Below 15 points: This is a wake-up call. Accumulate 30 minutes of moderate exercise over the course of a day, every day. This will help shed pounds, reduce stress, and reduce risk of certain types of cancers, heart disease, and other chronic illnesses.

Physical Fitness Answer Key—Beginner Level

1. T. She uses more calories.
2. T. He cannot participate for 20 minutes if he cannot breathe.
3. T. Strengthening exercises teach muscles to contract, thereby shortening them.
4. F. Static stretches are recommended to avoid injury.
5. F. Aerobic activity requires continuous motion with breath; football is not continuous.
6. T. The heart, lungs, arteries, and veins supply the body.
7. F. The heart rate of 220 beats per minute is the maximum heartbeat of a newborn.
8. F. Endurance is the ability to continue; tiring prevents endurance.
9. F. Physical activities are necessary to maintain health.
10. T. Raising your heart rate means you are doing an activity; physical activity reduces stress.

Extra Credit:

1. A
2. N
3. A
4. N
5. N

Physical Fitness Answer Key—Intermediate Level

1. T. More effort raises the heart rate.
2. F. A loss of flexibility can lead to muscle tears, ligament ruptures, and so forth.
3. T. $220 - 16 = 204 \times 65$ percent $= 133$ beats per minute, the minimum recommended rate.
4. F. Aerobics require continuous movement with breath; these are not continuous.
5. T. This is the 1997 minimum recommendation.
6. T. A set is the number of times one lifts the same weight without stopping.
7. T. It is the feeling you get when the muscle cannot lift a weight again without rest.
8. F. Performing an exercise incorrectly leads to injury.
9. F. Warm muscles stretch further than cold muscles.
10. T. Speed is not a function of fitness.

Extra Credit:

1. d
2. a.
3. e
4. c
5. b

Physical Fitness Answer Key—Advanced Level

1. T. Both people are moving 170 pounds.
2. F. Stretching reminds muscles to return to their full length, increasing the range of motion.
3. T. The formula, 220 – age (75%), yields those numbers. The differences are the ages.
4. T. Dancing is continuous (aerobic). The other activities start and stop (anaerobic).
5. T. Target zones are efficient both aerobically and for the cardiovascular system.
6. F. Cardiovascular benefits are derived by not being sedentary.
7. T. A baby has the highest resting heart rate.
8. F. Warm muscles stretch better and lower the risk of injury.
9. T.
10. F. The idea is to find some activity you love that will keep you healthy.
11. T. Both done recreationally are considered moderate activities.
12. T.
13. T. Tiredness, some muscle fatigue, and sweating is not always comfortable.
14. F. It is just the opposite
15. T.

Matching

1. C
2. B
3. E
4. D
5. A

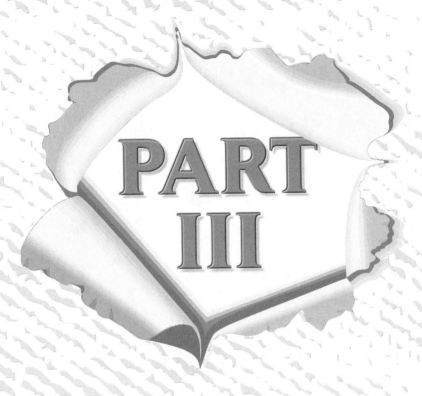

PART III

Lifetime Activities Unit Plans

chapter

5

Badminton

Unit Overview

1. Introduce one skill at a time:
   - Short serve
   - Overhead clear
   - Long serve
   - Underhand clear
   - Smash
   - Forehand and backhand drives
   - Directing shuttlecock from left to right
   - Hairpin shot

2. Teach rules of the game as the skill being taught is presented:
   - The serve—Teach serving rules: short, out-of-bounds, turn of service.

- Once game play begins—Teach scoring, boundaries, order of receiving, and positioning.
- Once tournament begins—Review all game rules, teach court strategies, teach skills strategies, for example, strategies for the smash.

  Teach the reliability of smashing from different distances.

  Go over the laws of trajectory and angles.

  Discuss the concept of probability with a net in the way.
- Doubles strategies
- Playing matches instead of games

Badminton

HISTORY

Badminton began about 2,000 years ago. Then, the game was the battledore and the shuttlecock, played in ancient Greece, India, and China. The name *badminton* came from the Badminton House in Gloucestershire, where the sport was played for many years. Gloucestershire is now home of the International Badminton Federation (IBF), which was founded in 1934.

FUN FACTS

→ One hundred thirty-one countries are members of the International Badminton Federation.

→ Badminton became an Olympic sport in 1992.

→ More than 1.1 billion people watched the Olympic debut of badminton on television.

→ China and Indonesia are two of the most successful badminton countries, winning 70 percent of all IBF events.

→ Badminton is the world's fastest racket sport (a shuttlecock can leave the racket at a speed nearing 200 mph).

BENEFITS OF PLAYING

1. By playing badminton you can burn .214 calories per minute per pound of your body weight. So, for example, if you weigh 120 pounds and you play badminton at a vigorous pace for 30 minutes, you will burn 770.4 calories (.214 $\times$ 120 $\times$ 30).

2. A badminton player may cover more than one mile in a single match.

3. You only need one other person in order to play. Thus, it is easier to get a game going than in other sports that require large numbers of players.

4. Badminton is a lifelong sport. You can play it when you are 5 or 75!

5. It's fun!

TIME TO SURF!

Web Site	Web Site Address
USA Badminton	www.usabadminton.org
The International Badminton Federation	www.intbadfed.org
The Badminton Association of England	www.baofe.co.uk/intro.html

From *Complete Physical Education Plans for Grades 7–12* by Isobel Kleinman, 2001, Champaign, IL: Human Kinetics.

Badminton Unit Extension Project

NAME _____ CLASS _____

Equipment needed to play badminton

Item	Where you would purchase it (be specific)	Cost

Where you would play badminton

Please explain where in the community you would play badminton. Be specific.

Health benefits of playing badminton

Please explain the health benefits of playing badminton. Include how much badminton you would need to play each week to gain these benefits.

Reflection question

Do you think badminton is an activity you would like to play as an adult? Why or why not?

From *Complete Physical Education Plans for Grades 7–12* by Isobel Kleinman, 2001, Champaign, IL: Human Kinetics.

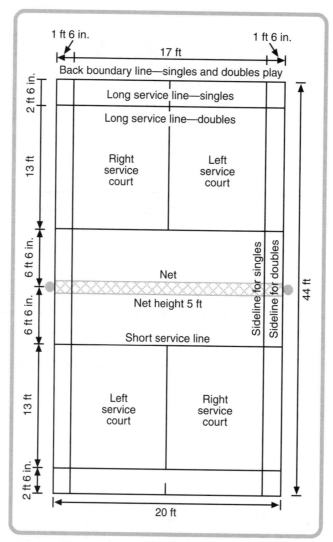

Figure 5.1—Badminton court dimensions.

Badminton Teaching Tips

1. Equipment for badminton is fragile and needs special care and attention. You must elicit the help of your students:
   - Explain the fragility.
   - Explain how best to make sure the rackets and strings are in one piece at the end of the unit.
2. Shuttlecocks do not travel the same way that balls do:
   - Explain the drop on descent and the reason for this.
   - Explain the weight and shape difference.
3. Generating power is more difficult in badminton:
   - Explain how the laws of momentum come into play with the lighter badminton racket.
   - Explain that less mass requires more velocity for the same force to be generated.
   - Explain how wrist snap can increase the velocity.

4. Because this game is indoors, space might be limited, preventing 100 percent of the students from playing 100 percent of the time. This is particularly true when practice drills are over. Since every student deserves equal court and game time, try a rotation, such as
   - assigning players A, B, and C to court 1;
   - dividing class time into three play periods;
   - setting up play period 1—player A plays B while C officiates;
   - setting up play period 2—player B plays C while A officiates; and
   - setting up play period 3—player C plays A while B officiates.

5. Allow noncompetitive practice time daily so students can improve their skills without performance pressure.

6. Each lesson should include some kind of contest that emphasizes the point of the lesson.

7. Students whose coordination makes learning the badminton serve difficult should be encouraged to forget the court and the net and work at a wall until they are able to drop the shuttlecock and contact it repeatedly without a problem. The wall, while not essential, will allow students to focus on contact and timing, not the flight of the shuttlecock. It will also allow easy retrieval, more repetition in a shorter time, and prevent students from worrying about whether the serve passes over the net and goes in the diagonal box. This way students' work on their timing for making contact with the shuttlecock will not be further compromised by fear of failure.

8. In the event of absentees: If a tournament is running, to keep its flow and its fairness, and to guarantee all prepared players a good daily experience, the following is suggested. The player whose partner is absent may
   - play the whole court by himself, or
   - officially lose the game (forfeit) but play anyway by asking one of the substitute officials to play in his partner's place.

9. If students are unable to participate fully in class activities, remember that they can be involved by coaching, officiating, keeping score, or conducting a research project.

Unit Setup

Facility

There should be a minimum of one court for every two sets of doubles partners. Courts should have nets and be marked with
- sidelines,
- service boxers,
- short lines, and
- long lines.

Equipment

One badminton racket for each person

One shuttlecock for every two people, with extras to replace shuttlecocks that get lodged on overhead rafters and basket backboards

A round-robin tournament chart and schedule. Examples can be found in appendix A.

Unit Timeline

There are two units, Beginner and Intermediate. Each has
   four to six lessons to develop skill enough to enjoy a game,
   two lessons on a game,
   six lessons for a class tournament, and
   three lessons for assessment.

Planning a Tournament

Round-robin tournaments are the best format for classes. If the class has a wide range of abilities, it is best to have separate round-robin tournaments running concurrently. That way, competition is even, students get to play on their own level with partners of their choice, the atmosphere is competitive, players still have to play their personal best, and there are more winners. See appendix A for tournament schedules and charts.

Unit Assessment

Observe students during each lesson to decide whether to go on and teach something new or to reemphasize what was taught. In the early lessons, moving forward should depend on whether the majority of the class is comfortable with the essential skill taught—in other words, in badminton the essential skills are the serve and the overhead clear.

TABLE 5.1   Badminton Student Portfolio Checklist

STUDENT NAME _____

- [ ] Knows the use and care of badminton racket and shuttlecock
- [ ] Knows and can perform the long serve and the short serve
- [ ] Knows the rules of service
- [ ] Is familiar with the court and all its markings
- [ ] Has learned and can perform the overhead clear
- [ ] Has learned and can perform the smash
- [ ] Has learned and can perform the underhand clear
- [ ] Has learned and can perform the overhead drop shot
- [ ] Has learned and can perform the hairpin shot
- [ ] Has learned and can perform the backhand clear
- [ ] Can direct the shuttlecock right or left
- [ ] Is able to play a game
- [ ] Knows the official rules of scoring in badminton
- [ ] Can play both singles and doubles
- [ ] Exhibits responsibility and sporting behavior during competition

From *Complete Physical Education Plans for Grades 7–12* by Isobel Kleinman, 2001, Champaign, IL: Human Kinetics

A student portfolio checklist is provided here for student use (table 5.1). Encourage students to track their progress as they master new skills. You can also assess the students by concluding the unit with a quiz. Students will also be evaluated on the basis of performance goals as outlined in the performance rubric for their grade and experience level. Further general assessment rubrics can be found in appendix B.

Additional Resources

Ainsworth, Dorothy, ed. 1965. *Individual Sports for Women*. Philadelphia: Saunders Co.

Miller, Donna, and Katherine Ley. 1963. *Individual and Dual Sports for Women*. Englewoodcliff, NJ: Prentice Hall.

Poole, Jon. 1996. *Badminton* (4th ed.). Prospect Heights, IL: Waveland Press.

Badminton Lesson 1   Beginner level

Lesson Setup

Facility

Courts marked with boundaries and short lines
Nets up

Equipment

One racket for each student
One shuttlecock for every two students
Extra shuttlecocks for replacements

Performance Goals

Students will

perform a short serve, and
take care with the equipment and return it.

Cognitive Goals

Students will learn

that equipment is fragile and needs special care,
the parts of the racket and the shuttlecock and how to hold both, and
some service rules:
  • The serve must be met below the waist.
  • The serve must clear the net.
  • The serve must pass a short line.

Lesson Safety

Practice wall areas are separated by a minimum of 10 feet per group.

Warm-Up

Students will

1. Perform sit-ups and push-ups
2. Complete agility footwork (short, quick change of direction steps—side to side, crossovers, backward and forward)
3. Perform specific mimetics
   - Snap the wrist forward and back several times, exaggerating the full range of motion.
   - Add a gentle forearm swing followed by a wrist snap.

Motivation

Badminton is a very popular game in Asia. People practice on the streets, in local parks, in any space they can find. A badminton racket is as common to the people of Shanghai as a softball glove is to the U.S. population. The racket is light and so is the object traveling through the air. Some people call it a "birdie," maybe because it should never land, but the official name is more peculiar than that: shuttlecock. Because it is light and not round, it does not play or fly like a ball. For those who play or watch tennis, racquetball, pickleball, or squash, the equipment and rules make badminton very different from other racket sports. Start by discussing how to get the shuttlecock in play legally.

Lesson Sequence

1. Discuss the following:
   - The lightness of equipment
   - Equipment use
   - Assigning students responsibility for preserving equipment
     Not throwing it
     Taking care not to unravel racket grips or pluck the strings
     Taking care not to break feathers or plastic feathers, or remove cork on shuttlecock
   - The proper gripping of the racket, and the shuttlecock (figure 5.2).
2. Demonstrate and teach the short serve:
   - Make lines and have the students practice dropping the shuttlecock before hitting it to

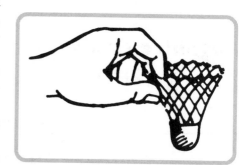

Figure 5.2—Holding a shuttlecock.

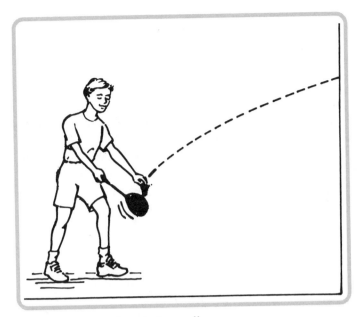

Figure 5.3—Serving to the wall.

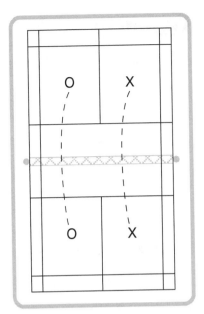

Figure 5.4—Serving over a net.

the wall. Do not rotate until they are successful two times. Go through the line a few times (figure 5.3).
- Have students pair off and try their serve over the net (figure 5.4).

3. Teach service rules:
- The shuttlecock must be met below the waist.
- The shuttlecock must clear the net.
- Players get one chance to serve it properly or they lose their turn of service.

4. Create a skill contest that relates to the serve. Some examples:
- Who can meet the shuttlecock with their racket every time they drop it?
- Who can get the shuttlecock to land in the service box?
- Report when you have been able to hit the serve over the net and into the service box three times.

Review

Review the rules of service and concerns about equipment.

Badminton Lesson 2   Beginner level

Performance Goals

Students will

improve their short serve, and
perform an overhead clear.

Cognitive Goals

Students will

learn the remaining service rules:
- The serve must be hit to the diagonal box.
- The service alternates from right to left and back again after a point is scored.
- The server gets one chance to direct the serve correctly or loses her turn of service.

understand that to hit up, they must contact the shuttlecock beneath it; and understand the reason for being able to hit shots with depth.

Lesson Safety

No more than four people at a time should be on one court.

Warm-Up

Students will

1. Perform sit-ups and push-ups
2. Complete footwork drills for agility
3. Complete specific mimetics
   - Practice the motion of the short serve
   - Learn and practice the motion of an overhead clear, with rackets if possible

Motivation

The building blocks of any game begin with how to get play started. After receiving the serve, students must learn how to play the shuttlecock back so they don't get into trouble. That means keeping their opponent back, away from the net. To do that they must hit the shuttlecock up. There is a skill called the "overhead clear," which is very much like the motion one uses in throwing, serving overhead in volleyball, spiking, or smashing. The difference is where one meets the shuttlecock. Discuss how to hit an overhead clear.

Lesson Sequence

1. Demonstrate and teach the overhead clear (figure 5.5):
   - Practice the full swing until the motion can be heard cutting the air.
   - In pairs, put the shuttlecock in play and have partners rally using the overhead clear.
   - Encourage full swings, with the shuttlecock traveling from baseline to baseline.

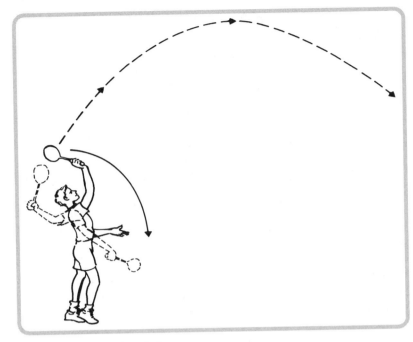

Figure 5.5—Overhead clear.

Figure 5.6—Serving on the diagonal.

2. Discuss the specific requirements of serving:
   - Being able to direct the serve diagonally—demonstrate follow-through
   - Strategy of keeping the serve low and short
3. Practice the short serve:
   - Aim for the diagonal box, as shown in figure 5.6.
   - Get the serve lower so partner cannot use the overhead clear.
4. Create a contest to prevent waning interest, such as the following:
   - Whose serve can keep their partner from hitting an overhead?
   - Which partners can rally from baseline to baseline?

Review

Ask students where they want the overhead clear to go.
Review why they have to swing so hard.
Ask if they want their short serves to be high or low.
Review what happens if they don't send their serves into the diagonal box.

Badminton Lesson 3   Beginner level

Performance Goals

Students will

be able to perform a short serve, overhead and underhand clears;

117

be able to perform forehand and backhand clears; and improve skills already introduced.

Cognitive Goals

Students will learn

that light things will not travel fast or deep without full swings, and the order of serving and receiving serve in doubles.

Warm-Up

Students will

1. Complete side-to-side stepping, running forward and backward
2. Practice all motions with a racket—the short serve, the overhead clear, and the motion for forehand and backhand underhand clears.

Motivation

Sometimes the shuttlecock drops too low to get under it so that one cannot clear it with an overhead shot. This is especially true if one's opponent has a good short serve. The solution is the underhand clear. Work on the clears with the students and go over the rules of serve and receiving serve. If there is time, maybe the players can start playing a short game.

Lesson Sequence

1. Demonstrate the backhand clear first. Have students practice in pairs.
2. Demonstrate the forehand clear and allow rallying practice in pairs.
3. Teach turn of service and receiving rules:
   - On an even score, the person serves on the right; odd score is from the left.
   - In doubles, both hands serve, except during the first turn of service at the beginning of the game.
   - Receivers must receive all serves that are intended for their box.
4. Play a short game if time remains.

Review

Ask students what the difference is in the motion between hitting a short serve and an underhand clear on their forehand side.
Review the objective of the underhand clear.
Ask what players should do differently if they're not getting enough depth.
Review the rules of service and concerns about equipment.

Badminton Lesson 4 — Beginner level

Performance Goals

Students will

learn the smash,
improve skills already introduced, and
play a short game.

Cognitive Goals

Students will learn

that hitting down instead of up depends on the contact point, and
that the motion for the smash and the overhead clear is the same.

Warm-Up

Students will

1. Practice with equipment before class begins during a free play period
2. Complete mimetics—practicing all motions of all learned skills with a racket in hand

Motivation

The past few lessons have warned of hitting up, encouraging players to hit deep so they won't get into trouble. The reason is that when someone hits up and short, she is vulnerable to a smashing return. Discuss the first attacking skill—the smash. It will clear the net when someone hits a high short serve or a weak clear. When they do, it is to one's advantage to step forward and smash the shuttlecock, because a smash travels fast and down and is very difficult to return. It usually wins the points. Have students learn how to do it.

Lesson Sequence

1. On the blackboard, show the differences between the point of contact for overhead clears and for smashes.
2. Demonstrate the smash (figure 5.7):
   • Self-toss and smash.
   • Partner toss and smash.
   • Have one partner hit short and high so they can smash it.
3. Play a game.

Review

Review what makes the difference between a short serve and a long serve.

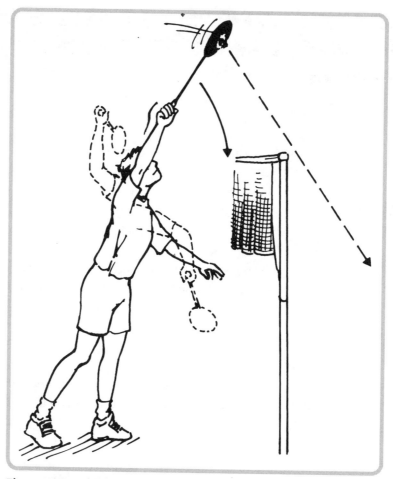

Figure 5.7—The smash.

Badminton Lesson 5 | Beginner level

Performance Goals

Students will

learn the long serve,
learn how to receive the different serves,
improve skills already introduced, and
play a game.

Cognitive Goal

Students will

learn that the wrist is the biggest factor between the long serve and the short serve, and
learn that different service situations require different strategies.

Warm-Up

Students will

1. Practice during a free play period (about five minutes). Encourage students with difficulty serving to see you for extra help during this time.
2. Complete footwork drills for moving up and back.

Motivation

Some books suggest that the first serve to learn is the long serve. Now that players have mastered the short serve, it may be time to learn how to fake out an opponent who expects a short serve and is waiting close to the short line to receive it. Of course, what is the problem with attempting a long serve that falls short? The opponent can smash it. Here's how to be effective.

Lesson Sequence

1. Show the differences between long- and short-serve swings, timing, and shuttlecock flight.
2. Have students practice long serves, aiming for everyone to have five successes before moving on.
3. Ask students to see if they can mix up their serves, long and short, spending a short time on this.
4. Bring the class together and discuss possible responses:
   - Change court positioning to be more central and ready to receive either serve.
   - Respond to the serve by using the overhead clear or the underhand clear.
   - Look for a bad serve and be ready to attack it by moving forward to smash.
5. Play a game.

Review

Review what makes the smash fast and low and the clear high and deep.

Badminton Lesson 6   Beginner level

Performance Goals

Students will

improve their skills, and
score a game.

Cognitive Goal

Students will learn what constitutes a point and official scoring.

Warm-Up

Students will

1. Participate in a free-practice period, with individual coaching
2. Complete footwork for agility—drill in quick starts and stops and changes of direction

Motivation

After all these lessons and practice periods, players are ready for full games. Some already may have picked up the rules on how to score, but in preparation for a tournament, scoring rules should all be reviewed so that everyone is at the same point. Go over scoring before getting started on competition.

Lesson Sequence

1. Show a diagram of a badminton court (see figure 5.1).
2. Review when a team wins a point or simply loses its serve.
3. Review how to handle a situation in which opponents serve illegally.
4. Review all boundaries, service rules, and receiving rules.
5. Teach when a game is over.
6. Have students choose a permanent tournament partner.
7. Allow play that duplicates tournament game conditions.

Review

Ask the class if any questions arose during practice games.

Assessment

Observe every court. See what problems the students are having with the rules and order of play and plan to reintroduce those items at the beginning of the next lesson even if you cover them fully during this lesson's summary.

Teacher Homework

Having allowed students to choose their own partners, divide the number of partner teams into 2 (or, if the class has 12 or more doubles teams, into 3) groups, and group teams by ability level. Once done, plan to have a tournament for each level of ability. This will work great using the round robin. Students from each ability level will play among themselves. Several small round-robin tournaments will run concurrently. In this way, the playing field has been leveled and players are given an opportunity to have a competitive game at their own level of ability.

Badminton Lesson 7 — Beginner level

Lesson Setup

Equipment

Posted round-robin tournament information (see appendix A for examples)

- Game schedules
- Team standings list

The best badminton equipment available for competition

Performance Goal

Students will play round 1.

Cognitive Goals

Students will

learn how to be responsible for themselves during a tournament:
- practice reading a tournament schedule,
- get to their court on time,
- play by the rules,
- demonstrate good sporting behavior,
- be responsible for reporting their scores,
experience reliance on a partner during a competitive experience.

Lesson Safety

Be vigilant about the emotional tone during competition. Be sure to address any psychologically unhealthy behavior as well as any physically unhealthy behavior that may erupt.

Warm-Up

Students will participate in a free-play practice period

Motivation

It's time to start a tournament. The more time on the court, the more time students will have to play. When both teams get to the court, give them a little warm-up time, practicing clears and maybe serves before scoring begins. Wish them luck!

Lesson Sequence

1. Post the tournament schedule. (See appendix A for a sample round-robin schedule and a round-robin team standing sheet.)
2. Teach students how to read it themselves.
3. If students are absent, explain the procedure:
   - Games go on.
   - If the present partner wants the game to count, he must play alone when his partner is absent.
   - If he wants a substitute partner, the game will be recorded as a default.
4. Move from court to court, giving helpful hints or positive comments.
5. Receive scores when the game is over.

Review

Ask if students have any questions.
Find out if everyone submitted their scores.

Assessment

Observe each group's ability to be self-directed. Be available for students who are having difficulty following the tournament schedule so their game time is not wasted by going to the wrong court or playing with the wrong opponent.

Badminton Lesson 8   Beginner level

Lesson Setup

Equipment

Rackets and shuttlecocks that are in good repair
A portable blackboard for posting the tournament schedule and court assignments
A chart of tournament standings

Performance Goals

Students will

continue improving skills, and
play the second round of the tournament.

Cognitive Goal

Students will continue to work on the goals from lesson 7.

Lesson Safety

If there are courtside officials, make sure they are between courts or at net poles.

Discourage inappropriate use of rackets to vent frustration.

Remind students not to run on someone else's court for any reason if the players are in the middle of a point.

Warm-Up

Students will

1. Participate in a free-practice period
2. Practice swings, with the racket in hand, taking full swings with a wrist snap and going through the whole motions of
   • the long serve,
   • the short serve, and
   • the overhead clear.

Motivation

After the first round of the tournament, announce the team standings. Wish students luck, and remind them to come to you if they have a rules question, need some help with their strategy, need to replace their shuttlecock, or anything else. The main thing is for them to go out there and have a good contest and have some fun.

Lesson Sequence

1. Update the posted tournament schedule.
2. Discuss, with the help of blackboard diagrams, how doubles players split the court responsibilities:
   • Diagram the up-and-back strategy.
   • Diagram the side-to-side strategy.
3. Remind students to take full swings with a wrist snap.
4. Move from court to court, giving helpful hints or positive comments.
5. Receive scores when the game is over.

Review

Ask students what happens if they try to clear the shuttlecock and don't take a full swing.

Review what they should be prepared for if their shot travels short.

Badminton Lessons 9-13   Beginner level

Lesson Setup

Equipment

Rackets that are in good condition for each player
Shuttlecocks for every court, plus some extras in case they are needed
An updated tournament schedule and standings
A posted performance rubric—either on blackboard or bulletin board, large
    enough to be read easily

Performance Goals

Students will

improve their skills,
play by the rules, and
complete a tournament.

Cognitive Goals

Students will

learn to follow the tournament routine and find their own court and opponent;
learn to demonstrate good sporting behavior during a competitive tournament;
learn to be responsible for their own games, scores, and standings; and
focus on different strategies each day to help their game play:
- Lesson 9—hit to open court.
- Lesson 10—exploit opponents' weakness.
- Lesson 11—where is their backhand? Hit to it.
- Lesson 12—keep them in the back of the court.
- Lesson 13—confusion helps; hit down the middle.

Warm-Up

Students will

1. Jog around the playing area
2. Practice swings, with the racket in hand, taking full swings with a wrist snap,
   and going through the whole motions of
   - the overhead smash,
   - the forehand drive,
   - the forehand clear,

- the backhand drive, and
- the backhand clear.

Motivation

After so many rounds of the tournament, announce the team standings. Tell students you have been watching their games and are impressed with how good they look—although most probably have never played the game before this class. Whatever the score in the tournament, they should be pleased with their skills. Furthermore, as Yogi Berra used to say, "It ain't over 'til it's over." So many things can change. In fact, discuss how the standings will change if so-and-so wins.

Wish the players luck, and remind them to call if they need help. Also remind them to warm up their strokes before they start scoring.

Lesson Sequence

1. Follow the posted tournament schedule until it comes to each natural end. The tournament should come to a natural end at the end of the unit.
2. Go over the strategy of the day, each day changing something:
   - Keep them deep.
   - Be ready to move up and put away any high, short shot.
   - Make them move by hitting to the empty court.
   - Play the weaker of the two opponents.
   - Concentrate so you cut down your errors.
3. Receive scores when the game is over.
4. Announce that the last day will begin with a short quiz. See the quiz for the beginner level on page 146.

Review

Ask if anyone has any questions.
Check that all the scores are in.
If something has come up that should be shared with the class, let students know that it should be discussed now.

Assessment

Observe the players, looking for standards as defined by the performance assessment rubric on page 130.

Teacher Homework

For the last lesson of the unit, remind students to bring a pen or pencil for a short quiz. After the quiz, they should plan to play against the opponents their team played when the tournament began.

Badminton Lesson 14 — Beginner level

Lesson Setup

Equipment

A posted beginner's performance rubric
Quizzes for everyone in the class
Some extra pencils

Performance Goals

Students will

take a written quiz lasting no more than 10 minutes;
sit quietly if finished early, stretching until everyone is done; and
play a rematch against earliest tournament opponents and see if the tables can be turned.

Cognitive Goals

Students will be responsible for proper behavior during a 10-minute quiz. They will

have a pen or pencil,
read carefully, and
demonstrate conceptual knowledge by doing well on the test.

Warm-Up

Students will jog around the playing area

Motivation

Now the students will go back up against the opponents they played when they were all still novices, and many will have improved a lot. This is their chance to see if their improvement can turn the tables. Tell the players to enjoy themselves, and while they're at work, they should know you'll be coming up with their skills grades based on the posted skills rubric.

Lesson Sequence

1. Students will pick up quizzes as they enter the gym and begin them right away.
2. Quizzes will be collected.
3. Do a general warm-up.
4. Announce the games and allow students to play for the remainder of the period.

Review

Inform students that they will get back their quizzes the next day.

Assessment

Grade assessments will be based on

the results of a written quiz, and
the level that students have achieved on the performance assessment rubric.

Badminton Lesson 15   Beginner level

Lesson Setup

Equipment

A posted skills rubric—either on blackboard or bulletin board, large enough to be read easily
Graded quizzes

Performance Goals

Students will

review each question, and
play a three-game match.

Cognitive Goals

Students will

learn what a match is, and
learn what they got wrong on their quizzes and what the right answers are.

Warm-Up

Students will participate in free play upon entering gym

Motivation

Now the students will play opponents who had almost the same record. That means they are playing their closest rivals. Because the competition will be close, you might have the period spent playing a real match. Mention that you haven't discussed much about matches, but in this case, a match means winning two out of three games. Have the students enjoy themselves while you finish their skills grades.

Lesson Sequence

1. Students will have free play, warm-up, and motivation segments.
2. Play will begin with the announcement of court assignments. Match challenges will be based on the standings in the tournament.
3. Quizzes will be returned and reviewed the last five minutes of the period.

Review

Review the quizzes, particularly the questions that had the most frequent incorrect responses.

Assessment

Complete the evaluation of skills based on the performance assessment rubric (table 5.2). For further general assessment rubrics, see appendix B.

TABLE 5.2 Beginner Badminton Performance Assessment Rubric

STUDENT NAME _____

	0	1	2	3	4	5
Serve	No effort	• Uses proper grip • Has correct stance • Holds shuttlecock correctly • Uses underhand swing	• Drops shuttlecock prior to swing • Makes contact below the waist • Uses wrist on swing • Redirects shuttlecock forward	• Makes contact using legal swing • Directs shuttlecock on the diagonal • Able to put shuttlecock in play	• Has developed consistent short serve • Aims the serve strategically	• Varies depth and height of serve • Short serve is low and offensive • Long serve is deep and high
Overhead clear	No effort	• Uses correct mimetics • Chooses to use overhead swing when shuttlecock is high	• Uses full practice swings that whip through air making sound • Redirects shuttlecock upward using overhead swing	• Moves to get under shuttlecock • Hits high	• Runs four steps or more and still directs high/deep hit • Receives from back line and clears shuttlecock past middle of opponent's court	• From deep in the court hits deep in opponent's court • Directs to either left or right purposefully
Underhand clear	No effort	• Uses correct mimetics • Correctly chooses underhand swing when shuttlecock is too short or low	• Practice swings whip the air • Able to redirect a low shuttlecock over the net	• Is capable of intentionally sending underhand swing up • Able to succeed redirecting on forehand side	• Redirects low shot upward on backhand and forehand sides • Clears the shuttlecock high off favorite side	• Clears shuttlecock high and deep • Clears off forehand and backhand swings • Able to send to left or right side of opponent's court

Badminton Lesson 1 — Intermediate level

Lesson Setup

Facility

Courts marked with boundary lines and short lines
Nets up

Equipment

One racket for each student
One shuttlecock for every two students
Extra replacement shuttlecocks

Performance Goals

Students will

be able to perform a short serve and a long serve, an overhead clear, and a smash; and
care for equipment.

Cognitive Goals

Students will

review the special care of equipment and be given responsibility for proper handling;
review the mechanical differences between swings that produce a
- long serve
- short serve
- overhead clear, and
- smash;

know service rules:
- The serve must be met below the waist.
- The serve must clear the net and pass a short line.
- The serve must start with the right and be directed to the diagonal box.

Lesson Safety

Practice areas should be separated by a minimum of 10 feet per group.
No more than four students should be assigned to any one court.

Warm-Up

Students will

1. Jog around the play area
2. Practice each swing using a racket so that the racket can be heard moving air.

Motivation

It may have been a while since the students have last touched a badminton racket. Before covering any new shots, get a feel for what they already know and see if they can improve on it.

Lesson Sequence

1. Discuss equipment use and care and responsibility for preserving equipment.
2. Demonstrate and evaluate. Ask students to pick up the mechanical differences between
   - long serves (figure 5.8):
     Opposite foot forward, knees bent
     Full back swing
     Forceful wrist snap
     Follow-through ending above the head, in line with point of aim

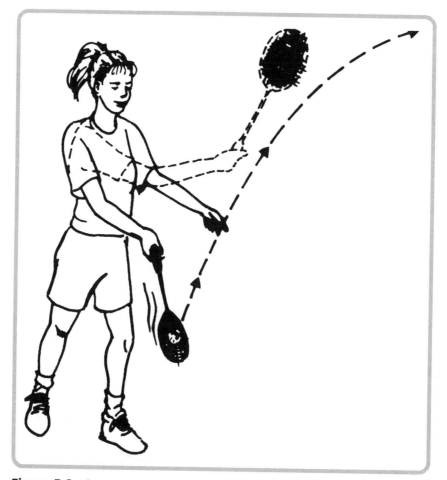

Figure 5.8—Long serve.

- and short serves:
    Feet and back swing the same as the long serve
    Slow wrist snap with no force
    Little follow-through
3. Allow practice of both serves.
4. Demonstrate and ask students to pick up the mechanical differences between the overhead clear and the smash. Allow them time to practice both.
5. Review service rules.
6. If there is time, allow a game with the opponents of choice.

Review

Review the rules of service and concerns about equipment.
Ask if the swing looks different in the smash and the clear.
Review the biggest difference between the two.
Ask if the swing looks different between the short serve and the long serve.
Review what makes one travel so much farther.
Tell students that when they arrive for their next class, they should get their equipment right away, find the first student dressed who is available, and practice the shot that still needs work after this lesson.

Badminton Lesson 2 — Intermediate level

Performance Goals

Students will

improve their overhead shots;
learn a new overhead shot—the overhead drop shot; and
play a short game.

Cognitive Goals

Students will

visualize and review the differences in preparation, contact point, follow-through, and the effect of the overhead swing when clearing and smashing;
learn the overhead drop shot—preparation, contact point, and follow-through; and
understand the strategy for having three different results though they all use the same preparation.

Lesson Safety

Practice areas should be separated by a minimum of 10 feet per group.
No more than four students should be assigned to any one court.

Warm-Up

Students will

1. Participate in free-play practice on the courts
2. Stretch
3. Complete sit-ups

Motivation

Now that the students are masters of their own skills, you can teach them how to be a little sneaky: using the overhead motion to have three different results. If they get really good at it, they can call it their legal method for making their opponents flinch. Here's how they can thoroughly confuse their opponents.

Lesson Sequence

1. Discuss body mechanics and techniques that cause differences between the overhead shots:
   - The point of contact
   - The wrist snap and follow-through
   - The drop shot's lack of follow-through, which results in a short, slow fall (figure 5.9)
2. Allow students to practice the drop shot first.
3. Encourage students to practice mixing up the shots.
4. Allow a game in the remaining time.

Review

Review the mechanics that lead to different shots, such as the following:

If the shuttlecock is directly over your head, what kind of shot will you take if you do not move and simply swing at it?
If you want to hit offensively, what could you do to change the shot?

Badminton Lesson 3 — Intermediate level

Performance Goals

Students will

improve their underhand shots;
learn a new underhand shot—the hairpin shot; and
play games.

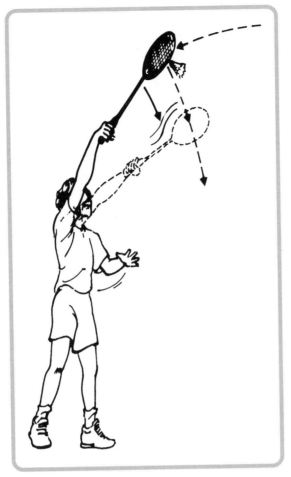

Figure 5.9—Drop shot.

Cognitive Goals

Students will

visualize and review the differences in preparation, contact point, follow-through,
and effect of underhand swing when clearing and driving;
learn the hairpin shot—preparation, contact point, and follow-through; and
understand the strategy for having three different results with the same preparation—the underhand clear.

Warm-Up

Students will

1. Participate in free-play practice on the court
2. Complete footwork drills. Either by voice or visual command, have students practice a sudden change of direction:

- Crossover steps going backward and sideways
- Small side-to-side steps, going left to right, and right to left
- Running forward, stopping, and running backward
3. Review (without a shuttlecock) the motions for overhead strokes and underhand strokes

Motivation

The sneakiness alluded to in the previous lesson can be accomplished with underhand shots, too. Let's see how, what the effect is, and if students can do it themselves.

Lesson Sequence

1. Discuss body mechanics and techniques that cause differences between the underhand clear and the hairpin shot (figure 5.10):
   - The same backswing
   - The same point of contact with a different wrist snap
   - Follow-through is minimal in a hairpin
   - Trajectory of the shuttlecock during a hairpin barely passes over the net
2. Allow students to practice the hairpin shot first.
3. Encourage students to practice mixing up the shots.
4. Allow a game in the remaining time.

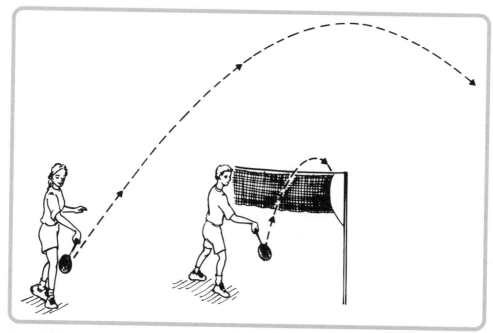

Figure 5.10—Underhand clear contrasted to the hairpin shot.

Review

Review the mechanics that lead to different effects.

Assessment

Observe each student's control and court coverage in preparation for developing a fair and competitive tournament to be designed for each level of play.

Identify the weaknesses that might need to be reviewed in the following lesson.

Badminton Lesson 4   Intermediate level

Performance Goals

Students will

improve their backhand shots, and
play games.

Cognitive Goals

Students will

understand and compensate for why people have difficulty with their backhand, and
review serving rules.

Warm-Up

Students will

1. Practice on the court
2. Complete backhand mimetics

Motivation

Most people avoid the shots that occur on their least dominant side. That is, the backhand. Mostly, their fear of the shot is usually a result of not using it as much as the one they learned first, the forehand. Unfortunately, they cannot always run around their backhand, and therein lies the rub. In this lesson, knowing that it will not feel nearly as uncomfortable if students practice it, take a little time out just for working on the backhand. Hopefully the efforts will give players some backhand confidence.

Lesson Sequence

1. Practice the backhand swing so that it is natural, like an opening-up motion that is smooth:
   - Without having to react to the shuttlecock
   - With the shuttlecock
2. Teach the strategy of aiming for an opponent's weakness: the backhand.
3. Practice the backhand a little more; this time, aim to the backhand of the person on the other side of the net.
4. Review service rules and allow time for a short game.

Review

Review the rules of service and concerns about equipment.

Badminton Lesson 5 — Intermediate level

Lesson Setup

Equipment

A clipboard
Paper and pencil for team sign-up

Performance Goals

Students will

choose their doubles partner for the day, and
improve all their skills while playing in a game situation.

Cognitive Goals

Students will learn

strategies for playing in a doubles tournament, and
how to divide the court up equally (figure 5.11 shows both positioning strategies):
- Up-and-back positioning
- Side-to-side positioning

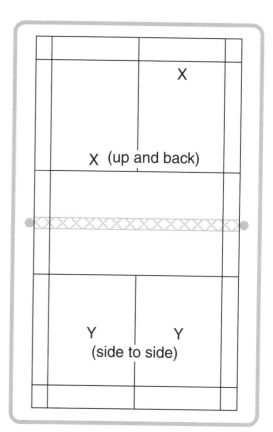

Figure 5.11—Doubles formation.

Warm-Up

Students will participate in free-play practice on the court

Motivation

It's time to put everything to good use. Start organizing a round-robin tournament. So far, the concentration has been on skills to use in a game. Students have been introduced to seven major skills, which is a lot. Have the players use what they are comfortable and consistent with; once the games start counting, they do not want to be giving opponents easy points because they tried something they really couldn't do.

Plus, when playing doubles, it is not just one's own skills that players need to worry about, but also how they and their partner can best cover the whole court without getting in each other's way and without leaving empty spaces for opponents to aim for. Badminton is a fast game and having good team positioning helps a lot.

Lesson Sequence

1. Discuss the attributes of a good partner, for fun and fair competition.
2. Teach the strategy of dividing the court:
   • Up and back
   • Side to side
3. Direct students to pick a partner and register their partnership with the "desk" or person holding the clipboard.
4. Have rotating games, asking students to come to you when they finish a five-point game.
5. Reassign players coming off to other teams so that they can get right on again and play someone different. Keep this going until the end of the period, matching winners with winners and losers with losers. (But do not call them "losers." The whole purpose of this is that they have a variety of people to play against, and you get to know on what level they play so you can draw up a better and more equitable tournament.)

Review

Ask if everyone has submitted their doubles team; if not, make sure they do before they leave.

Review the rules of scoring and the service order.

Comment about maintaining the equipment so that it is in the best shape for the tournament.

Teacher Homework

Look at the skill range of the class. Divide up the class so students with the most similar skills play each other. Create a round-robin tournament for each of the groups with a schedule, team names, and numbers.

Badminton Lesson 6 — Intermediate level

Lesson Setup

Equipment

A posted tournament schedule (see appendix A for an example)
A posted list of teams that will show standings as they come in

Performance Goal

Students will enter into competition by playing round 1.

Cognitive Goals

Students will

learn to read a tournament chart and schedule,
show up for scheduled games prepared and prompt,
record their scores before leaving, and
discuss the use of strategies
  • Who should serve first?
  • Who should take shots down the middle?

Lesson Safety

Assign no more than four students at a time to play on any one court.
Be vigilant about students' psychological safety as well as physical safety.
Be prepared to deal with poor sporting behavior and any psychologically abusive behavior that might come out during competition.

Warm-Up

Students will

1. Participate in free-play practice on the court
2. Complete footwork drills for agility and moving back

Motivation

It's the first round of the tournament. Wish the players good luck and tell them to ask you if they need any help.

Lesson Sequence

1. Post and discuss how to read the tournament schedule.
2. Review the expected daily procedure.
3. Focus on this lesson's strategy and decision making:
   - Who should serve first
   - Who should take the shot down the middle
4. Direct students to begin the tournament.

Review

Ask if anyone forgot to turn in their scores.
Have players point to the strongest server on their team.
Ask if that person began the game on the right-hand side.
Review who serves first.
Ask if the strongest server should begin on the left-hand side.

Badminton Lessons 7-11   Intermediate level

Lesson Setup

Equipment

Posted, updated team standings
Posted daily game and court assignment schedule

Performance Goals

Students will

follow the tournament routine responsibly, and
demonstrate good sporting behavior.

Cognitive Goals

Students will

have a different strategy to focus on each day,
learn to follow procedures expected of them daily, and
discuss the different strategies that will be each day's new focus before games:
   - Lesson 7—stepping up to short shots
   - Lesson 8—varying speed and depth
   - Lesson 9—identifying weaknesses in one's opponent and playing them
   - Lesson 10—varying serves
   - Lesson 11—staying focused so one does not cause one's own lost points

Lesson Safety

Be vigilant about students' psychological safety as well as physical safety. Be prepared to deal with poor sporting behavior and any psychologically abusive behavior that might come out during competition.

Warm-Up

Students will participate in free-play practice on the court

Motivation

After so many rounds of the tournament, announce the team standings. Wish the players luck. Ask them to call you over if they're having trouble with anything, need help getting a winning strategy, or have any questions during a game.

Lesson Sequence

1. Play a new round each day.
2. Focus on the day's strategy and decision making.
3. Direct students to begin games.

Review

Tell students that if someone on their team was able to execute this lesson's strategy, they should raise their hand. Ask if the strategy helped them, and to explain how.

When the round robin tournament concludes, tell students there will be a short quiz.

Assessment

Observe for performance standards in the intermediate performance assessment rubric on page 145. For further general assessment rubrics, see appendix B.

Badminton Lesson 12 — Intermediate level

Lesson Setup

Equipment

One quiz for each student (can be found on page 147)
Blackboard or poster of the performance rubric

Performance Goals

Students will

take a quiz, and
play the team whose ability is closest to theirs for the last games/match of the unit.

Cognitive Goals

Students will learn how to put their knowledge of the game into words.

Warm-Up

Students will participate in on-court practice

Motivation

Announce the final standings of the round robin. Tell students that you have planned the last competition of the badminton unit. Arrange an activity that they might enjoy to make the last day a little different. (Evaluate your class and decide, with their help or on your own, which approach would work best.) Some suggestions:

Playing the team with the closest score
Playing the team that finished in the same place but which played in a different round robin
A battle of the sexes
A day of singles play against the students' own partners

Lesson Sequence

1. Hand out quizzes as the students arrive; have them sit on the perimeter of the gym and begin immediately.
2. Collect the quizzes as they are done and allow students to begin their on-court warm-ups.
3. Announce the last match schedule and tell students that the skills grade will be based on the posted rubric.
4. Direct students to begin the games.

Review

Ask students if any questions on the quiz confused them.
Let them know that in the next class you will return and discuss the quizzes.
They also will finish their matches.

Assessment

Observation will determine the qualitative score for skills. It will be based on the performance goals in the assessment rubric. Knowledge grades will be based on the grades from the written quiz.

Badminton Lesson 13 — Intermediate level

Lesson Setup

Equipment

The graded quizzes
Blackboard or poster of performance assessment rubric

Performance Goals

Students will

finish the match they began last class, and
review their quizzes.

Cognitive Goals

Students will learn what they missed on their quizzes and what the right answers are.

Warm-Up

Students will participate in on-court practice

Motivation

It's time to review the quizzes with the class; there might be something on them that will help students play better for the last day of the tournament. Announce the standings of the matches that the students had begun. Have the players continue from where they left off. Continue to come up with their skills grades while they are playing. Suggest that they look over the things that you will be looking for, if they haven't already. The list should be posted on the blackboard. Remind the students that it is their last game and to enjoy it.

Lesson Sequence

1. Hand out the graded quizzes and review them.
2. Begin the games.

Review

Extend congratulations to the students with the best overhead, the best record, the most improvement, the best sporting behavior, the best ability to mix up opponents, the best ability to adjust in an emergency, and so on. Announce the tournament winners.

Assessment

Make observations, basing qualitative scores on the performance goals in the assessment rubric (table 5.3). For further general assessment rubrics, see appendix B.

TABLE 5.3 Intermediate Badminton Performance Assessment Rubric

STUDENT NAME _____

	0	1	2	3	4	5
Serve	No effort	• Legally begins play from one side of the court • Has correct stance • Holds shuttlecock correctly • Uses underhand swing	• Is capable of legally serving from both sides of the court	• Has consistent serve	• Has developed a good short serve • Aims the serve strategically	• Varies depth/height of serve • Is very consistent • Serve puts opponents on the defensive
Skills	No effort	• Uses at least one overhead stroke • Hits an underhand stroke on one side	• Clears often fall deep in opponent's court • Receives from back line and clears past middle of opponent's court • Varies depth occasionally	• Covers shots up to seven feet away • When possible moves up to hit a smash • Has occasional success with smash, drop, or hairpin shots	• Directs shuttlecock to open court • Chooses when to smash at proper moments • Is consistently able to change direction of play	• Uses variety of shots, speeds, and depth • Wins points by moving opponent or use of speed • Covers a large part of the court • Has mastered one offensive shot
Team play	No effort	• Arrives on court promptly, prepared and equipped • Takes the left side of court if weakest of two servers • Moves to shots within a four-foot radius	• Plays service and receiving rules properly • Assumes responsibility for own territory on court	• Switches sides with partner to keep court fully covered • Keeps score legally • Has occasional success at offensive strategy	• Uses offensive strategies: place/smash/fake out/exploit weaknesses • Backs up partner without taking over partner's position	• Is the best server on team • Detects opponent's weaknesses and sets team strategy to exploit them • Is very focused • Is ethical, competitive sports enthusiast

Badminton Quiz—Beginner level

NAME _____ TEACHER _____

DATE _____ CLASS PERIOD _____

This diagram represents a badminton court. Each number will give you a location of a player or an actual spot on the court. If the number is on a line, it refers to that line. If it is in a space, it refers to the general area. Based on the statement and the diagram, decide whether the statement is true or false and record your answers in the appropriate box in the column to the left of the statement.

True False

☐ ☐ 1. The Team X players are 2 and 9. Player 9 should serve first.

☐ ☐ 2. Server 2 is correct to serve to box 12.

☐ ☐ 3. Team Y's player 7 gains the serve. Her first serve travels to the line—11. Player 2 must return it.

☐ ☐ 4. A serve sent in by a player on Team X and landing in area 4 is a short.

☐ ☐ 5. If Team X wants to hit a good overhead clear, the shuttlecock should land near area 5.

☐ ☐ 6. If player 9 is the server, the area bounding box 12 is the only legal area she can serve to.

☐ ☐ 7. If player 2 hits a clear and it falls short, near area 7, the closest Team Y player should step up to it and smash it.

☐ ☐ 8. Team Y's player 7 serves. Team X players let it land. It lands on the line marked by 3. Team Y's score should increase by one point.

☐ ☐ 9. Attempting a smash when standing deep in the court, near area 5, will result in netting the shuttlecock.

☐ ☐ 10. If the shuttlecock has been hit between right-handed players, 2 and 9, it is best that Team X's player 9 leave it to her partner. That way, player 2 can return it with the forehand.

From *Complete Physical Education Plans for Grades 7–12* by Isobel Kleinman, 2001, Champaign, IL: Human Kinetics.

146

Badminton Quiz—Intermediate level

NAME _____ TEACHER _____

DATE _____ CLASS PERIOD _____

This diagram represents a badminton court. Each number will give you a location of a player or an actual spot on the court. If the number is on a line, it refers to that line. If it is in a space, it refers to the general area. Based on the statement and the diagram, decide whether the statement is true or false and record your answers in the appropriate box in the column to the left of the statement.

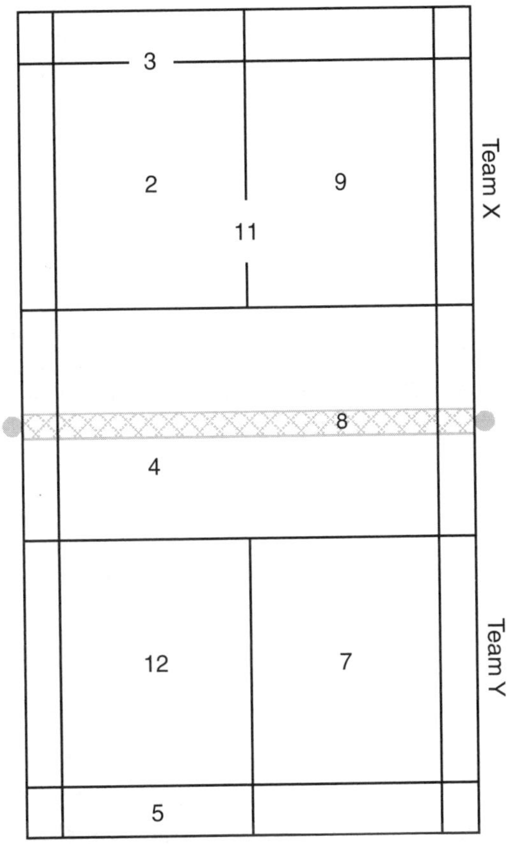

True   **False**

☐   ☐   1. Team Y wins the first turn of service of the game. When player 7 loses serve, player 12 becomes the next server.

☐   ☐   2. Server 2 is in a very good position to hit a successful smash.

☐   ☐   3. Team Y regains the serve. Player 12 becomes the first server for the Y team the second time it gets to serve.

☐   ☐   4. A good hairpin shot lands in area 4.

☐   ☐   5. The main difference between a shot that goes to area 4 and one that lands in area 5 is a wrist snap.

☐   ☐   6. If player 7 is the server, the serve most likely to be hit by a backhand is one directed to area 11.

☐   ☐   7. A good strategy, if your opponents are right-handed, is to hit the shuttlecock down your right so it goes to the left side of their court.

☐   ☐   8. Serves that land on the short line and on the line dividing the two service boxes are both considered good serves and should be returned to prevent the serving team from winning a point.

☐   ☐   9. Attempting a smash when standing deep in the court, near area 5, will result in netting the shuttlecock.

☐   ☐   10. The shot whose swing most looks like a hairpin shot is an overhead clear.

[Court diagram: Team X at top, Team Y at bottom. Numbers shown: 3, 2, 9, 11 (Team X side); 8 on the net line; 4 below net; 12, 7 (Team Y side); 5 at bottom.]

From *Complete Physical Education Plans for Grades 7–12* by Isobel Kleinman, 2001, Champaign, IL: Human Kinetics.

Badminton Answer Key—Beginner level

1. F. The server on the right, player 2, should serve first.
2. F. The server must serve to the diagonal box. In this case, player 2 must serve to player 7.
3. T. If the shuttlecock is allowed to land and it lands on the line, it is a good serve to player 2.
4. T. Area 4 indicates the area between the net and the short line.
5. T. Such a clear would be very deep but not out of bounds.
6. T. The area and its boundaries are in the diagonal that player 9 must serve to.
7. T. The Team X player has hit a weak shot that is a setup for a smash. Team Y should take advantage.
8. T. In not returning a legal serve, the team that serves gets a point.
9. T. If the net is the proper height, the angle of a smash that will stay in bounds will not clear the net.
10. F. If player 2 is forced to return the shot, she will have to use her backhand.

Badminton Answer Key—Intermediate level

1. F. The first team to serve gets one turn of service. When lost, the serve goes to the opponent in the right-hand box.
2. T. Player 2 is close enough to the net that smashing a shuttlecock dropping from overhead clears the net.
3. F. The first person to serve in doubles when winning the serve back is always the person on the right-hand side of the court.
4. T. A good hairpin shot is a very short shot.
5. T. Wrist snap, not arm swing, provides the power in badminton.
6. T. The serve must be returned by player 2, who would have to meet the shuttlecock on the left of his body.
7. T. The left side of a right-handed player is her backhand, notoriously the weakest of the sides.
8. T. The lines are good.
9. T. The smash will not clear the height of the net if the smash is hit from deep in the court. That is why deep shots are safe shots to hit: Your opponent cannot return a deep shot with a smash.
10. F. A hairpin shot is underhand, and an overhead clear is overhead. A hairpin is short and low; a clear is long and high.

Dance

Unit Overview

1. Teach background for motivation:
   - Value of dance historically and presently as a social outlet, an aerobic exercise, and an art
   - How local popularity has led to dance clubs for country-western, ballroom, swing, Latin dancing, and disco
   - How cultures have their own specialties such as samba, tango, mambo, and cha-cha

2. Teach terminology and how to match locomotion to words:
   - Basic locomotion—step, run, skip, slide, gallop
   - Basic dance formations:
     Line—single, double, differing directions
     Circle—facing in or out, moving counterclockwise or clockwise, single or double
     Square
     File
     Long-ways or contra formation
   - Basic dance positions—two hands joined and facing, promenade, varsouvienne, open social dance, closed social dance
   - Basic square-dance calls—circle, promenade, swing, do-si-do, allemande, grand right and left, star
   - Basic dance steps—two-step, polka, waltz, schottische, mazurka

3. Focus on the following directions:
   - Following calls
   - Following a line of direction
   - Synchronizing with large groups

4. Have students learn the importance of music and rhythm:
   - Staying on the beat
   - Picking up the rhythm of specific songs
   - Identifying folk dances

5. Assign partnering responsibilities—leading, following, going "home," counterbalancing.

6. Stress etiquette and courtesy.

7. Encourage an exploration of creativity once the fundamentals have been taught:
   - Creating one's own dance routine to favorite music
   - Creating a modern dance sequence
   - Taking movement sequence and playing with size, speed, and flow

Dance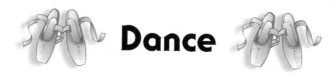

HISTORY

Dance was first observed in cave paintings found in Spain and France dating from 30,000 to 10,000 B.C. Ballet began in 1581. In the 1920s and '30s, the rumba, the tango, the samba, the cha-cha, the lindy-hop, and the jitterbug began mainstreaming. The 1940s popularized swing dancing and big-band music. The '50s introduced the twist, and the '60s brought on freestyle dance. The '70s consisted of disco dancing, while the '80s embraced break dancing. Finally, the '90s popularized hip-hop and line dancing, with a rediscovering of swing dancing and big-band music in the very late '90s.

FUN FACTS

→ In the Virginia Reel, dancers make their own music by clapping their hands and singing.

→ George Washington's favorite dance was the Virginia Reel.

→ Folk dancing is the oldest form of dance.

→ Tanko Bushi is a folk dance from Greece.

→ Balthazar de Beauthoyeulx put on the first ballet dance.

BENEFITS OF DANCING

1. Dancing is energizing.
2. Dancing can provide you with an excellent cardiovascular workout.
3. Dancing can improve flexibility.
4. Dancing can be done alone or with friends.
5. Dancing is an expressive way to have fun and learn about other cultures!

TIME TO SURF!

Web Site	Web Site Address
5678 Magazine	www.5678magazine.com
Dance Spirit Magazine	www.dancespirit.com
DanceTeacher Magazine	www.dance-teacher.com

Dance Unit Extension Project

NAME _____ CLASS _____

Equipment needed for dance

Item	Where you would purchase it (be specific)	Cost

Where you would dance

Please explain what type of dance you like best and where in your community you could go to participate in this type of dance.

Health benefits of dancing

Please explain the health benefits of dancing. Include how much dancing and what type of dancing you would need to do each week to gain these benefits.

Reflection question

Do you think dancing is an activity you would like to do as an adult? Why or why not?

From *Complete Physical Education Plans for Grades 7–12* by Isobel Kleinman, 2001, Champaign, IL: Human Kinetics.

A Special Message to Teachers With No Experience Teaching Dance

The list in front of you might look daunting. The range of dances per experience level might look impossible, but covering this unit is definitely worth it. Regardless of your qualifications, most of your students will find your effort endearing, if not wonderful, especially if you have the confidence to tell them where you are coming from, a person who cares to try but who is not quite sure about the dance you are teaching. If you have no colleagues who can help, rest assured, in almost every class there will be one or two, possibly more, students who will be willing to come to your aid, help you figure out how to fit the written instructions to music, and help you get through the first few lessons. Most classes will go along with the experiment in good humor. So go ahead with this program. Sure it takes some tackling, but it will be easier and even rewarding if you elicit the help of your best class and its dancing students to work it through.

Dance Teaching Tips

1. It is probably best to assume that students have little or no exposure to any kind of dance and that most of the males in class will be resistant. While many young men feel threatened by having to learn to dance, many cultures have strong male participation. Use explanations of cultural differences and the history of dance to motivate students and teach diversity. Explore the development of the tango and how widespread dance is in community social halls in Latin countries such as Argentina and Brazil. Discuss how dance marks cultural ceremonies—Native American prayer dances and dances for rain (which may be familiar to Native American students and students who have watched westerns). Explain how orthodox societies that separated boys and girls used dance as a way for them to flirt and show off their talents. Speak to the power of dance, such as Russian men doing lifts in ballet. Use films—*Saturday Night Fever, Fame, Flashdance, White Nights, Tap Dance, Shall We Dance?, Dirty Dancing, Strictly Ballroom*—in order to motivate your male students and find male role models.
2. Provide variety before worrying about accurate renditions of the dances you teach. Do this by using different songs, different formations, and different cultural influences.
3. Teach dances that originated in countries other than the United States and include background about the dance, its purpose, and how (or if) it is used today.
4. Try to introduce several new things a day while reviewing the dance activities learned before.
5. The unit should be planned to reach the skills level and experience of the group without treating students as if they are in elementary school, even though some elementary dances are introduced in early lessons.
6. Students should, regardless of their likes and dislikes, learn to be courteous and cooperative.
7. Students will not be changing to gym clothing during this unit. Dance typically is done in street clothing. Therefore, despite the fact that there is a good

chance they will be sweating, students will welcome the opportunity to wear their street clothes and you will welcome the fact that you have 10 minutes more with them before they have to leave. It is suggested you instruct them to wear clothing that will not be ruined by sweating and that they come to class with sneakers or special dance shoes so the dance floor will not be ruined.

8. The dance unit is the most taxing on a teacher's voice and body of any unit I have taught. You will be dancing with every class and giving dance cues while the music is on until the students learn the dances themselves. As I have gotten older and have found five classes of dancing a day too wearing on my body and vocal cords, I have learned to look for students to lead the class who have learned the dance already, are on beat, and are not thrown off by those who aren't—students who can be the dance model for those not quite able to remember the dances themselves. This has served several purposes very well: It not only has been good for my voice, body, and knees, but it has been wonderful for the students who are doing great work. Frequently, they are the students who do not shine during the sports units. Singling them out for the job of teacher boosts their self-esteem, which has seemed to generate such good feelings of trust and camaraderie that once the dance unit is over and class is back to sports, those standouts in dance try harder in sports and do even better than they had before.

9. Use scrimmage vests to identify who does the girl's or boy's role when there is not an equal number of girls and boys to partner off. It cuts down on the confusion of who should be inside, where the corner is, and who is supposed to go in which direction on the grand right and left.

10. Students who ask to be excused should, if possible, work through all dance instructions as they are given. If students are unable to participate fully in class activities, remember that they can be involved by helping run equipment (starting and stopping music, changing the music) or by conducting a research paper.

Unit Setup

Facility

A clean and well-ventilated room.

A slick, clean floor.

A room large enough so each student can move freely and small enough that the acoustics do not get lost.

Preferably, a room with a mirrored wall. This would be the best to use; it gives students who are standing in the back many more angles where they can move to see your demonstrations. A mirror also facilitates your feedback. You can pace the lesson better if you can pick up where your directions are falling short by immediately seeing when the kids are having difficulty keeping up.

Equipment

A music library on record, tape, or compact disc (CD) that can be available at all times once you start the unit

A phonograph, cassette player, or CD player to play the music in the library
Detachable speakers that can be moved in front of the microphone, with voice-over microphone features on the amplifier, and a microphone with a long lead (cordless would be great)
A teacher's resource with specific dance instructions
Scrimmage vests

Unit Timeline

There are three units in this chapter. Each grade level has 8 to 10 lessons.

Unit Assessment

A student portfolio checklist is provided here for student use (table 6.1). Encourage students to track their progress as they master new skills. There is also a performance assessment rubric for each grade level, and a quiz is available for each grade level at the end of this chapter. For further general assessment rubrics, see appendix B.

Additional Resources

Record inserts and record jackets usually include dance instructions.

Harris, Jane A., ed. 1999. *Dance a While: Handbook of Folk, Square, Contra and Social Dance*. Boston: Allyn and Bacon.

Kraus, Richard. 1964. *Folk Dance*. New York: Macmillan Publishing Company.

Krauss, Richard. 1950. *Square Dances of Today: How to Teach and How to Call Them*. New York: A.S. Barnes.

TABLE 6.1 Dance Student Portfolio Checklist

STUDENT NAME _____

- ☐ Is able to move on the beat and stay in rhythm
- ☐ Can perform basic locomotion—stepping, running, hopping, jumping, skipping, sliding, galloping
- ☐ Has developed a vocabulary of basic dance steps
- ☐ Has learned a variety of dance formations
- ☐ Has learned to move in different directions while in formation
- ☐ Has learned a variety of dance positions
- ☐ Can dance with a partner
- ☐ Has learned basic square-dance calls
- ☐ Has learned to appreciate the cultural diversity and history of dance
- ☐ Has internalized proper social etiquette
- ☐ Has explored creative choices in dance choreography

From *Complete Physical Education Plans for Grades 7–12* by Isobel Kleinman, 2001, Champaign, IL: Human Kinetics

Folk Dance Lesson 1   Beginner level

Lesson Setup

Equipment

Records, tapes, or CDs for the Grand March, the Pata Pata, and the Savila Se Bela Loza

Performance Goals

Students will

learn to walk to a beat, and
identify right from left.

Cognitive Goals

Students will learn

to identify rhythm,
how marching can be dancing, and
that different countries use different rhythms.

Lesson Safety

When dancing line dances, students who lead must learn to take their lines to open spaces in the room and move so that they are not racing or dragging the line behind them. They should be discouraged from doing what for some come naturally—trying to crash, running through other lines, or racing ahead of the music.

Warm-Up

The general following of dance instructions will be considered the warm-up. It is a gradual introduction to the movements of the day and serves the warm-up purpose. This can be assumed for the dance unit in total, because the dances do not start at top speed or ask for movement extremes.

Motivation

Explain to the class that it is starting a unit that will be an introduction to the way that countries around the world played and socialized in earlier times. Their music is different. Their styles and their costumes are different. Over the course of the next few weeks, students will learn dances from England, Scotland, Mexico, the Caribbean, Israel, Serbia, and Yugoslavia, and they will get a sampling of how dance developed in the United States.

Because this is the one unit in which students normally wear their regular street clothes or, if trying to demonstrate the costume of the period they will wear traditional dress, you will not have them dress in gym clothes. Instruct them to choose school clothes that will not be ruined by dancing and sweating. Ask them to leave their valuables in the locker room and come to class with sneakers or special dance shoes.

Lesson Sequence

1. Have students march in place with no music, just cadence:
   - Get everyone to begin with their left foot and stay on the called cadence.
   - Ask them to chorus your cadence: Left. Left, right, left.
2. Line up the class and instruct students to march forward, toward you. As they get there, give them directional cues—about face, right turn, halt, and so forth. Begin with no music, and then try it again with music and instructions.
3. Teach the Pata Pata:
   - Teach one part at a time, calling out the instructions with no music.
   - Add music for one part at a time.
   - Add parts until it is finished.
   - Dance with the class and the music, calling out instructions for the first four repetitions.
   - Discuss where the class thinks the dance came from. Is it old?
4. Teach the Savila Se Bela Loza, which will look like figure 6.1 once all the class lines are dancing independently:
   - Introduce its country of origin, Serbia, and a little of its history.
   - Introduce the idea of a line dance, demonstrating how each person follows the leader and how the change of directions is just to retrace steps.
   - Teach the steps and walk through it.
   - Put music on and ask students to listen for when the musical phrases change.
   - Dance with them, leading one line and calling out instructions.
   - When done, ask how, in a culture where the boys had to stay away from the girls but were still interested anyway, they could dance and show their interest.

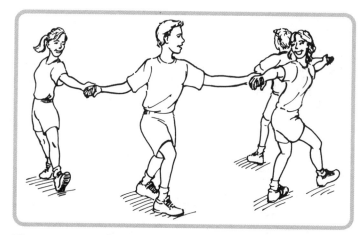

Figure 6.1—Savila Se Bela Loza.

Review

Ask students which dance reminded them of the West Point Military Academy.
Ask which seemed like it might have been done a hundred years ago.
Ask which seemed like the slow music encouraged a little hip action.

Assessment

Observation will determine how quickly to move forward. If students are able to follow instructions, having them experience a variety of dances is much more important at first then their acquiring expertise. If they are hopelessly lost, however, subsequent lessons should be delayed. This will remain true for several lessons.

Folk Dance Lesson 2   Beginner level

Lesson Setup

Equipment

The music for the Seljancica Kolo, the La Raspa, and the Hora

Performance Goals

Students will

learn the schottische and use it in dances:
- La Raspa
- Seljancica Kolo
- Hora
move in a circle.

Cognitive Goal

Students will identify these dances as popular folk dances of Mexico, Israel, and Yugoslavia.

Motivation

This lesson teaches students the first basic dance step—the schottische. It is used in dance more often than most other steps. Let the class know that in searching through the 100-year-old dances that you have the music for, you could find a lot of dances with the schottische and fewer with the other basic steps. The schottische is simple. It is just three steps and a hop—try it.

Lesson Sequence

1. Begin with requests from the floor. Allow one or two before beginning to teach something new.
2. Teach the schottische step first. Play music while students do the schottische forward, sideways, and back.
3. Teach Seljancica Kolo:
   - Begin with a little history of Yugoslavia.
   - Teach the steps with no music.
   - Try it again with music and instructions.
4. Teach La Raspa:
   - Begin with the location and history of La Raspa—in Mexico.
   - Teach one part at a time, calling out instructions with no music.
   - Add music for one part at a time.
   - Add parts until it is finished.
   - Dance with the class and the music, calling out instructions over the music.
5. Teach the Hora:
   - Introduce its country of origin, Israel, and a little of its history.
   - Introduce the idea of dancing in an unbroken circle, what that means symbolically, how the carousel effect in live music makes the dancers fly if they stay connected, and how energetic this dance is.
   - Teach the steps and walk through it.
   - Put music on and dance the dance through with the students.
6. If time remains, use it as a chance to review what was learned before. Ask for student requests.

Review

Ask students which dance made them tired, and if they could imagine doing it in a hot climate.

Review what the schottische step is.

Folk Dance Lesson 3 | Beginner level

Lesson Setup

Equipment

Records, tapes, or CDs for Bingo, Greensleeves, and Electric Slide

Performance Goals

Students will

learn to partner,

learn the grand right and left, and
learn Bingo and Greensleeves.

Cognitive Goals

Students will

learn what a mixer is,
identify these as partner folk dances, and
identify dances from the United States and England.

Warm-Up

Allow students, once class is assembled, to choose a dance or two that they learned in previous classes to warm up to before starting the new lesson.

Motivation

The social mixer is a tradition in dance; sometimes simple instructions are done with partners. This lesson's dance will follow the traditional route. Have partners spend a bit of time together, but promise them you won't marry anyone off in the class! Partners will change from time to time. Ask them to listen to the instructions and follow the best they can. If they get through what is planned, you can teach the popular disco line dance, the Electric Slide.

Lesson Sequence

1. Let students dance to one class request before starting something new.
2. To establish partners begin the instruction with the Grand March.
3. When everyone is partnered off, teach the grand right and left.
4. Teach Bingo:
   - Demonstrate how the dance goes from a double to a single circle to couples facing each other for the grand right and left.
   - Sing the words as the dance is danced.
5. Teach Greensleeves:
   - Begin with explaining its original location, England.
   - Teach formation first, then the number of walking steps.
6. Teach the Electric Slide:
   - Teach it in two parts, getting the class in rhythm without music.
   - Add the music as each part is completed.
   - Dance with the class, calling out instructions over the music for the first four repeats.
7. As time permits, review what was learned before and ask for student requests.

Review

Tell the class that the grand right and left is a square-dance call. Sometimes it is called a "chain" because even though they are going in the same direction, they have to weave in and out of everyone coming their way.

Folk Dance Lesson 4   Beginner level

Lesson Setup

Equipment

Records, tapes, or CDs for the Electric Slide and polka music

Performance Goals

Students will

improve on working with a partner;
review the grand right and left;
learn the polka step; and
review or learn a dance they can do at parties, the Electric Slide.

Motivation

Mention to the class that you have been moving them right along, and some may feel as if they don't really know the material. Can they believe that they've already learned nine different dances? Slow things down in this lesson. Review the Electric Slide, since the students probably will have the opportunity to do it at the next dance they attend.

Lesson Sequence

1. Ask students what they would like to start with. Review it quickly and put on the music.
2. Review the Electric Slide.
3. Review the grand right and left and redo the Bingo.
4. Teach the rhythm to the polka. Allow the class to dance the polka independent of any complicated instructions.
5. Ask for student requests and review each dance request by walking through the instructions if the dance has not already been done twice.

Review

Tell the class that in the next lesson, they will use the polka step in a popular folk dance called the Jessie Polka, and they will use the grand right and left in a square dance.

Folk Dance Lesson 5 — Beginner level

Lesson Setup

Equipment

Records, tapes, or CDs for Jessie Polka and Red River Valley

Performance Goals

Students will

partner up for a square dance;
perform the grand right and left as part of a square dance;
use the polka step in a traditional folk dance, the Jessie Polka; and
review and improve the performance of dances previously learned.

Cognitive Goal

Students will learn some rules of square dance and its vocabulary.

Motivation

You might mention to the class that these are some of your favorite dances (if they are). "Let's learn them!"

Lesson Sequence

1. Have the class dance to one request before teaching something new.
2. Teach the Jessie Polka:
   - Teach the heel-toe part (which I call the "heelie") first.
   - Since the students already know the polka step, all they have to do is count four of them before the "heelie" part begins again.
   - Have students get in groups of three to six, with arms around each other's waists, leaning back together. A heel goes forward, as shown in figure 6.2, and they perform the whole dance through, with the groups following a line of direction, counterclockwise, performing in unison.
3. Teach some square dance terms, concepts, and rules:
   - A square has four walls.
   - How to find a partner, corner, and opposite.
   - How to respond to calls.
   - The "home" and the male/lead partner's responsibility to put his partner on the right and bring her home.
   - Red River Valley.
   - How to regroup after a mistake wipes out the square.
   - Put music on and allow students to make their own mistakes.

161

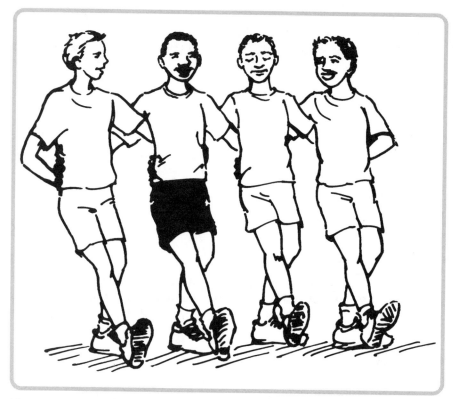

Figure 6.2—Dancing the Jessie Polka.

4. Ask for student requests:
   - Review the dances that have not already been done twice.
   - Ask if those that have been done twice need to be reviewed.

Review

Since square dance was developed hundreds of years ago and it has certain rules that always have the men taking their partners "home," ask students if that tells them how strong the American male's role was. Review whether that says something about the good old homestead and how important it was to go home. Square dance and the habit of the man taking the woman home suggests that to you. It sort of seems like an inside look to an old way of life.

Folk Dance Lesson 6 — Beginner level

Lesson Setup

Equipment

Record, tape, or CD for Virginia Reel

Performance Goals

Students will

learn the Virginia Reel,
learn more square-dance calls and be able to dance to them, and
review and improve performance of dances previously learned.

Cognitive Goal

Students will increase their dance vocabulary.

Motivation

Tell the class that they have learned 11 different dances. Mention that you have so much to teach them but it is time to give them a chance to slow down and enjoy what they already have learned. So, in this lesson, they'll learn just one new dance. It is a popular though traditional American dance: the Virginia Reel.

Lesson Sequence

1. Begin with a request.
2. Teach the Virginia Reel:
   - The long-ways position.
   - Specific calls: cast-off (figure 6.3), sashay, reel.
   - If possible, use "Turkey in the Straw" music and call the dance yourself.
3. Ask for student requests, but throw in a dance that they haven't asked for in a while. Review it first.

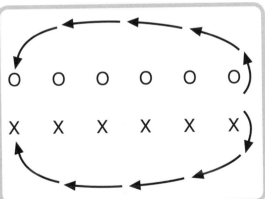

Figure 6.3—Casting off in the Virginia Reel.

Review

Ask students what sliding down the set is called. (Note that a *set* refers to a group in formation. Here the set is in longways position with space between the two lines.)
Have them describe a reel.
Ask what side the boy always should be on when dancing with a partner.

Folk Dance Lesson 7   Beginner level

Lesson Setup

Equipment

Records, tapes, or CDs for Grand March, Pata Pata, Sevila SeBela Loza, Seljancica Kolo, La Raspa, Hora, Bingo, Greensleeves, Electric Slide, Jessie Polka, Red River Valley, and Virginia Reel
The posted performance assessment rubric

Performance Goal

Students will learn more square-dance calls and be able to dance to them.

Cognitive Goal

Students will review and improve performance of dances previously learned.

Motivation

Tell students that they have learned 12 different dances. Suggest that they see how many they can do before the period ends. Ask who has a favorite they want to start with.

Lesson Sequence

1. Ask for student requests.
2. Throw in a dance that they haven't asked for in a while, and review it first.

Review

Ask the class if anyone can tell you the name of the dance in which no one holds hands.
Ask what the circle dance with the joined circle is.
Review what happens when the four couples in a square join their hands.
Ask which dance is like a spoke on a wheel.
Tell students that at the end of the unit they will be taking a little quiz on what they have learned. Suggest they also review the things you will be looking for when you grade them, and tell them those criteria are posted.

Assessment

Student evaluations are from the posted standards of the performance assessment rubric. The last day of the dance unit will begin with a short quiz. Student assessment will begin in the next class.

Folk Dance Lessons 8-10 — Beginner level

Lesson Setup

Equipment

Records, tapes, or CDs for Road to the Isles and Saturday Night Fever Walk, both of which are optional

Performance Goal

Students will review and improve performance of dances previously learned.

Cognitive Goals

Students will

be able to identify a dance when they hear the music, and
decide whether they want to add to their dance repertoire and learn something new.

Motivation

Tell the students that you have two more dances you are willing to teach to the best of your classes. One is from Scotland and the other is a dance that made John Travolta famous. Ask who wants to learn more.

Lesson Sequence

1. Ask for student requests. Throw in a dance that they haven't asked for in a while and review it first.
2. If students choose so, teach the Saturday Night Fever Walk in lesson 8 and the Road to the Isles in lesson 9.
3. Take the liberty to choose the dances that students avoid and review their importance.
4. Give the quiz during lesson 10. The quiz can be found on page 196. It should take only 10 minutes.

Review

Announce the upcoming quiz and review all the items that students should know: the head couple, counterclockwise, the definitions of polka and schottische, the difference between a line and a circle, the definition of grand right and left, what foot marches start on, which dances have no partners, and which countries traditionally avoided having girls and boys dance together.

Assessment

Evaluate students by observation, based on the beginner performance assessment rubric (table 6.2). For further general assessment rubrics, see appendix B.

TABLE 6.2 Beginner Dance Performance Assessment Rubric

STUDENT NAME _____

	0	1	2	3	4	5
Directions	No effort	• Faces correct direction • Moves in line of direction • Changes line of direction after seeing others	• Knows left from right • Joins group formation • Gets into lines, circles, or longways sets on verbal command	• Anticipates a direction change • Joins hands if requested • Do-si-dos, elbow swings, and promenades home	• Changes direction at the appropriate times • Partners pleasantly • Able to sashay, cast off, and reel • Knows, in the partner dance, that the leader/boy is on the left	• Remembers instructions for all dances repeated more than three times • Leads others • Recognizes dance by music • Does the grand right and left
Footwork	No effort	• Steps, hops, runs, slides, and jumps on cue • Knows left from right	• Leaps, skips, and gallops on cue • Goes left or right on cue • Counts steps	• Knows the schottische • Performs basic steps in any direction • Counts steps so direction changes are on time • Corrects self by following other	• Combines footwork patterns without pause • Knows the polka step • Begins direction change on correct foot • Steps flow into one another	• Acts as class role model • Correctly does all dances taught • Keeps flowing motion despite change of direction or formation • Performs proper footwork after a verbal cue only
Rhythm	No effort	• Claps or stomps on the beat	• Identifies tempo changes and can clap to them • Able to walk, run, jump, hop, and slide on the beat	• Combines slow and quick steps • Identifies musical phrases • Stays in sync with other dancers doing the same pattern	• All footwork is on the beat • Counts steps • Follows square-dance calls on cue	• Able to keep rhythm without a musical accompaniment • Able to use other body parts in rhythmical way • Sets strong model for others in class

Folk and Social Dance Lesson 1 — Intermediate level

Lesson Setup

Equipment

Records, tapes, or CDs for Grand March, Bingo, Pata Pata, Sevila SeBela Loza, Hora, Saturday Night Fever Walk, Virginia Reel, La Raspa, Greensleeves, Jessie Polka, Seljancica Kola, Red River Valley, and Road to the Isles

Records, tapes, or CDs for Mayim, Oh Johnny Oh, and Limbo Rock

Scrimmage vests to designate male and female positions

Performance Goals

Students will

choose several dances they remember and then review and repeat them, and learn three new dances:

* A Latin ballroom dance step, the mambo
* An Israeli rain dance, the Mayim
* An American dance, the Oh Johnny Oh

Motivation

Like the previous dance unit, you are mixing up the kinds of dances they will learn by teaching dances from different countries, with different tempos, and that are typical of different time periods. Tell the class that you will continue to give them background in dance from other regions of the world and lots of variety. You hope that, by the time they finish their second lesson, they all will feel that what they've learned has been enjoyable. Express hope that their experience here will allow them to go out dancing socially and that some will even find an outlet in dance that keeps them physically fit. Promise them that, if they bear with you for a little while and do the best they can to get over whatever apprehensions they may have, they eventually will love this unit if they don't already.

Lesson Sequence

1. Begin with requests from the floor. This will set a positive tone and get the class moving quickly. Review a few measures for everyone; the dance has not been done in a year. After being sure most students are comfortable with the steps, put the music on.
2. Introduce the Mayim (figure 6.4), walking the students through the steps while they are in a circle:
   * Begin with no music.
   * Have students dance through it, along with the music and instructional cues from you.

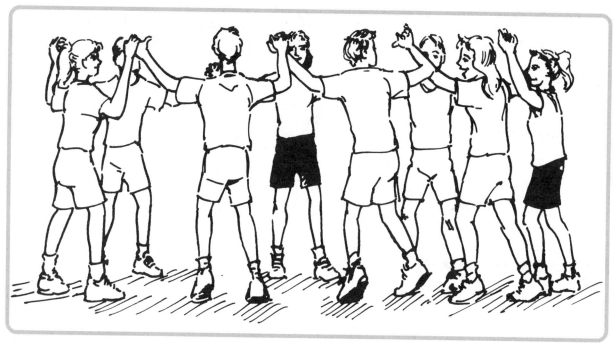

Figure 6.4—Mayim.

3. Teach the Oh Johnny Oh in a circle with partners:
   - Review what a mixer is.
   - Review where to find one's partner.
   - Review where to find one's corner.
   - Teach the dance "lost and found" rule: Tell students if they lose a partner they must get a new one during the promenade and before the set is called over again.
   - Discuss what to do if, on the promenade, one is left standing alone: go to the center of the circle to find a new partner.
   - Have the class walk through the dance three or four times.
   - Put the music on and allow anything to happen.
4. Teach the Limbo Rock:
   - Introduce its origin—the Latin American influence. (See students doing the Brazilian limbo in figure 6.5.)
   - Introduce the mambo step of the Limbo Rock first.
   - Then teach the other two sections of the dance, one at a time, having students do it in rhythm.
   - Put the music on and ask students to listen for when the musical phrases change.
   - Dance the dance through, calling out instructions.
5. If time permits, fill other requests from the previous year.

Review

Ask the class which dance uses hips a lot.
Ask which dance is a prayer for rain.
Discuss which dance made some students get lost.

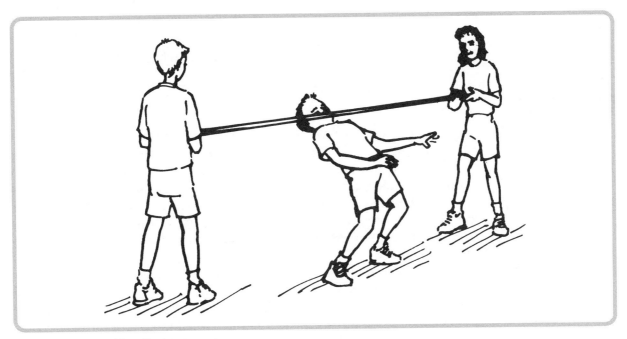

Figure 6.5—Brazilian limbo.

Remind students to come to class with sneakers or special dance shoes and to be prepared to remove their sweaters and jackets during the lesson.

Assessment

Observe students' ability to keep up with the pace of the class. Is the lesson too fast? Too slow? Should you review more, or less? What common dancing weakness exists? Adjust the next lesson to your knowledge of the class.

Folk and Social Dance Lesson 2   Intermediate level

Lesson Setup

Equipment

Record, tape, or CD library, specifically for Miserlou, mambo music from *Dirty Dancing* or another source, and for Achy Breaky Heart or other country line dance

Performance Goals

Students will

review and repeat new dances learned;
learn a traditional Greek dance that still is used today, the Miserlou;

learn to use the mambo in a variety of directions—forward, back, and sideways; and

learn a country-western line dance, the Achy Breaky Heart.

Motivation

Ask the class if anyone has gone to any weddings, bar mitzvahs, or confirmation parties lately. The fact is, most parties with live music always have a time during the evening when the band leader tries to get everyone up and moving and always uses traditional dances to do so. In the previous year, students learned the Hora, which, though Israeli, frequently is performed at social functions, whether Jewish or not. The Hora is an example of an old, traditional dance that has some popularity today. This lesson will cover a traditional but still popular Greek dance called the Miserlou.

Tell the class that you also will begin to develop their ability to … dirty dance. Just kidding! But for those who have seen the movie *Dirty Dancing*, remind them of that great scene in which Jennifer Grey's character is trying to learn to replace Patrick Swayze's dance partner, and they are out in the woods trying to get the beat. That is what the class will do—get the beat of the mambo.

Lesson Sequence

1. Begin with requests from the floor and do a quick review.
2. Introduce the two-step as a basic dance combination step before showing how it is used in a dance:
   • Teach the Miserlou, walking the class through the steps.
   • Begin with no music, talking the students through the whole A section and bringing them up to rhythm.
   • Have students dance through it, with the music, on instructional cues.
3. Review the mambo step:
   • Teach students how to go forward four steps and backward four steps.
   • Walk through the entire song—forward four mambo steps and back four—using no partners.
4. Teach the Achy Breaky Heart:
   • Introduce its origin in American country-western dance.
   • Walk through each section, slowly putting together the parts until the next turn.
   • Add music, and use cues while everyone is dancing to the music.
5. If time permits, fill other requests from the previous year.

Review

Ask the class which dance is American.
Inquire which has the most traditional music they've heard.
Put the mambo step into words.
Ask students how the mambo step is different from the two-step.
Put the two-step into words.

Folk and Social Dance Lesson 3 — Intermediate level

Lesson Setup

Equipment

Record, tape, or CD library, especially for Nebesco Kolo and Sicilian Tarantella

Performance Goals

Students will

review and repeat dances learned in this unit;
learn a traditional Italian dance, the Sicilian Tarantella;
learn the two-step and the pas de bas; and
learn a Slavic line dance that uses the two new steps—the Nebesko Kolo.

Motivation

In this lesson, tell the students that they will use the dance building block, the two-step, in another way. It's worth spending more time on the two-step since it can be done in many kinds of dancing—in traditional dances that are more than a hundred years old, or in modern social dance forms from ballroom to country-western dance. It can be used in a slow dance or a fast dance.

Inform the class that this lesson's dance is a fast line dance that uses a new step called the pas de bas. It is called the Nebesko Kolo and is a Yugoslavian line dance. Mention that Yugoslavia is a country that was created after World War II. In the 1990s, a civil war broke it up. The Sevila SeBela Loza, the dance from the previous unit, is from the Serbian portion of Yugoslavia, but the literature doesn't indicate exactly what part of Yugoslavia this lesson's dance came from. Just knowing the region will have to be good enough, unless anyone in the class wants some extra credit to do a search for its origins.

After the line dance, have students pay a little attention to the Italian heritage of some of their classmates and learn a Sicilian folk dance as well.

Lesson Sequence

1. Begin with requests from the floor. Review a few measures for everyone if the dance has not been done in this unit or if it has been newly learned. After being sure most students are comfortable with the steps, put the music on.
2. Introduce the pas de bas:
   • Start slowly but build up to the fast pace of the two-step used in this dance.
   • Teach the sequence of moves by section and walk it through a few times.
   • Put the music on and dance it through, reminding students when to turn.

171

3. Teach the Sicilian Tarantella as a simple, flirtatious Italian dance:
   * Review the do-si-do and the star, and then teach each sequence.
   * Walk through the entire song, pointing out its similarity with calls learned in square dance and the previous year's Greensleeves.
4. Review or teach the Achy Breaky Heart (if not already done in warm-up).
5. If time permits, fill other dance requests.

Review

Ask the class which dance is Italian.

Ask students which dance has music they've heard before.

Review the difference between a pas de bas and a two-step:
   * Is the rhythm the same or different?
   * Is it reminiscent of Irish dancing?
   * Is the pas de bas French or English?
   * Can anyone translate?

Folk and Social Dance Lesson 4   Intermediate level

Lesson Setup

Equipment

The music for Texas Star and Stepping Out

Performance Goals

Students will

review and repeat dances learned in this unit;

learn a 1940s American soft-shoe novelty dance, Stepping Out;

learn some basic tap-dance steps; and

learn to use the star in a square dance—the Texas Star.

Motivation

Let students know that they are going to do two American dances in this lesson. The two are very different: One comes from our traditional barnyard hoedown and the other derives from our tap-dance heritage.

Lesson Sequence

1. Begin with requests from the floor. Allow one or two before beginning to teach something.
2. Introduce Stepping Out:
   * Teach the first part in two parts and then put them together, first without music and then with music.
   * Teach the second part without music.

- Have the class walk through the first part twice, the second part once, and then the first part again.
- Add the music.
- Explain the challenge and then dance the whole dance through.
- Do the whole dance through a second time.

3. Have the class get into squares:
- Review the grand right and left.
- Walk through the Texas Star instructions (figure 6.6).

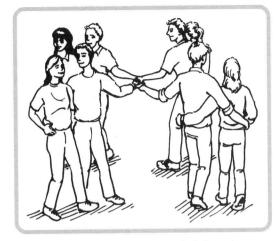

Figure 6.6—Square dance—left-hand star.

4. Before allowing the squares to break up, review the Red River Valley.
5. If time permits, fill other dance requests.

Review

Ask the class which dance is the oldest, the Texas Star or Stepping Out.
Ask which dance has music one would expect to hear when people are in jeans and boots.
Discuss what makes it difficult to move without music.
Ask what the students did during the silent passage in the song Stepping Out.

Folk and Social Dance Lesson 5   Intermediate level

Lesson Setup

Equipment

Records, tapes, or CDs for a dance library, especially for To Ting

Performance Goals

Students will

review and repeat dances learned in this unit;
learn the waltz and how to move to three-quarters timing;
learn a pivot turn; and
do a Danish dance that changes rhythm, the To Ting, using three-quarters and two-quarters timing.

Motivation

Tell students that they have learned steps that are considered basic to dance—the polka, the schottische, and the two-step. In this lesson, they will learn another—

the waltz. A waltz is a dance step done to three-quarters timing. As with all fundamental steps, the waltz is a building block. The only thing necessary is that the music be three-quarters timing. As with other steps, dancers can do them alone and move in any direction they choose. In this lesson students might try and build up to something more refined, a little more sophisticated musically, and a little more adult socially.

Perhaps they have seen films with ballroom dances with people dressed formally, behaving with an elegance typical of "good breeding," and dancing in smooth, flowing circles around the floor. This is typical of an old-world elegance, made famous in Vienna by wonderful Strauss music. The waltz is not necessarily formal and elegant, however. People in Cajun country, usually dressed in their cleanest sportswear, dance the waltz whenever a Cajun band plays a set.

The To Ting, an old, traditional Danish dance, includes a waltz, stepping to three-quarters timing. Most students are very familiar with disco, which generally plays everything in four-quarters timing. The interesting thing about this dance is that it does something very rare: It changes tempo from three-quarters time to two-quarters time. Inform the students that they'll learn the steps alone and then combine them so they are dancing the To Ting.

Lesson Sequence

1. Begin with requests from the floor. Allow one or two, before beginning to teach something new.
2. Introduce the waltz:
   - Practice in the open dance position.
   - Practice in the social dance position (figure 6.7).
3. Have the class choose partners and get into a double circle facing counterclockwise:
   - Walk through the first part of the To Ting.
   - Walk through the second part, pointing out the rhythm change.
   - Take some time to teach and practice the pivot turn.
   - Dance the whole dance through.
4. If time permits, fill other dance requests.

Review

The waltz differs from other dances because of its timing. Ask the class what the timing of the waltz is.

If a couple is dancing and the leader goes forward, ask students what direction the partner should go in.

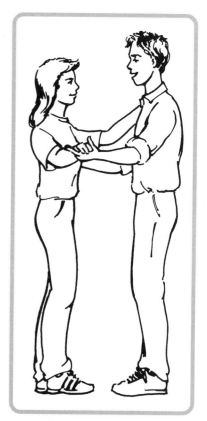

Figure 6.7—Couples in the social dance position.

Dance

Discuss whether dancers turn more easily if their weight is leaning away from or close to the center of the couple.

Folk and Social Dance Lesson 6 — Intermediate level

Lesson Setup

Equipment

Record, tape, or CD library, especially for Teton Mountain Stomp

Performance Goals

Students will

review and repeat dances learned in this unit;
learn to use the pivot turn again in an American folk dance, the Teton Mountain Stomp; and
improve the performance of the dances they usually do not select.

Motivation

Tell the students that this lesson will stick to American dances. Ask how many dances they remember from this unit that are American. There are Oh Johnny Oh, Achy Breaky Heart, Texas Star, and Stepping Out. And from the previous dance unit? Bingo, Saturday Night Fever Walk, Virginia Reel, and Red River Valley.

Lesson Sequence

1. Begin with requests from the floor that are American only.
2. Teach the Teton Mountain Stomp:
   • Review how to find a partner in a partner-changing dance.
   • Review the pivot turn.
3. Review the names of American dances and fill dance requests for American dances only.

Review

Ask students which dances they like better, those with partners or those without. Ask if they prefer those with instructions or those in which one has to remember the instructions. Do they like a square or a circle?
Find out if they think it is neat to get to dance with everyone.
Discuss which dances allow them to switch partners.
Review in which dances they were alone.

Folk and Social Dance Lesson 7   Intermediate level

Lesson Setup

Equipment

Record, tape, or CD library, especially for Salty Dog Rag
The posted intermediate performance assessment rubric

Performance Goals

Students will

review and repeat dances learned in this unit;
perform the schottische step in a variety of dances, one of which is a new one, the Salty Dog Rag; and
review the Teton Mountain Stomp and select others of their choice.

Motivation

Tell the class that this lesson is an all-schottische day. Ask students what the schottische is, and what dances they have learned in this unit that have the schottische in them. The Miserlou is one. And in the previous dance unit? The Sevila SeBela Loza, Seljancica Kolo, and Road to the Isles. (See students dancing Road to the Isles in the Varousvienne dance position in figure 6.8.)

Tell students that the new dance of the day is called the Salty Dog Rag, and you think they'll love it. The whole dance is based on the schottische, so they should have no trouble picking it up.

Lesson Sequence

1. Begin with requests from the floor that are schottische only.

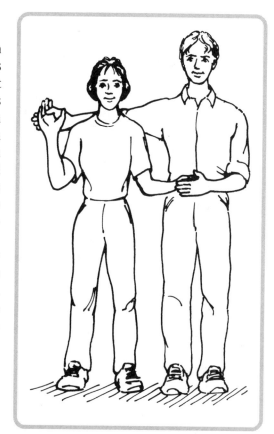

Figure 6.8—Dancing in the Varsouvienne position doing the Road to the Isles.

2. Teach the Salty Dog Rag:
   - Show the skater's section part (figure 6.9)—without music first, but on rhythm.
   - Teach the "heelie" section—without music first.
   - Combine the whole thing.
3. Do the Salty Dog twice.
4. Review other dances with the schottische.
5. If time permits, allow other requests from the floor.

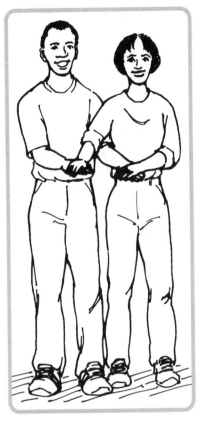

Figure 6.9—Skater's dance position.

Review

Ask students which dance is the most energetic.

Ask which dance does the schottische to the side.

Ask which does the schottische as if one is skating on a pond.

Ask which does the schottische in a line.

Let the class know that the end of the unit is nearing, which means you will be coming up with grades. Tell them you have posted the standards you will use and advise them to take a look. Invite any questions the class may have at any time.

Assessment

Observation will be based on posted standards. The intermediate performance assessment rubric on page 181 can be enlarged and posted for students to see.

Folk and Social Dance Lesson 8   Intermediate level

Lesson Setup

Equipment

Records, tapes, or CDs for the full library of dances already taught
Records, tapes, or CDs for a full library of new dances

Performance Goals

Students will

review and repeat dances learned this year,
perform a variety of folk dances from the Middle East and Greece, and
improve dances already learned.

Cognitive Goal

Students will learn how they will be graded.

Motivation

In the past couple of dance units, students have learned 24 dances. Tell them there is no way you would expect them to do all the dances 100 percent correctly, although it would be great if they could. Answer any questions they might have on what exactly you are looking for in your grading. If they don't have questions, ask them if they want you to read out the standards for them or if they are just as happy to go on with the lesson and check it out themselves.

Take some time to review dances from eastern Europe and northeastern Africa before getting to the dances students request. Ask if anyone can identify where the Hora, Mayim, the Miserlou come from.

Lesson Sequence

1. Begin with requests from the floor. Allow one or two before beginning to teach something new.
2. Go over the Salty Dog Rag.
3. Review old dances from the Middle East—Hora and Mayim—and from Greece—Miserlou.
4. If time permits, allow other requests from the floor.

Review

Conduct questions and answers in preparation for evaluation. If you decide not to use the rubric as defined, you and the students can decide how they should be graded:

On how they dance several dances—if so, which ones?
Or, on how they learn a new one

Assessment

Performance assessment will be based on observation and standards as written and posted in the performance assessment rubric for 9th and 10th grades.

Folk and Social Dance Lesson 9 — Intermediate level

Performance Goals

Students will

review the mambo and create a 16-measure pattern with a partner, and focus on dances they choose to be graded on.

Motivation

At the very beginning of this unit, the class learned the mambo, a Latin social dance step. Tell students that the mambo is done in dance clubs. It is very useful for them to not only feel comfortable doing it but to realize that they can create their own dance. Review the mambo and then, with a partner of their choice, have them spend 15 minutes creating and practicing a 16-mambo-step routine that they can do together.

Lesson Sequence

1. Begin with requests from the floor. Allow one or two before beginning to teach something new.
2. Review the mambo.
3. Review dances for grading.

Review

Have students watch half of the class mambo at a time. Ask them whose routine they like enough to learn.

Announce that in the next class they will take a short quiz. Ask them to bring something to write with. Let them know they will dance after the quiz.

Assessment

Observation will be based on the posted standards in the performance assessment rubric on page 181.

Folk and Social Dance Lesson 10 — Intermediate level

Lesson Setup

Equipment

A quiz for each student
Pens or pencils

Performance Goal

Students will dance to final floor requests.

Cognitive Goals

Students will

take a quiz, and
be graded on dances the class has agreed on.

Motivation

Tell students they've done a great job. Let them know it's the last day of the dance unit, and after the quiz, they can choose any dances they want to end the unit with.

Lesson Sequence

1. Test the class with a quiz (on page 197) and then for skills.
2. Allow one warm-up dance.
3. Take requests from the floor.

Review

Ask students what they think would improve the unit.
Ask them what they think would have improved themselves.

Assessment

Students will be assessed by their graded written quizzes and their performance as based on the standards predefined to the class in the intermediate performance assessment rubric (table 6.3). Further general assessment rubrics can be found in appendix B.

Folk and Social Dance Lesson 1   Advanced level

Lesson Setup

Record, tape, or CD library to include all dances from all prior grades: Grand March, Bingo, Pata Pata, Sevila SeBela Loza, Hora, Saturday Night Fever Walk, Virginia Reel, La Raspa, Greensleeves, Jessie Polka, Seljancica Kola,

TABLE 6.3 Intermediate Dance Performance Assessment Rubric

STUDENT NAME _____

	0	1	2	3	4	5
Directions	No effort	• Gets in single and double circle • Knows clockwise from counter-clockwise • Follows a line • Joins hands when requested	• Knows the position of a square • Knows partner • Knows corner • Knows inside from outside • Forms a square	• Takes social, skater's, or Varsouvienne dance positions • Has mastered basic square-dance calls	• Has mastered the grand right and left, allemande the corner, and courtesy turns • Is always on the correct side of partner • Has learned the star	• Remembers instructions for all dances repeated more than three times • Leads others • Recognizes dance by music • Is unfazed by direction changes
Footwork	No effort	• Has mastered basic locomotion • Has mastered skipping, leaping, and galloping • Knows the scottische	• Has mastered the polka and two-step in the line of direction • Stays on beat when the tempo speeds up	• Knows the waltz in the line of direction • Performs a pivot turn alone • Begins on the correct foot	• Has learned how to lead/follow when dancing with a partner • Uses combination steps while turning • Steps flow into one another	• Able to polka, pivot turn, or waltz with partner • Ably does all dances taught • Performs proper footwork after a verbal cue
Group work	No effort	• Joins the group formation on request • Follows established class rules	• Follows the line of direction but needs to watch • Is on beat with the music	• Follows the accepted etiquette • Anticipates the next steps and direction changes • Does not drag others	• Accepts responsibility for leading or following • Able to keep rhythm without a musical accompaniment	• Knows all the dances well enough to lead • Has synchronized and cooperative partner work

Red River Valley, Road to the Isles, Mayim, Oh Johnny Oh, Limbo Rock, Miserlou, mambo music from *Dirty Dancing* or other source, Achy Breaky Heart or other country line dance, Nebesko Kolo, Sicilian Tarantella, Texas Star, Stepping Out, To Ting, Teton Mountain Stomp, Salty Dog Rag
Record, tape, or CD for Doudlebska Polka

Performance Goals

Students will

choose several dances they remember from prior years, review, and repeat them;
review the polka step and the Jessie Polka; and
learn the Doudlebska Polka.

Motivation

In this unit the plan is to bring students' dance skills to a more social level than before. They will be partnering a lot. Tell them that you have planned things to teach, but you also will give them the opportunity to ask for more emphasis on things they want to learn about in dance. This lesson is polka day.

Lesson Sequence

1. Begin with requests from the floor. This will set a positive tone and get the class moving quickly. Review a few measures for everyone before putting the music on.
2. Review the polka step and, in rhythm, have the class do polka steps around the room.
3. Review the Jessie Polka:
   * Review the heel-and-toe part.
   * Have students get in threes, fours, or fives, reviewing the heel-and-toe section with them locked together, arms around waists, bodies leaning forward and back.
   * Announce that the part just practiced is preceded by four polka steps; put the music on and dance.
4. Teach the polka in couples:
   * Introduce the ballroom dance position.
   * Introduce the reciprocity of footwork between male and female.
   * Teach how to move as a couple:
     The male's job is making sure the dancers do not crash into walls or each other.
     Try to get students to lean away from their center, while holding onto their partner.
   * Associate holding on and leaning away with centrifugal force.
   * Explain that leaning away and holding on enables turning.
5. Teach the Doudlebska Polka:
   * Where it is from
   * That it is a mixer
   * The circle formation of the second section of the dance
   * The mixer part
   * Listening to the music cues
   * Dancing the dance, with you calling out reminders for the first few repeats of the dance

Review

Ask students how many had more than three different partners.
Ask which partner felt easier to move with, the one who was firm and leaned away or the one who was limp.

Discuss laws of physics and their relevance in dancing. Ask which law applies here and how important it is.

Ask the class to explain what a mixer is.

Assessment

Observe class progress. Most students should be having no trouble with the basic polka step, and the activity level of the class should be high. If not, evaluate what needs more review and plan it for the next lesson.

Folk and Social Dance Lesson 2 — Advanced level

Lesson Setup

Equipment

Records, tapes, or CDs for Doudlebska Polka, Texas Two-Step, and Cajun two-step music

Performance Goals

Students will

choose several dances they remember, review, and repeat them;

review the Doudlebska Polka;

review the two-step and a dance they learned in the previous year that includes it—the Nebesko Kolo; and

learn the Texas Two-Step folk dance and the two-step to Cajun music.

Motivation

The two-step is done with lots of music. As the music changes, so does the style. Tell students that this lesson will review a dance they learned before, and then they'll learn two kinds of dances that use the two-step. One is called the Texas Two-Step, also known as the Texas Shuffle. The other is really just a music change, the Cajun two-step.

Lesson Sequence

1. Begin with requests from the floor. Allow one or two before beginning to teach something new.
2. Review the Doudlebska Polka in rhythm; put the music on and dance the dance.
3. Review the two-step and the pas de bas:
   - Review specific parts of the Nebesko Kolo: the two-step, balances, pas de bas, stomp.

183

- Walk once through this line dance without music.
- Put the music on and dance.

4. Teach the Texas Two-Step:
   - Quick, quick, slow; slow in long, gliding steps
   - A closed dance position
   - The girl's left hand either on the boy's arm (not shoulder) or hooked in his belt
   - The line of direction—everyone moving counterclockwise
   - Emphasis on the boy leading, the girl following

5. Change to Cajun music and instruct everyone to change partners:
   - Begin the same way.
   - Teach a break—the boy turns the girl under his right arm.

6. If time permits, ask if anyone remembers a Texas line dance. Review the Acky Breaky Heart and do it.

Review

Ask the class to describe the differences among the dances that use a two-step.
Ask which is the line dance.
Review which dance glides smoothly.
Ask which is more funky.
Describe the timing of a two-step.

Folk and Social Dance Lesson Plan 3 — Advanced level

Lesson Setup

Equipment

Records, tapes, or CDs for Doubleska Polka, Texas Two-Step, Cajun two-step, Oh Johnny Oh, and Virginia Reel

Performance Goals

Students will

choose several dances they remember, review, and repeat them;.
review the Doubleska Polka and the Texas or Cajun two-step;
learn a second break for the two-step;
review common square-dance calls; and
dance using common square-dance calls.

Motivation

Once one learns the footwork, the two-step differs when the tempo changes, when the partner changes, and if the leader chooses to do something new. Mention to students that they know how to go counterclockwise, how to turn the girl under the arm, and how to turn as a couple. In this lesson they'll learn a new break.

Lesson Sequence

1. Begin with requests from the floor. Allow one or two, before beginning to teach something new.
2. Review the two-step.
3. Teach the break in rhythm and making sure turns take place during the quick step:
   - Walk through the instructions.
   - Try it to music.
   - Suggest that everyone do four basics, one girl's turn, four basics, and a new turn.
   - Emphasize the boy leading, the girl following.
4. Make a circle, review the corner, partner, and promenade. Do the Oh Johnny Oh.
5. Straighten the circle, breaking into long-ways sets, four to six couples:
   - Review the castoff, sashay, and reel.
   - Do the Virginia Reel.
6. If time permits, fill requests.

Review

Ask the class, which dances result in a change of partner.
Ask which is in longway position.
What about Oh Johnny Oh reminds them of square dancing?
What makes Oh Johnny Oh definitely not a square dance?

Assessment

Observe for the ability of the majority of the class to move along with the lesson tempo. If that is not happening, slow down and give more repetition without the music and then more repetition of each step with the music, before letting the music play through and expecting everyone to dance to the end.

Folk and Social Dance Lesson 4   Advanced level

Lesson Setup

Equipment

Record, tape, or CD for Ve' David

Performance Goals

Students will

choose several dances to review and repeat them,

review the Doubleska Polka and the Texas or Cajun two-step, and

learn a third break for the two-step.

Cognitive Goal

Students will review the reason for a mixer and use a new mixer to find a new partner.

Motivation

In this lesson, the class will learn another break for the two-step and a new mixer. Discuss the mixer they are about to learn. It is quite simple; the only thing in it that they haven't learned before is the *buzz turn* (figure 6.10). You'll be warming them up and then teaching the buzz turn and the Ve' David, a folk dance from Israel.

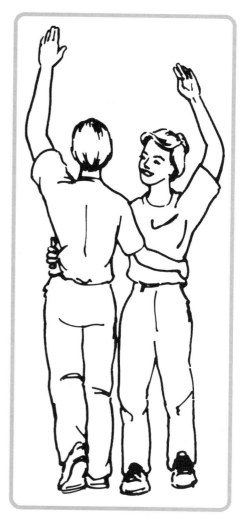

Figure 6.10—Buzz Turn.

Lesson Sequence

1. Begin with requests from the floor.
   Allow one or two, before beginning to teach something new.
2. Teach the buzz turn:
   • Demonstrate without a partner, just working on keeping one foot as the anchor and pushing with the other to get around it.
   • Teach the arm position and how partners are side to side.
   • Show how centrifugal force, pulling away but holding on, helps the swing.
3. Teach the Ve' David in sequence:
   • Walk through the instructions.
   • Remind students where to go if they lose a partner ("lost and found" in the middle of the circle).
   • Put the music on, and with verbal cues over the music, do the dance through.
4. Do the Texas Two-Step.
5. Do the Doubleska Polka as a mixer.
6. Teach a new break for the two-step, using Cajun music this time.
7. If time permits, fill requests.

Review

Ask if anyone is sweating.

Discuss whether dancing can be a good activity for improving fitness, and why.

Folk and Social Dance Lesson 5 — Advanced level

Lesson Setup

Equipment

Record, tape, or CD for Hot Lips

Performance Goals

Students will

choose several dances to review and repeat;

review one dance with the two-step in it, but they can choose which one; and

learn a novelty dance that is based on the swing, Hot Lips.

Motivation

Ask the class if anyone knows what popular dance came after the Charleston and before the twist. A hint: the teenagers started it, it was fast, became athletic, and was done to big-band sounds. It was. . .the swing. Tell students that the dance they are going to learn is as specific as a hundred-year-old folk dance in that it repeats itself and has a set of steps that go with each phase of the music. Though it follows folk dance trends, it is an offshoot of swing, which is relatively modern, 50 or a little more years old. Comment that you don't know why, but it is called Hot Lips. It has a few breaks in it that also can be used in the Cajun or Texas two-step.

Lesson Sequence

1. Begin with requests from the floor.
2. Teach Hot Lips in sections:
   - Have students choose partners and get in a double circle, with partners facing each other, in the social dance position.
   - Have them move so their joined hands are facing counterclockwise and the couples are in the open dance position, as shown in figure 6.11. In that position, couples begin by taking two two-steps and four walking steps forward:

     Walk it through each section first, with no music.

     Add the music as each section is learned, to keep the learning process in rhythm.

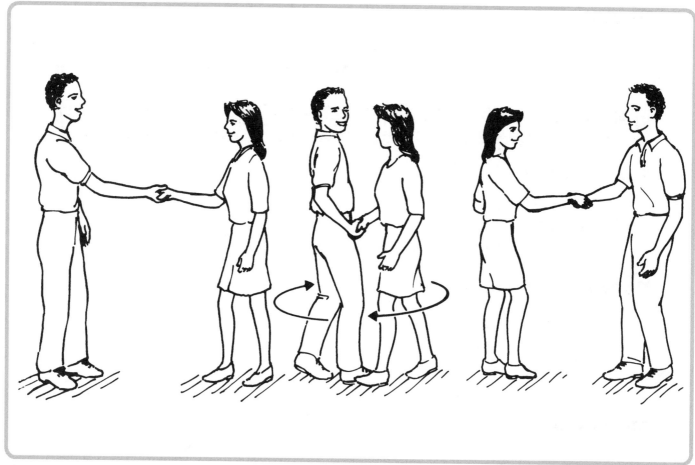

Figure 6.11—Open dance position.

- Teach the first break and then the change of direction—clockwise. In Hot Lips, which is done with couples in a circle, the partners face each other so that the man's back is to the center of the circle and his partner is facing him. Their right hands are joined. To exchange positions, they walk forward, pass right shoulders without letting go of their hands, reach the side their partner has been on, and, without letting go, turn to face each other. Now the girl has her back to the center of the circle. The couple is still in the same general place in the circle, but the boy is now on the outside and the girl on the inside.

    Walk it through with no music.

    Add music to keep the turn in rhythm.

    Follow this procedure with each section.
- Teach the second break, being careful to explain the change of sides in the circle and the change of direction.
- Complete the dance via the instructions, walking it through a few times.
- Dance it through to the music.
3. Do a mixer so students get new partners.
4. Have them do Hot Lips again with a new partner.
5. If time allows, fill requests.

Review

Ask the class what dance Hot Lips is based on.
Review what dance step in Hot Lips is used the most frequently.

Folk and Social Dance Lesson 6 — Advanced level

Lesson Setup

Equipment

Record, tape, or CD for cha-cha music

Performance Goals

Students will

choose several dances to review and repeat;
review one folk dance with a Latin rhythm in it—the Limbo Rock; and
learn a Latin ballroom dance form—the cha-cha.

Motivation

Brazil favors the samba, Argentina favors the tango, in Costa Rica and Cuba the mambo is the most popular dance. Somehow in our country, the cha-cha has survived. Tell students that in this lesson, you are introducing them to the cha-cha.

Lesson Sequence

1. Begin with a review of the mambo and the Limbo Rock.
2. Teach the cha-cha:
   - Teach the footwork without students partnered up.
   - With a partner, the boys leading, teach the basic step in rhythm:
     Walk it through without music at first.
     Add music to keep them learning on rhythm.
   - Teach a break, in rhythm, with no music first, then adding music.
3. Do a mixer so students get new partners.
4. Have them do Hot Lips with a new partner.
5. If time allows, fill requests.

Review

Ask the class to tell you, using the words "slow" and "quick," the rhythm for the footwork in the mambo and in the cha-cha.
If they want to turn their partner, ask students if they do it on the slow or the quick steps.

Announce that the next lesson will be a hoedown—an American dance all the way. Instruct students to dress down for square dancing.

Folk and Social Dance Lesson 7   Advanced level

Lesson Setup

Equipment

Records, tapes, or CDs, specifically for Red River Valley, Oh Johnny Oh, Texas Star, Promenade the Ring, Arkansas Traveler, and Gents Star Right
The posted advanced performance assessment rubric for 11th- and 12th-grade dance students
Scrimmage vests

Performance Goals

Students will

do a variety of square dances—up to six dances; and
use as many previously learned square-dance calls as time permits:
- The shuffle—a light walk
- The do-si-do—walking forward, passing right shoulders and backing out to one's place
- The promenade—hands joined in a skater's position, shuffling
- The swing—two turns around, couples leaning away from each other
- The allemande left—left forehand grasps while turning around each other
- The grand right and left—chaining the opposite gender, by extending one's right hand to the first person, passing her by, left to the next, passing her by, and so on
- The right-hand star—right hands join in the center, in a counterclockwise line of direction

Motivation

Suggest to students that it should be up to them on how they want you to grade their performance. Tell them that you have posted the performance assessment rubric you thought you might use, and ask them to look it over (page 195). In the next class they can decide whether they want you to use it or if they would prefer some other method. You could grade their performance on any of the following choices:

Three specific dances learned in the unit
One dance of each type—folk, social, and square
The ability to perform, on cue, a specific instruction
The ability to create one's own dance

On to the current lesson: let students know that they just have to listen and follow directions immediately after they hear them. Tell them to be ready to move the minute they hear the instructions.

Lesson Sequence

1. Have students form squares:
   - Review the head couple and the side couple.
   - Review going halfway around.
   - Review the counterclockwise line of direction.
   - Review the promenade.
   - Tell students to listen, wish them luck, and put on Promenade the Ring.
2. Review the swing:
   - The position of couples—that they lean away.
   - The direction of the corner and the partner.
   - What to do when one is told to promenade while dancing with someone who is not one's partner.
   - Put on an oldie but goodie, Oh Johnny Oh.
   - Put on a new one, Arkansas Traveler.
3. Review the social fun of square dancing:
   - Dancing with everyone in the square.
   - The rule of when the male goes home with the partner he started with.
   - When he must take the new partner home, with the new one becoming his partner until the next partner change.
4. Review by doing each of the following calls as they are needed in the dances:
   - Walk through the allemande left—grasping left forearms.
   - Walk through the grand right and left.
   - Review the call "head couple head down the valley."
   - Put on another oldie but goodie, the simple version of Red River Valley.
   - Review the distinction between "head couples head down the valley" and "side couples head down the valley."
   - Put on the more complex version of Red River Valley, in which everyone is dancing all of the time.
5. Review a star:
   - Discuss what going halfway means in a square-dance call.
   - Put on Gents Star Right.
   - Review and walk through the star promenade.
   - Put on Texas Star.
6. If time allows, fill requests.

Review

Ask the class whether a girl's corner is to her right or her left.

Discuss what happens when a square is told to join hands.

Ask, if couple three is told to go left, which couple it is headed to.

Review, when beginning a grand right and left, whom the dancer reaches out her right hand for.

Announce that in the next class you will teach some new calls.

Assessment

Post your standards for grading skills and start to observe for them. This may be done by using the performance assessment rubric at the end of this unit (page 195).

Folk and Social Dance Lesson 8   Advanced level

Lesson Setup

Equipment

Records, tapes, and CDs for Red River Valley, Oh Johnny Oh, Texas Star, Promenade the Ring, Arkansas Traveler, Gents Star Right, Split the Ring and Around Just One, Bend It Tight, and Four in the Middle
Microphone

Performance Goals

Students will

do a variety of square dances,
learn up to three new square dances using the new calls, and
review general rules of square dance:
  • Movement is continuous. If waiting for a call, keep feet moving.
  • Calls are ahead, so while executing one call, listen for what you have to do next.
  • Keep the square a normal size.
  • If inactive while other couples are moving on the outside of the square, move in.
  • Unless specifically told to promenade a fraction of the way around, boys take their dancing partner home.
  • The dance will end with the dancers at home.
  • If there is a mix-up in your square, everyone should go home and pick up the call after the promenade ends.
  • React to instructions by going to the position in the square, not to the person you expect is supposed to be in it. Remember, the caller is moving everyone around—for example, allemande left means turn to your corner, a set position in the square.
  • When a call is made to take a girl, the call is directing the boy to take the girl.

Lesson Safety

Be sure there is enough space for each square to move without hitting an obstruction.

Motivation

Announce that in this lesson you will try to get to more advanced calls. You will teach the calls first, and then it is up to their listening skills to dance the dance once you put the music on. But first, you'll have students do two dances they already know, but they'll use some new procedures that are not called but are done at the option of the male dance partner. They are the twirl and the courtesy turn. Suggest that students try these if they are feeling good about the dance.

Lesson Sequence

1. Teach the twirl:
   - Have students get a partner and form a circle.
   - Demonstrate the boy moving in a line of direction while twirling his partner under his right arm.
   - Let the class practice with their partner.
   - Have them practice with new partners and take care that the girl does not get dizzy.
2. Have students form squares:
   - Review the grand right and left:
     Point out how the girl has to turn back to the counterclockwise direction.
     Teach the reason for the courtesy turn and how to do it.
     Have them do the grand right and left again, concluding it with the courtesy turn.
   - Let students request which square dance they want to do, instructing them to use the twirl during the promenade and the courtesy turn when the girl's direction must change.
   - Choose another square for this practice.
3. If the dances from the previous lesson were not done, complete the lesson.
4. Teach a new call—"split the ring." Call and walk it through for each couple.
5. Teach a new call—"around just one." Call and walk it through for each couple.
6. Put on Split the Ring and Around Just One:
   - Help students anticipate the sequence by walking through it.
   - Remind them how to handle a square when dancers in the group get mixed up.
   - Put the music on and allow it to play through, unless everyone is confused:
     If they are, stop the music and walk them through it again.
     If they still are, you should stay with the square that is confused and ask the dancers who are in the know to reach for the ones who are getting confused, so they can keep them going in the correct direction.
7. Teach a new call—the "pass-through." Have the class walk through it for the side couples and then the head couple.
8. Teach a new call—"bend the line." Have the class walk through it for the side couples and the head couple.
9. Put on Bend It Tight:
   - Ask if students want a walk-through since they already know the calls.
   - Put the music on, stopping only if everyone is confused.
10. Put on Four in the Middle, a new dance that uses all of the calls just learned:
    - Ask if students want a walk-through.
    - When they are ready, put the music on in its entirety and leave it on until it's over unless there are problems.
11. If time allows, fill requests.

Review

Ask students to draw a map in the air of their path for "split the ring and go around one."
Review what the boy does while twirling.

Ask why a boy courtesy-turns his partner.

For the next lesson, request the students to dress for dancing, but to also bring a pen or pencil for a quiz.

Folk and Social Dance Lessons 9-10   Advanced level

Lesson Setup

Equipment

A quiz for everyone

Pens and pencils

Performance Goal

Students will do a variety of dances, as many as possible within the period.

Cognitive Goal

Students will begin the 9th lesson with a short quiz and the 10th reviewing it.

Lesson Safety

Be sure there is enough space for each square to move without hitting an obstruction.

Motivation

Tell students that they have learned a lot. Now it's time to discuss how to evaluate it. Within the next two lessons you will be giving them a grade. Ask how they would prefer to be evaluated.

Lesson Sequence

1. Give the written quiz in lesson 9. It can be found on pages 198-199.
2. Receive requests for the warm-up.
3. Once students have decided how they want to be evaluated, teach what they want.
4. Keep the music on, trying to keep the class moving the whole period.
5. Observe and grade the class.

Review

Tell students that you are glad they dressed for dancing in this unit. Ask how many found themselves sweating more than they ever did for badminton, volleyball, or softball.

Ask what that tells them about the fitness potential of dance.

Tell students that they'll have to go back to their regular gym clothing for the next unit. You'll miss having that extra time with them, since now they'll have to take time to change their clothes.

Assessment

Complete the assessment based on the goals that you and the students agreed to in an earlier lesson based on the performance assessment rubric (table 6.4). For further general assessment rubrics, see appendix B. There's also the written quiz.

TABLE 6.4 Advanced Dance Performance Assessment Rubric

STUDENT NAME _____

	0	1	2	3	4	5
Directions	No effort	• Takes the assigned formation on cue • Follows the line • Follows a line of direction • Joins hands when requested • Knows inside, outside and left, right	• Knows the head couple and side couple in square dance • Identifies partner and corner • Able to take social, skater's, or Varsouvienne dance positions	• Has mastered basic square-dance calls • Does not get lost in the square • Is always on correct side of partner	• Has mastered the grand right and left, allemande the corner, and stars • Has learned to safely dance in partners at random • Has learned new square-dance terms and done them three times	• Remembers instructions for all dances repeated more than three times • Leads others • Recognizes dance by music • Is unfazed by direction changes
Footwork	No effort	• Has mastered basic locomotion, basic movement combinations, and basic steps in the forward direction	• Uses the correct foot • Stays on the beat through tempo changes	• Has mastered dancing with a partner in the line of direction • Has step flow into one another	• Turns when dancing with a partner • Uses combination steps while turning	• Turns use centrifugal force to keep flowing • Ably does all dances taught • Performs proper footwork after a verbal cue
Group work	No effort	• Gets into position or formation on request • Follows established class rules • Follows line of direction but still needs to watch	• Follows the rules of etiquette • Follows directions during a mixer • Able to keep rhythm without a musical accompaniment	• Does not cause the square or mixer to malfunction • Works with partner to learn new breaks • Random couple dancing is safe for others in room	• Works with others to accomplish the shuffle, split the ring, and pass-through • Practices with a partner without being told	• Knows all the dances well enough to lead • Partner work is synchronized and cooperative • Dances smoothly with the flow

Dance Quiz—Beginner level

NAME _____ TEACHER _____

DATE _____ CLASS PERIOD _____

True or False: Read each statement below carefully. If the statement is true, put a check under the True box in the column to the left of the statement. If the statement is false, put a check under the False box in the column to the left of the statement. If using a grid sheet, blacken in the appropriate column for each question, making sure to use the correctly numbered line for each question and its answer.

True **False**

☐ ☐ 1. Marching begins with the left foot.

☐ ☐ 2. The "grand right and left" begins by facing your partner, joining right hands, walking forward until passing right shoulders, and extending your free hand to the next person.

☐ ☐ 3. The polka is three steps—skip, run, run—and is done to four beats of music.

☐ ☐ 4. If the first polka step begins with the left foot, the next also begins with the left foot.

☐ ☐ 5. In its time and place, Sevila SeBela Loza was probably as popular as the Electric Slide is today.

☐ ☐ 6. John Travolta made great acting success by dancing the Virginia Reel.

☐ ☐ 7. Traditional Serbian and Yugoslavian dances were done in lines.

☐ ☐ 8. A schottische is a basic dance step whose proper execution requires four steps and a hop.

☐ ☐ 9. An Israeli circle dance requiring high energy is the Hora.

☐ ☐ 10. "Promenade home" instructs the boys to walk around the square until returning to their own side and to take whomever they are dancing with as their new partner.

From *Complete Physical Education Plans for Grades 7–12* by Isobel Kleinman, 2001, Champaign, IL: Human Kinetics.

Dance Quiz–Intermediate level

NAME _____   TEACHER _____

DATE _____   CLASS PERIOD _____

Multiple Choice: Read each question and each answer carefully. Be sure to choose the best answer that fits the statement preceding it. When you have made your choice, put the appropriate letter on the line to the left of the numbered question.

_____1. Dances in which the instructions are typically sung with the music are
    a. partner circle dances
    b. European folk dances
    c. square dances
    d. country-western dances

_____2. The male partner always should
    a. bring his partner home
    b. put his partner on the right
    c. start with the left foot
    d. all of the above

_____3. The "grand right and left"
    a. is a human moving chain
    b. is a way for the girls to meet and join hands momentarily with all the boys
    c. starts with the right hand, passing right shoulders, then the left, passing left shoulders, then the right, passing right shoulders, and so on
    d. all of the above

_____4. The waltz is
    a. "quick, quick, slow"
    b. three equal steps
    c. only done forward
    d. done only in the social dance position

_____5. The pivot turn taught in class while learning To Ting is
    a. four equal steps
    b. done in a couple
    c. done to four-quarters time
    d. all of the above

_____6. The mambo step
    a. was influenced by Latin music
    b. is a step, step, and close and hold
    c. is used in the Limbo Rock
    d. all of the above

_____7. Which of the following is *not* a traditional folk dance?
    a. Miserlou
    b. To Ting
    c. Achy Breaky Heart
    d. Texas Star

_____8. Which of the following does *not* require that you have a partner?
    a. Texas Star
    b. Limbo Rock
    c. Salty Dog Rag
    d. Oh Johnny Oh

_____9. Choose the dance with a silent musical passage:
    a. Nebesco Kolo
    b. Sicilian Tarantella
    c. Stepping Out
    d. all of the above

_____10. If you were designing an aerobic unit with the dances you learned and you wanted to have an energetic dance that would significantly raise one's heart rate, which one would you choose?
    a. Salty Dog Rag
    b. Mayim
    c. Stepping Out
    d. Achy Breaky Heart

From *Complete Physical Education Plans for Grades 7–12* by Isobel Kleinman, 2001, Champaign, IL: Human Kinetics.

Dance Quiz–Advanced level

NAME _____ TEACHER _____

DATE _____ CLASS PERIOD _____

True or False: Read each statement below carefully. If the statement is true, put a check under the True box in the column to the left of the statement. If the statement is false, put a check under the False box in the column to the left of the statement. If using a grid sheet, blacken in the appropriate column for each question, making sure to use the correctly numbered line for each question and its answer.

True   False

☐   ☐   1. If a square-dance caller sings, "Swing your corner, and promenade home," you must return to your partner to promenade home.

☐   ☐   2. If the head couple is supposed to be closest to the music, in a square they would be standing with their backs to the music.

☐   ☐   3. The Ve' David, Texas Star, Oh Johnny Oh, Teton Mountain Stomp, and Doubleska Polka all are mixers.

☐   ☐   4. When "splitting the ring," head couples separate their opposites and then walk around the square in opposite directions.

☐   ☐   5. When a boy, in the closed dance position, leads with his left foot, the girl should move back with her right.

☐   ☐   6. The two-step is the basic dance step used in the Doubleska Polka.

☐   ☐   7. To get the best swing, couples should lean away from each other.

☐   ☐   8. The polka is the predominant basic dance step used in the Hot Lips.

☐   ☐   9. When a group of dancers put their left hands in the center of the group, they are "starring left" but walking right.

☐   ☐   10. A boy's corner is always on his left because his partner is always on his right.

Matching: Read one item at a time from the left-hand column. Look at the column on the right and read all the choices. Pick the one that most closely matches the left-hand item. Write the letter that represents your choice on the blank space to the left of the column, next to the appropriate item.

_____ 1. Hop, step, close, step

_____ 2. Quick, quick, slow (or) step, step, step/hold

_____ 3. Step, step, step

_____ 4. Couples with their right hands joined in front

_____ 5. Couples with their left hands joined in front and right hands joined behind

_____ 6. Boy's left hand holding girl's right, boy's right arm across girl's back, girl's left hand on boy's shoulder

_____ 7. Everyone's hands joined

_____ 8. Facing to the right of the center of a circle

_____ 9. Girls go opposite their partners, taking right hand, pass by, extend left hand to the next boy they see, pass by, and so on

_____ 10. Walking

a. A circle

b. Shuffling

c. The skater's position

d. The grand right and left

e. Social or closed dance position

f. The two-step

g. Counterclockwise

h. The polka

i. The Varsouvienne position

j. The waltz

From *Complete Physical Education Plans for Grades 7–12* by Isobel Kleinman, 2001, Champaign, IL: Human Kinetics.

Dance Answer Key—Beginner level

1. T
2. T
3. T
4. F. Each polka step begins on the alternate foot.
5. T
6. F. He danced the "walk" to disco music from the sound track of the film *Saturday Night Fever.* "Turkey in the Straw," the music used to dance to the Virginia Reel, is hundreds of years old.
7. T
8. F. A schottische is three steps and a hop, not four steps and a hop.
9. T
10. T

Dance Answer Key—Intermediate level

1. C. Square dances are called, and good callers attempt to call in tune.
2. D
3. D
4. B
5. D
6. D
7. C. Square dance is considered a traditional American folk dance.
8. B. The Limbo Rock is the only dance done without joining anyone's hands.
9. C. The nonmusic is the challenge to ending this soft-shoe dance.
10. A. It is the most energetic of all the dances listed.

Dance Answer Key—Advanced level

True/False

1. F. You must promenade your corner home.
2. T
3. T. In each dance there is a partner change.
4. T
5. T
6. F
7. T. By leaning away, centrifugal force helps them turn.
8. F. Hot Lips uses the two-step.
9. T
10. T

Matching

1. H
2. F
3. J
4. C
5. I
6. E
7. A
8. G
9. D
10. B

Chapter

7

Golf

Unit Overview

1. Teach the history and value of playing golf:
   - Physical benefits from hitting the ball and walking the course
   - Using golf carts limits cardiovascular benefits

2. Teach the accessibility of golf:
   - Public and private courses
   - Driving ranges
   - Pitch and putt courses

3. Teach the economics of golf:
   - Cost of equipment
   - Cost of course fees

4. Teach golf basics:
   - Proper grip and swing
   - Proper stance and weight transfer
   - Proper pitch, chip, putt, and drive

5. Teach golf terminology: fore, green, fairway, lie, rough, teeing up, divots

6. Teach the rules of scoring.

7. Teach golf courtesies.

Golf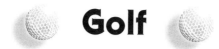

HISTORY

Golf began on the coast of Scotland in the 1400s. In 1888, America's father of golf, Scotsman John Reid, established the St. Andrews Golf Club in New York. In 1894, the Amateur Golf Association of the United States was formed. It later was renamed the United States Golf Association (USGA). In 1916, the Professional Golfers' Association (PGA) of America was founded. Finally, in 1950, the Ladies Professional Golf Association (LPGA) was established.

FUN FACTS

→ The PGA is the largest sports organization in the world.

→ There are about 40 million golfers worldwide.

→ Yale won the first collegiate golf championship.

→ In 1999, 13-year-old Aree Wongluekiet became the youngest winner in USGA history by capturing the Girls' Junior championship.

→ Walking 18 holes of golf is the equivalent of 4.5 miles.

BENEFITS OF PLAYING

1. If you walk while you play golf, you can get a good workout.
2. Golf is a great stress reducer.
3. Playing golf can help you with your flexibility, especially if you stretch before and after you play.
4. When you play golf with friends, you can socialize with them as you walk from one hole to another.
5. Golf is fun!

TIME TO SURF!

Web Site	Web Site Address
United States Golf Association	www.usga.com
Professional Golfers' Association	www.pga.com
Ladies Professional Golf Association	www.lpga.com

From *Complete Physical Education Plans for Grades 7–12* by Isobel Kleinman, 2001, Champaign, IL: Human Kinetics.

Golf Unit Extension Project

NAME _____ CLASS _____

Equipment needed to play golf

Item	Where you would purchase it (be specific)	Cost

Where you would play golf

Please explain where in the community you would play golf. Be specific.

How much does it cost to play?

How much does it cost to play golf, based on the course on which you'd most want to play? Select either 9 or 18 holes.

Health benefits of playing golf

Please explain the health benefits of playing golf. Include how much golf you would need to play each week to gain these benefits.

Reflection question

Do you think golf is an activity you would like to play as an adult? Why or why not?

From *Complete Physical Education Plans for Grades 7–12* by Isobel Kleinman, 2001, Champaign, IL: Human Kinetics.

Golf Teaching Tips

1. Every effort should be made for enjoyment, repetition, and lots of walking to get the balls.
2. Allow noncompetitive practice time with equipment.
3. Use as much golf technique as possible (swing, pivot, head down, knee bend) during warm-ups.
4. If students are having trouble staying focused, include a contest at the end of the lesson that emphasizes the point.
5. When students begin to learn the swing, have a little contest that asks, when addressing the ball, who could make 10 contacts in 10 swings, or how many swings it took to contact the ball 10 times.
6. When practicing putting, mark all first putt positions and count the number of putts it takes to drop the putt in the hole. The winner has the lowest score.
7. When practicing chips, set up a target. You can lay an archery target on the ground or use cones, or paint a circle and score a point when the chip lands within a designated area around the target—and with each student using the same number of balls, score their hits on the target. You will need to be creative!
8. Develop a short tournament.
9. Plan a field trip to a local driving range, a pitch and putt golf course, a par-3 golf course, or a regular golf course.
10. If students are not able to participate fully in class activities, remember that they can be involved by keeping score or conducting a research project.

Unit Safety

Safety is an issue that must be clearly addressed before anyone swings a golf club. The teacher must set up rules for

moving around a driving range,
where to stand and how to behave while people are hitting the ball, and
complying with the signals for ball retrieval.

The safety issues on a golf course should be included in part of the general instruction.

Unit Setup

Facility

This outdoor activity may have to be accommodated to smaller spaces and to coming indoors.

Defined areas must be set aside for
- full swings,
- putting, and
- chipping.

A putting green must be bought or created.

When outdoors, lay out a short golf course of at least four holes, with
- tee-off areas, and
- putting greens.

Find a local driving range and golf course that will work with the school. Explore public and private courses within a dedicated radius, get driving instructions, greens fees, and so forth.

Equipment

One club for pitching, putting, and driving for each student (9 iron, 5 iron, 2 iron, putter, 2 wood)

A minimum of six practice balls per student work station (yarn, paper, plastic)

Real golf balls for putting

Rubber doormats

Rubber and wood tees

Carpet for an indoor golf green

Hang cloth or golf cage

Cups for the golf holes

Targets for pitching, putting, and chipping to the green

Round-robin tournament schedules and charts (see appendix A)

Golf scorecards

Unit Timeline

There is one introductory unit of golf. It has
- 10 lessons for developing skill competency, scoring, terminology, and course courtesies; and
- 2 to 4 lessons for a class tournament.

Unit Assessment

A student portfolio checklist is provided here for student use (table 7.1). Encourage students to track their progress as they master new skills. A performance assessment rubric is also available to assess students' progress (page 226). A quiz at the end of the chapter tests their knowledge of the sport.

Additional Resources

In addition to these resources, the Internet is an excellent source of information for golf. In any search engine, type "golf" and go. National and regional golf associations are also helpful sources.

Hogan, Ben. 1989. *Ben Hogan's Five Lessons: The Modern Fundamentals of Golf.* New York: Simon & Schuster.

Jones, Bobby, Ben Crenshaw, Robert Yre Jones, and Martin Davis. 1997. *Classic Instruction.* New York: Broadway Books.

TABLE 7.1 Golf Student Portfolio Checklist

STUDENT NAME _____

- ☐ Is able to grip any golf club
- ☐ Can swing while transferring weight
- ☐ Can take proper stance to the ball
- ☐ Can consistently contact the ball
- ☐ Understands the differences among drives, pitches, putts, and chips
- ☐ Can use approach shots
- ☐ Can putt
- ☐ Can play a short game
- ☐ Is able to follow golf etiquette and common courtesy
- ☐ Has learned and follows the rules on the tees and the greens and for scoring
- ☐ Understands common golf terminology, value, and history
- ☐ Has identified local areas that provide a golf experience
- ☐ Assumes responsibility for equipment and appreciates care of equipment

From *Complete Physical Education Plans for Grades 7–12* by Isobel Kleinman, 2001, Champaign, IL: Human Kinetics

Golf Lesson 1 — Beginner level

Lesson Setup

Facility

Designated hitting stations in a clear area, set off from spectators, observers, and traffic

Equipment

Music
5 iron for each student
Six practice golf balls (plastic) for each student
Mat, if the unit is held inside

Performance Goals

Students will

grip a 5 iron properly,
learn the golf swing:
- Without the club
- With the club but without the ball
- With both the club and the ball
and get and return their own equipment.

Cognitive Goals

Students will learn

some history of golf,
the value of playing golf for fitness into old age,
to respect the reason for safety around golf clubs,
the value of a proper grip, and
why a natural pendulum swing is important.

Lesson Safety

The facilities must be set up to minimize accidents.
Practice areas should be separated by a minimum of 15 feet per station.
There should be a clearly defined waiting area.
Students must learn correct habits that will protect their safety.
Teachers must set up clear rules and procedures for retrieving balls.
Students must understand that they can only take full swings with their clubs
   in specified areas.

Warm-Up

Students will

1. Complete standard exercises (jumping jacks, sit-ups, push-ups, stretches) to music
2. Use the same rhythmical background to teach the progression of a golf swing from a windmill-like movement to a pivot and weight transfer

Motivation

Some people think golf isn't a physically challenging sport. If there is no running, how can one get fit? Well, there is a lot of walking when one plays on a full 18-hole golf course. Remind the class that players could be walking for upward of three hours. They can get good and tired playing a full round of golf when they walk and carry their own clubs. Tell a personal story of a golf outing that wore you out, or feel free to use my story.

The first time I was invited to play golf on an 18-hole course in Eisenhower Park, I grabbed my tennis racket and bathing suit, because I was sure that when I was done playing golf I would want to really move! We played the first nine holes and stopped for lunch. Thank goodness! I was really hungry. Then, we played the back nine. When I said good-bye, I went straight to my tennis club, put on my swim suit, swam a few laps, and sat down to dry off. The lounge where I sat is where I promptly took my first nap since I was 5 years old!

Golf became a very talked-about sport in 1997 because of one starting professional who not only broke the race barrier but scored incredible grand-slam victories his first year on the circuit: Tiger Woods.

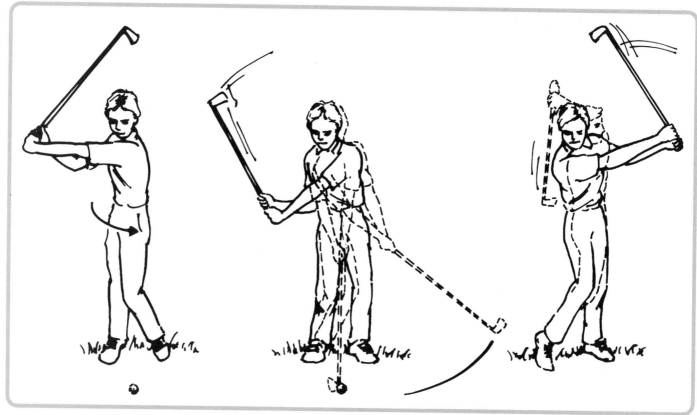

Figure 7.1—Full swing.

Lesson Sequence

1. Teach safety of being in an area with everyone swinging golf clubs.
2. Teach and check the proper grip.
3. Teach, demonstrate, and allow practice of a full swing without a ball:
   - The job of the left hand
   - The job of the right hand
   - Both hands together
4. Introduce the ball, and the golf stance relative to it, for the typical 5-iron shot (figure 7.1).
5. Have students use each of their balls before anyone is allowed to retrieve them and start again.

Review

Tell the class that the most important thing any golfer can learn is to have a smooth, rhythmical, consistent swing. Once that comes, the rest is easy.
Ask the class which hand is the power hand.
Review which hand controls the club head.

Ask students what number iron has been used.
Ask where they should stand in relation to the ball.

Golf Lesson 2 — Beginner level

Lesson Setup

Facility

Designated hitting stations in a clear area

Equipment

Music

Performance Goals

Students will

swing the golf club smoothly without the ball,
contact the ball with a 5 iron, and
direct the ball to a target.

Cognitive Goals

Students will learn

the parts of the golf club—head, shaft, and grip;
the distance a typical 5-iron shot travels;
how to address the ball; and
the proper stance.

Lesson Safety

Reemphasize safety rules and ball retrieval procedures before beginning practice. Do this each lesson until the behavior has become routine.

Warm-Up

Students will

1. Complete standard exercises (jumping jacks, sit-ups, push-ups, stretches) to a rhythmical background
2. Progress from a windmill to the pivot and weight transfer of a golf swing, still using the music as an accompaniment for practicing the swing without a club

Motivation

If golf players knew that when they addressed and swung at the ball it would go exactly the way it was supposed to, straight and at the estimated distance, they also would know that they would probably win the round. Something always interferes; usually it is the head. Tell your students that their job throughout the lesson is to get their swing nice and smooth. If they have a smooth, relaxed swing, they will hit the ball every time, straight every time, and at the same distance every time.

Lesson Sequence

1. Have students practice their swing:
   - With the left hand, emphasizing the relaxed drop of the pendulum—the club head
   - With both hands together
2. Remind the class about safety.
3. Teach and demonstrate the stance again.
4. Have students use each of their balls before anyone is allowed to retrieve them and start again.
5. Compliment players for the following:
   - A good, smooth swing
   - A good, solid contact
6. Set a target and compliment students for the following:
   - Reaching the target
   - Making repeated contacts with the target (how many out of their six shots hit?)
   - Trying it as a contest

Review

Remind the class that the most important thing any golfer can learn is to have a smooth, rhythmical, consistent swing and that once that comes, the rest is easy.

Ask students where they should stand in relation to the ball.

Ask if anyone noticed problems once they were aiming for a target.

Ask if anyone started looking at the target before they actually hit the ball.

Discuss what would happen if they took their eye off the ball before hitting it.

Golf Lesson 3   Beginner level

Lesson Setup

Facility

Designated hitting stations in a clear area for working with a 5 iron
A completely separate area for the putting greens

Equipment

Putters for each student
Three balls each for students working on putting
Practice green with holes

Performance Goals

Students will

putt at a variety of distances, and
continue working with the 5 iron.

Cognitive Goals

Students will learn

the different grip, stance, and swing for a putt; and
some golf terminology: green, lie.

Lesson Safety

Teach a new safety rule: No swinging in the area of the green.

Warm-Up

Students will

1. Complete standard exercises (jumping jacks, sit-ups, push-ups, stretches) to a rhythmical background
2. Practice mimetics of a golf swing using music as an accompaniment

Motivation

Most players love to practice their drives, hitting the ball as hard and as far as they can. What more than likely separates people in golf is how they play their short game. Ultimately, no matter how far a player can hit the ball, he still has to get it to drop in the hole. Once on the green, if students cannot play the surface and feel how much of a tap or swing they need, they will not be able to get the drop. Tell the class that this skill is called putting. Everything changes for most people—the club, even the way they hold the club, and most assuredly, the swing. Teach them how to do it.

Lesson Sequence

1. Introduce putting: the need for it, its difficulty, focus, nature of the green, what a lie is.
2. Teach grip and stance, and demonstrate (figure 7.2).
3. Have everyone in class aim at the same target, halfway to the same target, and a quarter of the way to the same target.

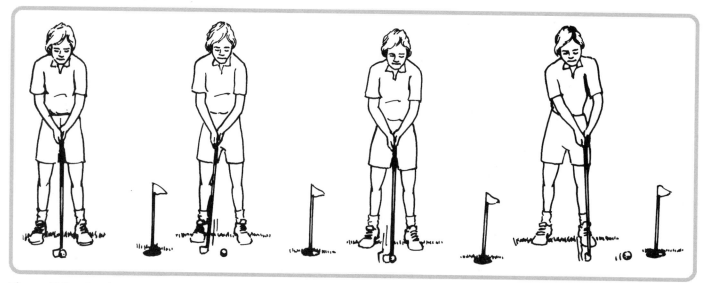

Figure 7.2—Putting.

4. Emphasize safety.
5. Divide the class into teaching stations:
   • One station for putting
   • A second station for rotation of practicing the 5 iron
6. Compliment students for repeated contacts with the target when using the 5 iron.
7. Talk to the students, before they leave, about a special area on the putting green with a 16-foot putt. Ask who can drop the putt in three strokes, two strokes, and one stroke.

Review

Ask the class what the difference is between the back swing in a drive and in a putt.

Ask students what they would do differently if they were 30 feet away than if they were 5 feet away.

Discuss what helpful hint would get them to line up properly for the putt.

Review what "watching the lie" means.

Ask what a golf green is.

Golf Lesson 4   Beginner level

Lesson Setup

Equipment

Music
A scorecard or sheet and golf pencil

Performance Goals

Students will

putt for a score, and
work with the 5 iron.

Cognitive Goals

Students will

learn putting terminology:
  • Eagle
  • Par
  • Birdie
learn golf scoring.

Lesson Safety

Reemphasize safety before practice: There is to be no swinging in the area of the green.

Warm-Up

Students will

1. Complete standard exercises (jumping jacks, sit-ups, push-ups, stretches)
2. Practice mimetics for the golf swing

Motivation

Tell students that in this lesson they will learn how to score, which is easy. Every time a player addresses and strokes at the ball, she gets a point. In golf, each stroke counts, and, unlike the rest of the games the students have played, the player who play her rounds with the least number of strokes—or what one would consider points—is the winner.

Lesson Sequence

1. Introduce scoring and golf-scoring terminology: par, birdie, eagle, bogey
2. Teach students the routine before starting a contest:
   • Lining themselves up
   • Practicing the swing or approach
   • After addressing the ball, counting the swing as a stroke
3. Teach the contest:
   • Where to stand for the first stroke
   • The order of targets or holes
   • When to consider the hole complete
   • How to record the score

4. Provide feedback to students for individual things that they might be doing wrong:
   - Not lining up properly
   - Forgetting their follow-through
5. Emphasize safety.
6. Compliment the following:
   - Good safety
   - A smooth swing
   - Remembering to write the score
   - Concentration

Review

Ask the class who was able to sink a putt in one stroke, and what that is called. Discuss how many putts are allowed for par once on the green.
Ask students how many of them had a hole where they were able to make par.

Golf Lesson 5 | Beginner level

Lesson Setup

Facility

Designate a third area for pitching, as shown in figure 7.3.

Equipment

Music
9 iron or pitching wedge

Performance Goals

Students will

pitch (figure 7.4),
take full swings using the 5 iron, and
putt.

Cognitive Goals

Students will

learn terminology—pitch, chip, and divot;
understand what is meant by an approach shot; and
learn the courtesy of replacing a divot.

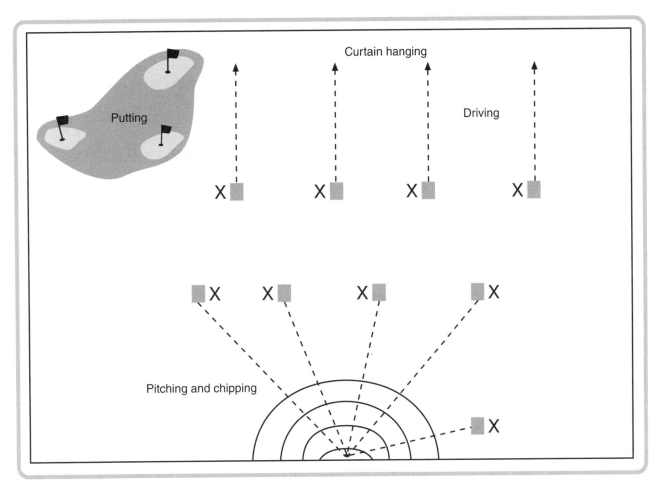

Figure 7.3—Three practice stations.

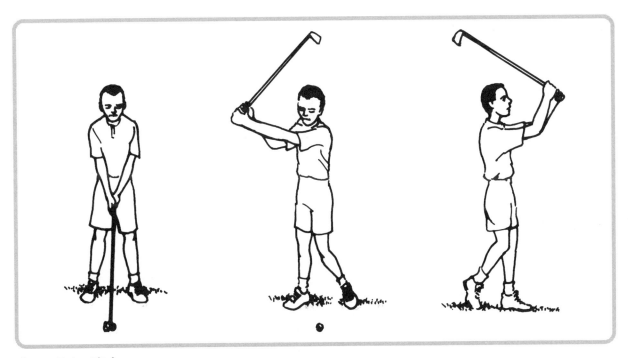

Figure 7.4—Pitch.

Lesson Safety

Announce that there now are three practice stations. Students at each should remain at their area until instructed to switch. Students must be careful to use their equipment only in designated stations.

Warm-Up

Students will

1. Complete standard exercises (jumping jacks, sit-ups, push-ups, stretches)
2. Practice mimetics for the golf swing

Motivation

Ask students if anyone ever goes to a pitch-and-putt course, which can be a lot of fun. These courses have holes that are between 50 and 85 yards to the green, not the 230-plus yards that are at major golf courses. Ask if students can imagine that the only shot they have sends the ball 120 yards away, like when they use their 5 iron, but they need to go 75 yards. That short shot is called an approach shot. It is the shot that is supposed to get them on the green.

Sometimes actually getting to the green can be frustrating. Tell students a personal story of your frustration with this, or feel free to use my story. The first time I ever played on a golf course, I got 30 yards from the green, took another stroke, and landed 40 yards past the green. In fact, it took four strokes to get my ball on the green so I could putt. It was frustrating. Tell the class you'll try to help them cut down on that kind of frustration if they learn to pitch the ball to the green.

Lesson Sequence

1. Introduce pitching to a target.
2. Demonstrate the use of the 9 iron for pitching.
3. Emphasize safety.
4. Divide the class time into three time units so students can practice pitching as well as all other previously learned skills.
5. Provide feedback.
6. Compliment good safety, a smooth swing, remembering to write the score, and concentration.

Review

Ask the class if anyone remembers what a divot is.
Ask if anyone took a divot while pitching.
Ask students if they saw divots that have not been replaced.
Review what one should do when taking a divot.
Discuss the difference between driving the ball and pitching the ball.
Ask if the backswing is different.
Ask if the foot one's weight is on is different.

Discuss which will go further when a player is pitching, a 5 iron or a wedge, and why.

Golf Lesson 6 — Beginner level

Lesson Setup

Facility

Three designated stations for driving, putting, and pitching.

Performance Goals

Students will

use a 2 iron,
try chipping, and
practice putting.

Cognitive Goals

Students will learn

that ball position varies when working with longer irons,
the difference between the chip and the pitch, and
how to decide where to place the ball for each iron.

Warm-Up

Students will

1. Complete standard exercises (jumping jacks, sit-ups, push-ups, stretches)
2. Perform mimetics for a pitching swing, a putt, and the full golf swing

Motivation

Sometimes, when golfers are not teeing off, they still must go for distance. Inform the class that the 2 iron is longer and the club head has angle; therefore, it is a good club to use when distance is still a factor. The feel will be different—show the class what is different.

Lesson Sequence

1. Introduce the 2 iron:
   - When it would be chosen for use
   - How to position the ball
2. Explain the difference between the last lesson on pitching and this lesson—the chip. Demonstrate.

3. Emphasize safety.
4. Divide the class time into three groups so students can practice driving, chipping (not pitching), and putting for an equal amount of time.
5. Provide feedback.

Review

Ask students when they would choose to use a 2 iron and not a wood.

Golf Lesson 7   Beginner level

Setup

Facility

A hitting station, putting station, and pitching station

Equipment

Scorecards and pencils

Performance Goals

Students will continue

to use a 2 iron,
to chip, and
to putt.

Cognitive Goals

Students will learn

courtesy on the golf fairway:
- *Honoring* who goes first
- Where to stand once leaving the tee, as foursomes take approach shots
- The meaning of *fore*
how to score a lost ball.

Warm-Up

Students will

1. Complete standard exercises
2. Practice mimetics for all swings

Motivation

In this lesson, tell your students you would like to see all of them contacting the ball with confidence and a smooth swing. Tell them of a time you didn't contact the ball well and wound up in an embarrassing situation. Or, feel free to use my story. During one particular golf outing, I was so nervous to make a good impression and so scared I would top my shot and have it wind up in the water below our tee-off area, that I sliced the ball and it wound up in the woods. I had never lost a ball before. Not only did I not have a second ball, but I had no idea how to score that shot.

Embarrassing plays do happen, and players may get nervous. It happens to everyone. Tell students they should be prepared for the event of losing a ball: not only should they have another ball, but they should acknowledge how, if they are playing a properly scored game, to score when they've lost the ball and where to take their next shot from.

Lesson Sequence

1. Teach fairway courtesies and how to deal with the lost ball.
2. Divide the class time into three groups so students have equal time to practice driving, putting, and chipping.
3. Emphasize safety.
4. Provide feedback to students.

Review

Ask students what they should do when they hear someone call out, "Fore!"
Ask why they should carry more than one ball.
Review which person takes his second shot first when leaving the tee.

Golf Lesson 8 — Beginner level

Lesson Setup

Equipment

Woods and tees

Performance Goals

Students will

use a driving tee and a designated driver, and
continue chipping and putting.

Cognitive Goals

Students will learn

the ball position for a wood,
how and where to set up a tee, and
the differences between using a wood and an iron.

Warm-Up

Students will complete standard exercises and golf swings

Motivation

Tell the class that woods are lighter and feel easier to swing, but some people have trouble with them because woods are longer than irons. Players have problems because they lose control coming through the ball with the longer shaft. The longer shaft makes the club head farther from the ball.

Lesson Sequence

1. Teach the use of woods and tees.
2. Divide the class time into three time units so students can practice driving as well as all other previously learned skills.
3. Emphasize safety.
4. Provide feedback.

Review

Review with the class when golfers are allowed to raise the ball off the ground.
Ask students what the ball rests on when raised.
Discuss what makes using woods different.

Golf Lesson 9   Beginner level

Performance Goals

Students will

continue using the woods and tees,
practice putting, and
vary pitching with chipping.

Cognitive Goals

Students will

learn about local driving ranges, and
learn the differences between hitting a practice ball and a golf ball.

Warm-Up

Students will complete standard exercises and golf swing

Motivation

Tell students it wouldn't be practical for you to teach them something they never could use on their own. Ask if any of them ever go to driving ranges. Discuss their locations, what players bring there, and how much a bucket costs.

Lesson Sequence

1. Talk about local areas at which to practice.
2. Divide the class time into three time units so students can practice driving as well as all other previously learned skills.
3. Provide feedback to the class and emphasize safety.

Review

Review what students can learn about their drives at a driving range that they could not learn at school.

Ask what they expect the difference to be between the flight of a real golf ball and one that is plastic and full of holes.

Tell students that in the next two weeks, you would like them to go to a driving range on their own. While there, they will get a bucket of real balls and be able to get an idea of how far their swing carries a real ball as opposed to the plastic practice balls.

Tell students that for the next lesson, they will meet at a golf course (if you decide to take them to one) dressed in street clothes. Otherwise, tell them they will be playing on a golf course you set up on school grounds.

Golf Lesson 10 — Beginner level

Lesson Setup

Facility

A short course of four holes should be set up before the students arrive. Each hole should vary in distance from the tee-off area to the putting green.

Equipment

A 9 iron, putter, and practice ball for each student
Four scorecards and four pencils

Performance Goal

Students will compete, using golf skills for the entire lesson.

Cognitive Goal

Students will learn to play in a competitive golf situation.

Warm-Up

Students will

1. Complete standard exercises that allow students to remain standing
2. Practice mimetics of each golf swing

Motivation

Announce that there are four holes for the class to play. Instruct students to tee off in a foursome, as they do at golf courses, score, and play the ball out before proceeding to the next hole. The scorecard will tell them the approximate distances to the green. Tell them to enjoy themselves.

Lesson Sequence

1. Provide students with a scorecard when they arrive. Encourage the foursomes to begin immediately.
2. Have each group begin at a different hole so there is no waiting.

Review

Mention that in this lesson, students had to use golf courtesies and scoring. Ask if anything came up that left them puzzled.

Ask how many students found themselves waiting before they could tee off.

Ask if anyone heard, "Fore!"

Discuss whether they remembered to replace their divots.

Ask who in their group had the "honor" most.

Tell the students that you hope they will be able to use all their skills and courtesies on a public course before the unit is over. If they can go on their own, that would be great.

Ask them to go to a driving range within the next two weeks, so they can get some experience with a real ball.

Tell students that for the next lesson, they will meet at a local driving range, a local golf course, or a course set up on school grounds. They will wear street clothes.

Assessment

Grade student skills based on performance standards, such as those listed in the performance assessment rubric on page 226. For further general assessment rubrics, see appendix B.

Golf Lessons 11-12   Beginner level

Lesson Setup

Facility

Short four-hole course

Equipment

9 iron, putter, and practice ball for each student
Four scorecards and four pencils

Performance Goal

Students will play a course.

Cognitive Goal

Students will learn to use their golf knowledge in a golf course-playing situation.

Warm-Up

Students will

1. Complete standard exercises that allow students to remain standing
2. Practice mimetics for all golf swings

Motivation

As students continue to play some golf rounds, it might be fun to see if they could par (two putt, approach shot if short hole). Tell the class that anyone who can par a hole will get an "A" for the day. Ask them what they think is the greatest difficulty in getting par—putting or approaching the hole? Suggest they don't answer now—that question will be answered at the end.

Lesson Sequence

1. Provide foursomes with a scorecard when they arrive. Encourage them to begin immediately.
2. Assign groups to start at different holes so there is no waiting to tee off.

Review

Ask students to tell you what courtesies they had to use in this class.
Discuss any questions on scoring.

Ask if anyone achieved par on one hole—or two, three, or all four.

Tell students you hope they will be able to use their newly acquired skills on a public course before the unit is over.

Assessment

Have students take a written quiz (see page 227). Grade students' skills based on the performance standards listed in the performance assessment rubric in table 7.2.

TABLE 7.2 Beginner Golf Performance Assessment Rubric

STUDENT NAME _____

	0	1	2	3	4	5
Chip	No effort	• Uses proper grip • Has correct stance • Ball is in proper position	• Uses correct swing • Contacts ball • Selects high number iron	• Uses proper body pivot • Consistently contacts ball in the square • Occasionally reaches target	• Reaches a variety of targets up to 30 yards • Takes and replaces divot	• Has a smooth swing • Has good body rotation on longer chips • Able to control depth of shot
Drive	No effort	• Has correct stance • Positions ball correctly	• Keeps head down on practice swings • Has good back swing • Has good follow through swing • Has proper hip rotation without ball	• Frequently meets ball • Has a smooth full swing • Keeps head down with ball in place	• Has many straight shots • Able to project ball 75+ yards • Contacts ball using a wood	• Drives ball 100+ yards • Rarely tops ball • Shots go down fairway straight
Putt	No effort	• Uses proper stance and grip • Keeps head down • Reaches for putter	• Aligns self correctly • Follows through to cup	• Inconsistent success on a flat surface • Follows proper etiquette on green	• Is developing touch • Reads dips and dives and compensates • Able to two putt all 5-yard shots	• Has frequent success in one putt at 5 yards • Is accurate approach on flat surfaces

Golf Quiz—Beginner level

NAME _____ TEACHER _____

DATE _____ CLASS PERIOD _____

True or False: Read each statement below carefully. If the statement is true, put a check under the True box in the column to the left of the statement. If the statement is false, put a check under the False box in the column to the left of the statement. If using a grid sheet, blacken in the appropriate column for each question, making sure to use the correctly numbered line for each question and its answer.

True   **False**

☐ ☐ 1. During the swing, control comes from the upper hand of the golf grip.

☐ ☐ 2. Taking your eye off the ball changes your swing.

☐ ☐ 3. Player A scored 87 and player B scored 85. Player B won the round.

☐ ☐ 4. The backswing would make the most difference in a 30-yard shot and a 55-yard shot, because you would use the same club for each.

☐ ☐ 5. The "lie" is the way the green slopes.

☐ ☐ 6. Long and short courses allow two putts for par.

☐ ☐ 7. If you hear someone shout, "Fore!" cover your head and duck because a ball is heading your way.

☐ ☐ 8. Taking a divot adds a penalty stroke to your score.

☐ ☐ 9. When good golfers need to gain more distance, they should swing harder on the downstroke.

☐ ☐ 10. Typically, a golfer tees off with a 9 iron.

From *Complete Physical Education Plans for Grades 7–12* by Isobel Kleinman, 2001, Champaign, IL: Human Kinetics.

Golf Answer Key—Beginner level

1. F. The upper arm is the power arm; control comes from the lower hand on the grip.
2. T. Looking up causes the shoulders to lift, thereby changing your swing.
3. T. The lowest score wins.
4. T. At these close and specific distances, only a 9 iron or a wedge would be used.
5. T.
6. T. Getting to the green in the acceptable number of strokes and two-putting will give a golfer par.
7. T. If a ball is hit on the wrong green, the golfer who hit it is supposed to alert everyone that they might get hit with a ball they were not expecting to come their way.
8. F. A divot is the expected result of a good shot. Courtesy has you find it and place it back where it came from.
9. F. Altering one's swing is the single most destructive thing a golfer can do.
10. F. Typically, woods—the 1, 2, and 3—are used to tee off.

Handball

Unit Overview

1. Combine some game aspect with each lesson.

2. Introduce one skill at a time: the serve, right-hand swing, left-hand swing, clearing shot, rollout (killer)

3. Teach strategies as students get more involved in the game:

   • Positioning—taking the center of the court
   • Hitting—to the open court, to the weaker side
   • Passing shots—down the line, over the head

4. Teach the rules of the game as the skill being taught is presented:

   • The serve—long, short, turn of service, order of service
   • Scoring rules when getting students into games
   • Interference and blocking when teaching students to take the center

5. Allow noncompetitive practice time daily so students can improve their skills without performance pressure.

6. Conclude lessons with a contest that emphasizes the point of the lesson.

7. Develop a short tournament.

229

Handball

HISTORY

The origins of handball can be traced back to ancient times, when handball was played in Egypt, Greece, Rome, and China. Ancient ball courts have also been found in the southwest United States, Mexico, and South America. The first national USHA tournament was held in 1959 and has been played annually except for two years.

FUN FACTS

→ In the 1930s, New York city built hundreds of handball courts throughout the city. Today, they have more than 2,000 courts.
→ The first women's tournaments were played on beaches.
→ Original handballs were made of tightly rolled pieces of cloth sewn together.

BENEFITS OF PLAYING

1. Handball provides you with a great workout.
2. Handball is super for hand-eye coordination.
3. Handball is a fast-paced game that keeps you on your toes.
4. Playing handball helps you with your agility and your reaction time.
5. Handball is fun to play with friends.

TIME TO SURF!

Web Site	Web Site Address
United States Handball	www.ushandball.org
Handball	www.streetplay.com
ICHA	www.icha.org
Manitoba Handball Association	www.escape.ca/~handball/

From *Complete Physical Education Plans for Grades 7–12* by Isobel Kleinman, 2001, Champaign, IL: Human Kinetics.

Handball Unit Extension Project

NAME _____   CLASS _____

Equipment needed to play handball

Item	Where you would purchase it (be specific)	Cost

Where you would play handball

Please explain where in the community you would play handball. Be specific.

Health benefits of playing handball

Please explain the health benefits of playing handball. Include how much handball you would need to play each week to gain these benefits.

Reflection question

Do you think handball is an activity you would like to play as an adult? Why or why not?

From *Complete Physical Education Plans for Grades 7–12* by Isobel Kleinman, 2001, Champaign, IL: Human Kinetics.

Making a Case for Handball

Since the advent of team handball, there has been some confusion about handball. This unit introduces handball the dual sport, popularly played in many urban areas. Handball is included here because it is a lifetime sport with many advantages. You can feel good about teaching handball as one of your lifetime sports because it is the safest of the wall games, has movement patterns similar to the racket sports, can be modified to almost any flat wall, costs almost nothing to run, is extremely rigorous, and can be relatively easy to play at the beginner level.

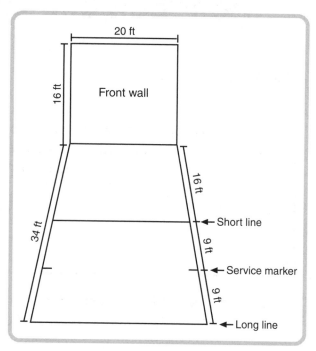

Figure 8.1—Handball court dimensions.

Unit Safety

Handball is played in close quarters, which makes safety an issue. The fact that opponents have to learn to run around each other safely, and that one's court is either adjacent to other courts or closed in by walls or fences, makes collisions probable. Collisions should be minimized. Once learning to play safely during one-wall handball, players have made headway toward being able to play safely in other wall games such as racquetball, squash, and four-wall handball. Clearly, problems decrease when players use only their hands and not a racket.

Unit Setup

Facility

This one-wall game can be accommodated indoors as well as out. Courts should be marked with sidelines, short lines, and long lines.

Equipment

One light ball for each student
Round-robin tournament schedules and charts (see appendix A)

Unit Timeline

Four lessons to develop skill enough to enjoy a game
Six to eight lessons for a class tournament

Unit Assessment

A student portfolio checklist is provided here for student use (table 8.1). Encourage students to track their progress as they master new skills. A performance assessment rubric and a quiz are also available for assessing your students.

Additional Resource

Lowy, Lance. 1991. *Handball Handbook: Strategies and Techniques.* American Press.

TABLE 8.1   Handball Student Portfolio Checklist

STUDENT NAME _____

- ☐ Is able to serve
- ☐ Has knowledge and can follow the rules of safety
- ☐ Can follow the game rules for singles or doubles
- ☐ Can score
- ☐ Has learned the rollout or kill shot
- ☐ Has learned the clear
- ☐ Is developing some sense of strategy for handball
- ☐ Can play a short game

From *Complete Physical Education Plans for Grades 7–12* by Isobel Kleinman, 2001, Champaign, IL: Human Kinetics

Handball Lesson 1   Beginner level

Lesson Setup

Facility

A wall with no obstructions

Performance Goals

Students will

swing and hit the ball with their right hand, and
learn to serve.

Cognitive Goals

Students will learn

service rules,
that the swing begins from the shoulder, and
that stepping into the ball and transferring their weight forward improves power.

Lesson Safety

Practice wall areas should be separated by a minimum of 10 feet per group with a ball.

Warm-Up

Students will

1. Jog around the playing area
2. Swing arm from back to front, adding jumps and side steps
3. Learn and repeat (several times) the pivot, taking a step forward as the body turns right
4. Combine pivot to right with arm swing on the right

Motivation

Mention to the class that handball is one of the best games for recreational play. All players need to find is a wall, an opponent, and a simple ball—and they can set up a game anywhere. Tell students that if they have seen kids at school hitting a ball against the school wall, they are playing some form of handball. You will be teaching them the competitive type that uses many of the same rules as paddleball and racquetball.

Lesson Sequence

1. Teach and demonstrate the serve: allow enough practice until the entire group can swing at the ball and hit the wall.
2. Teach service rules: send students back for more practice so that serves are legal.
3. Teach and demonstrate using the right hand to return the ball to the wall after it rebounds from the wall: allow five minutes more of practice.
4. Call the class together to encourage the following:
   - Consecutive hits so students start moving to the ball
   - Reacting to low and high balls
   - Throwing the ball up to themselves and hitting it
   - Throwing it high at the wall and hitting it
5. If the class seems to be losing interest, create some kind of skills contest, asking, for example, the following:

- Who can hit the ball five times in a row on one bounce or less?
- Who can hit it back to the wall so it goes high three times? How about five times?

Review

Ask the class to point to the short line.

Review the importance that the short line and the long line have for the server.

Discuss what happens if the serve does not land on the ground between the two lines.

Handball Lesson 2 — Beginner level

Performance Goals

Students will

be able to swing and hit the ball with the nondominant hand, and respond to an opponent's shot.

Cognitive Goals

Students will learn

rules that apply to the receiving team, and
safety rules applying to blocking and interference.

Lesson Safety

Game areas should be separated.

Court sidelines should be clearly marked so that one game does not overlap another at the same wall.

The playing rules that emphasize safety must be taught, understood, and practiced during every game.

Warm-Up

Students will

1. Complete sit-ups and a short jog
2. Swing arm from back to front, adding jumps and side steps, using the left hand
3. Repeat the pivot, stepping forward as the body turns left
4. Combine the pivot with the left-arm swing

Motivation

Tell students that, in this lesson, they will spend a little time recognizing that everyone favors one arm and not the other. But, since they need to be able to defend themselves in the game by athletically reacting to balls on either side, they need to learn to use their other hand so when they cannot reach the ball by running to hit it on their favorite side, they still can keep it in play. Their nondominant arm may feel spastic at first. But after some practice, it won't feel nearly as bad. Announce to the class that after students practice, if there is time before the period ends, they will use the game rules learned to date and try a little game.

Lesson Sequence

1. Allow practice of the hit on the left side, following the procedure in lesson 1 for the right hand.
2. Emphasize safety:
   * The need for concern
   * The rules that try to eliminate the danger of collisions—blocking and interference
3. Teach the remaining game-playing rules:
   * Receiving the serve
   * Alternating teams on the return after one bounce
4. If there is time, allow a short, five-point game.

Review

Ask the class why there is a blocking rule.
Ask what interference is and when it is called.
Review what should be done after interference is called.
Ask if players got in their opponents' way.
Ask the class, if one is returning serve and allows the ball to bounce twice, who serves the next point.
Discuss who serves the next point if the serve goes out of bounds.

Assessment

Observe to see if students are physically ready to go on to the game. If they are not, delay the game and its rules and stick to practicing skills. If they seem disinterested in practicing, make their practice into a contest. If they are ready, move on to the game, observing each court's ability to play safely. React accordingly.

Handball Lesson 3 — Beginner level

Performance Goals

Students will

hit "killers"; and
play a short, modified game in which the hitters alternate.

Cognitive Goals

Students will learn

the strategy of a kill shot and when to use it appropriately, and
the difference between a kill and a pinch.

Lesson Safety

Review blocking and interference rules and who is responsible for stopping play
when situations arise.

Warm-Up

Students will

1. Complete sit-ups and push-ups
2. Perform stretches
3. Perform semi-knee bends with a swing on either side
4. Pivot while bending down and stepping forward as turning right

Motivation

Ask students if they want to know how to end the point before their opponent
has the chance to end it for
them. The most winning
shot in handball is the "kill."
Tell them you will teach
them when they can try it
without causing their own
error and how to get the
ball to roll out.

Lesson Sequence

1. Demonstrate the point
   of contact and the flat
   arm swing necessary
   to get a killer.
2. Teach the rules that
   treat a pinched shot
   and a kill differently,
   and explain.
3. Review court posi-
   tioning:
   • Taking the middle
     (figure 8.2)
   • Interference
   • Block
4. Allow five-point games.

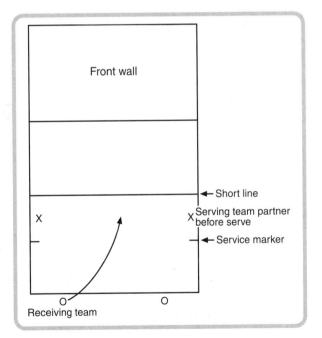

Figure 8.2—Taking the middle.

Review

Ask students at what point after the ball bounces they want to hit the kill.
Ask if anyone can explain why a player wants to "take the middle."
Review whether it is wise to go for a kill shot from deep in the court.
Discuss how far from the wall one should be when going for it.
Ask whether a swing that has a player's hand swinging from high to low gives her the effect she wants.

Handball Lesson 4   Beginner level

Performance Goals

Students will

hit a high shot, and
play a game.

Cognitive Goals

Students will

learn the strategy of getting the ball cleared, and
increase their knowledge about cause and effect when it comes to the direction of a ball and the path of their swing.

Lesson Safety

Continue to put emphasis on court enforcement of blocking and interference rules.

Warm-Up

Students will

1. Complete sit-ups and push-ups
2. Perform semi-knee bends

Motivation

Tell the class that everyone on the court has clustered near the wall, each trying to out-"kill" the other. Discuss what one could do to get them away from the wall: hit a clear, a high ball that cannot be played from the wall. Have students learn how.

Lesson Sequence

1. Demonstrate the point of contact and the arching arm swing necessary to get a clear.

2. Explain the following:
   • High shots are a solution to moving opponents out of the middle.
   • A follow-through must go up (figure 8.3).
3. Have students practice long enough for them to be successful five times.
4. Before sending students to play their games, remind them about back boundary lines.
5. Allow 11-point games and switch opponents if there is time.

Review

Ask the class what the purpose of a clear is.
Discuss whether it is best to use it when everyone is back or when they are all near the wall.

Teacher Homework

Prepare the draw for several small-group round-robin tournaments, basing each of the small tournaments on the level of skill displayed to date, placing only the teams that would be competitive together. See a sample round-robin tournament schedule in appendix A.

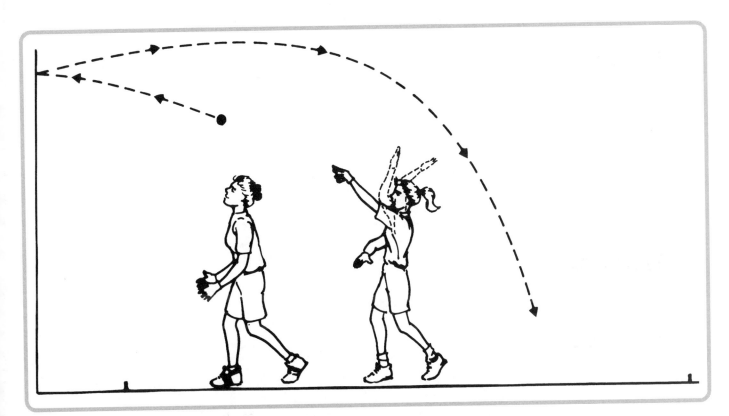

Figure 8.3—Using a high shot to clear the middle.

Handball Lesson 5 — Beginner level

Lesson Setup

Facility

Game areas with boundary lines, one area for every four students

Equipment

A round-robin tournament chart (see appendix A)

Performance Goals

Students will

improve their skills in a game situation, and
play doubles.

Please note that doubles play is more complex but less rigorous. It is a compromise when classes are too large to accommodate everyone in singles. If your facilities are adequate and you can run singles, save this doubles lesson to the end of the unit as a special culminating event (figure 8.4, a-b).

Cognitive Goals

Students will learn

the service rules for doubles,
the length of a game (time or score), and
how to proceed in the class tournament:
- How to find out who and where they play and get there daily
- What to do if one's opponent is absent
- What to do if one's partner is absent
- How to report scores

Warm-Up

Students will jog and stretch

Motivation

Tell students that you have divided the class up into several round-robin tournaments. Each tournament will have its own winner. Let them know that a round robin means that they will get to play each person in their tournament once. If they'd like, at the end of the tournament, they can have play-offs in which they can meet and play the other draw's team that placed the same bracket as their team did. Announce that the day's games are posted. They will learn how to read the schedules so they can get into their games as fast as possible in the future.

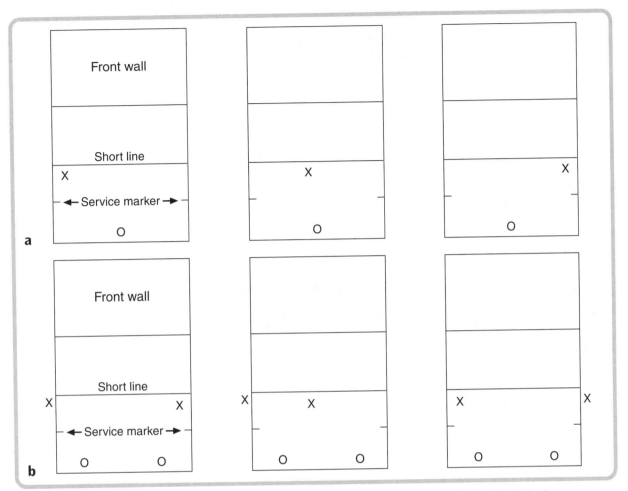

Figure 8.4—Server and receiver options for the serve: *(a)* during a singles game and *(b)* during a doubles game.

Lesson Sequence

1. Explain doubles:
   - The serving rotation
   - Court positioning for the nonserver on the serving team (see figure 8.4 a-b)
2. Post an enlarged round-robin tournament chart and explain it.
3. Post and explain how to read the game schedule and how to report scores.
4. Go over the reasons for daily attendance and preparation:
   - Explain what to do if one's partner is absent:
     The attending partner has to play the two opponents alone, or
     The attending partner can request a substitute and play the game two against two, but he forfeits his chance of winning the match in the tournament.
   - Explain what to do if one's opponent is absent—game goes on, either officially with opponent playing alone, or as a tournament forfeit. The single student can act as a substitute partner.

5. Have students vote on whether they want to start the tournament in this class and have the games count.
6. Explain what to do when the game is over and how to report scores.

Review

Ask the class if there are any questions.
Find out if anyone still has scores to report.

Teacher Homework

Post the round-robin standings and update them daily.

Handball Lessons 6-12   Beginner level

Lesson Setup

Equipment

A posted tournament schedule
Updated round-robin standings

Performance Goal

Students will play doubles.

Cognitive Goals

Students will compete with emphasis on

maintaining good sporting behavior;
playing by the rules; and
not hurting—physically or psychologically—their opponents.

Students will assume responsibility for

getting to the assigned court for a game,
returning equipment, and
reporting their scores.

Warm-Up

Students will jog and stretch

Motivation

Announce the standings after so many rounds of the tournament—first place, second place, and so on. Tell the class that if a certain player wins, that person will get out of a particular place, and explain how the standings will change.

Lesson Sequence

1. Post the game and court schedules.
2. Post team records.
3. Discuss court advantage and other possible strategies.

Review

Review common problems. Ask if there are any questions.

Assessment

Grades will be based on standards outlined in the performance assessment rubric (table 8.2). For further general assessment rubrics see appendix B. There also will be a short quiz at the conclusion of the unit.

TABLE 8.2 Beginner Handball Performance Assessment Rubric

STUDENT NAME _____

	0	1	2	3	4	5
Hands	No effort	• Hits ball to wall off self bounce with either hand	• Meets slow-moving object and redirect it to wall after it bounces with strong hand	• Meets slow ball after the bounce with weak hand • Reacts well to all balls on strong hand side	• Meets ball on the run on strong side • Handles volley • Returns low fast balls on strong side	• Hits return with purpose • Chooses correctly between volley and swing • Able to control depth or vary speed
Serve	No effort	• Clears the short line occasionally • Serves from the correct position on the court	• Serves underhand • Sometimes puts the ball in play • Tries to avoid shorts and longs	• Consistently puts the ball in play • Does not drive the ball back into self	• Serves can be driven • Does not drive serve into partner • Controls left or right serves	• Varies speed, depth, and direction of serve • Gets into a good position immediately after the serve
Play	No effort	• Tries to return the ball hit nearby	• Covers all plays to the forehand side • Remembers to keep score	• Covers plays within the one-step backhand side • Covers half court to the forehand side	• Feet react to shots on all sides • Avoids a hinder or block • Moves to the center	• Gets opponents out of the center • Uses strategic placement • Developing a killer

Handball Quiz—Beginner level

NAME _____ TEACHER _____

DATE _____ CLASS PERIOD _____

Multiple Choice: Read each question and each answer carefully. Be sure to choose the best answer that fits the statement preceding it. When you have made your choice, put the appropriate letter on the line to the left of the numbered question.

_____1. Opposing players must return the ball when
    a. the server serves the ball so that it bounces outside the sideline
    b. the server serves the ball so that it passes the short line
    c. the server serves the ball so that it hits herself
    d. all of the above

_____2. A *kill shot* is
    a. a shot that hits the opponent
    b. a shot that hits the lowest part of the wall and rolls back
    c. an ace serve
    d. all of the above

_____3. The reason players try to get to the center of the court is that
    a. it enables them to block all other players from getting to the ball
    b. they have the best chance of getting more open space in which to play
    c. they can more easily reach the shots their opponents hit
    d. all of the above

_____4. When the ball is served behind the long line, the following should occur:
    a. The opponents should take over the serve.
    b. The server should begin taking his second serve.
    c. The server gets a point.
    d. The ball is in play and no one gets a point until the point is played out.

_____5. A ball is sent out of bounds by the serving team. The game stops. The opponent
    a. gets a point
    b. takes over the serve
    c. gives the ball back to the server for another try
    d. takes over the serve and gets a point

_____6. The ball is served. The opponents allow the ball to bounce twice before they try to return it. They hit a killer. The score was 8 for the serving team to 7 for the receiving team before this point was played. The score should now be
    a. 8 to 8
    b. 9 to 7
    c. 8 to 6
    d. 9 to 6

_____7. The ball is served so that the server is blocking her opponent's ability to get to it. The correct thing for the server to do is to
    a. claim the point, declaring that the shot was too good for the opponent to get
    b. replay the point without anyone getting a point
    c. end the game because it is not right to be told to get out of the way
    d. all of the above

_____8. To hit a *kill shot*, you should
    a. hit the ball just before it bounces the second time
    b. hit the ball when it is at the height of the bounce
    c. wait for a time when you are near the wall
    d. do both A and C

_____9. The following is true of handball:
    a. It is an expensive game to play since so much equipment is necessary.
    b. You need many people to organize in order to play a game.
    c. You can set up a game on just about any wall you can find.
    d. All of the above.

_____10. Sometimes the best strategy is to
    a. aim for a killer on every shot
    b. stay near the long line
    c. hit the ball to the left side of the court when your opponent is a righty
    d. wait for the ball to bounce twice

From *Complete Physical Education Plans for Grades 7–12* by Isobel Kleinman, 2001, Champaign, IL: Human Kinetics.

Handball Answer Key—Beginner level

1. B. All other examples are illegal.
2. B. The only reason it is called a killer is that no one can get it after it bounces.
3. C. The center of the court is equidistant from every possible shot the opponent can hit.
4. B. The server is allowed one long or one short serve. If he has one, he gets a second chance.
5. B. Sending a ball out of bounds ends the point. Since the server sent it out, she loses her turn of service. No one gets any points on this play.
6. B. The score is 9 to 7; the serving team wins a point in this situation because the receivers let it bounce twice.
7. B. Blocking is not a legal strategy. The point must be replayed.
8. D. Aiming for a winning shot should be done when you will make the least amount of errors. If you accidentally hit a pinch, your opponents will win the point. Wait for the right moment.
9. C. The other statements are the opposite of what they should be: it is the least expensive, and a game requires the fewest opponents.
10. C. All the other statements will make success either difficult or impossible.

Pickleball

Unit Overview

1. Introduce the use of the paddle and its grip and encourage success by teaching beginning skills at a wall, then at close distances with a partner, and then over the net.

2. Teach the forehand, backhand, serve, and volley.

3. Explain that pickleball is called "slowed-down tennis" because some of its rules duplicate tennis and others don't. Teach the rules of pickleball:

   • A player cannot allow the ball to bounce twice before returning it.

   • A player must follow the service rules:

     The serve must go over the net into the diagonal box.

     The serve must pass the short line before bouncing.

     The server must change sides of the court, serving each point to alternate boxes.

     Each team player serves before the opponents take over the serve, except for the first service of the game.

   The first server of a team is always the person standing in the right-hand box.

   • Players must follow the receiving rules:

     The receiver must return all serves directed to her box if they are good serves.

     The receiver must allow the ball to bounce before returning it.

4. Teach the two-bounce rule (unlike any rule in tennis): The ball must bounce on each side of the court before any player can run to the net to volley.

5. Teach the short-line rule: No player can hit a ball on a fly if he is closer to the net than the short line (again, unlike any rule in tennis).

6. Introduce double positioning and have students play doubles games.

247

Pickleball

HISTORY

In 1965, in the state of Washington, U.S. Congressman Joel Pritchard invented a family game—pickleball. The name *pickleball* came from the family dog, Pickle, who used to chase the balls all over the yard. What was once a backyard game played by few is now a game played in thousands of schools, recreation centers, and homes. Pickleball is played in the United States as well as Canada, Japan, Singapore, and Western Europe.

FUN FACTS

→ There are more than 100,000 pickleball enthusiasts worldwide.

→ The United States Pickleball Association (USAPA) was founded in 1984.

→ In 1999, the USAPA released its Official Pickleball Tournament Rulebook.

→ In 1999, the State Games of Oregon included pickleball as a sport.

BENEFITS OF PLAYING

1. Pickleball is great for hand-eye coordination.
2. Pickleball helps you to build self-esteem.
3. It can be played when you are 5 or 85.
4. It can be played indoors or outdoors.
5. It is a ton of fun!

TIME TO SURF!

Web Site	Web Site Address
United States Pickleball Association	http://www.usapa.org/
Singapore Sports Council	http://www.ssc.gov.sg/ltppbs2.htm
Pickleball Study Guide	http://www.jisedu.org/ms/pe/ studyguide/pickleball.html

From *Complete Physical Education Plans for Grades 7–12* by Isobel Kleinman, 2001, Champaign, IL: Human Kinetics.

Pickleball Unit Extension Project

NAME _____ CLASS _____

Equipment needed to play pickleball

Item	Where you would purchase it (be specific)	Cost

Where you would play pickleball

Please explain where in the community you would play pickleball. Be specific.

Health benefits of playing pickleball

Please explain the health benefits of playing pickleball. Include how much pickleball you would need to play each week to gain these benefits.

Reflection question

Do you think pickleball is an activity you would like to play as an adult? Obviously there are very few organized adult pickleball leagues available, but it can be played with just one other person and a small investment in equipment.

From *Complete Physical Education Plans for Grades 7–12* by Isobel Kleinman, 2001, Champaign, IL: Human Kinetics.

Pickleball Teaching Tips

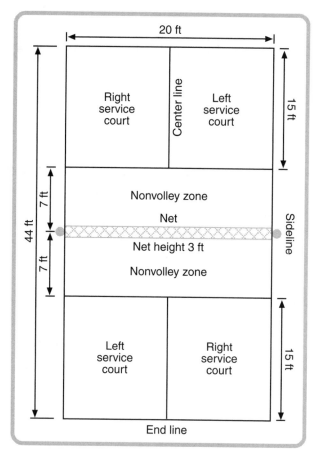

Figure 9.1—Pickleball court dimensions.

1. To maintain interest and foster more activity, create a balanced, round-robin doubles tournament. If classes are small enough to allow 100 percent participation, plan for singles instead or a combination of both.

2. The fun of involvement is a priority. Every student can enjoy this game because it is easy to pick up. It is important that they get as much court time as possible.

3. Though all students can be successful in this game, dramatic skills-level differences should be taken into account. As a result of some students' power, speed, reflexes, and general game sense, competition can become boring for the athlete and frustrating for players unless they can enjoy this game on their own level. Develop multiple tournaments to try and keep the competitions equal. Allow for multiple winners.

4. Because this game is indoors, space might be limited, preventing 100 percent of the students from playing 100 percent of the time. This is particularly true when practice drills are over. Since every student deserves equal court and game time, try a rotation, such as the following:

    Assign players A, B, and C to court 1.
    Divide the class time into three playing periods.
    In playing period 1, player A plays player B, and player C officiates.
    In playing period 2, player B plays player C, and player A officiates.
    In playing period 3, player C plays player A, and player B officiates.

5. In the event of absentees, the player whose partner is absent can
    • play the whole court by himself, or
    • officially lose the game (forfeit) but play anyway by asking one of the substitute officials to play in his partner's place.

6. If students are unable to participate fully in class activities, remember that they can be involved by coaching, officiating, keeping score, or conducting a research project.

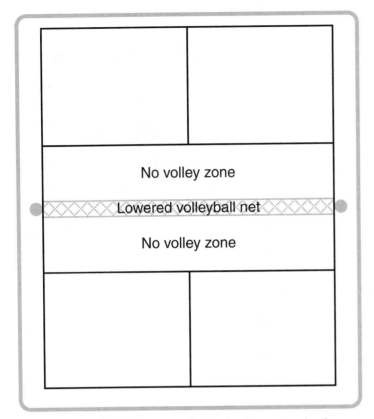

Figure 9.2—Pickleball court fitting inside a standard volleyball court.

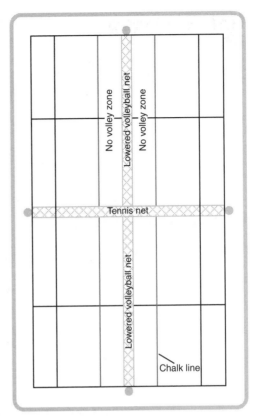

Figure 9.3—One typical tennis court makes two outdoor pickleball courts.

Unit Setup

Facility

Volleyball courts are easily converted by dropping the net and simply using the 10-foot line as the short line (figure 9.2). However, the difference in standard court size between pickleball and volleyball should be noted. Official dimensions are 20 feet by 44 feet, the no-volley zone 7 feet from the net, and the 2 service boxes split the area behind the no-volley zone. A standard volleyball court is 26 feet, 6 inches by 59 feet, with a 10-foot attack line.

It is possible to convert one tennis court into two pickleball courts, as shown in figure 9.3.

Courts can use volleyball standards and nets. The nets must be dropped to floor level.

Extra lines must be placed that divide the service box and indicate the short line. Tape can be placed where needed.

Preferably, there should be one court for every four students. Have specified practice areas if courts are not available.

Equipment

One paddle for each student (figure 9.4)
One ball for every two students
Extra paddles if needed

Unit Timeline

There is one introductory unit, with

10 lessons to develop skill competency and basic tennis scoring and terminology, and

4 to 8 lessons for a small class tournament.

Unit Assessment

A student portfolio checklist is provided here for student use (table 9.1). Encourage students to track their progress as they master new skills. Students will conclude the unit with a quiz, and performance will be assessed on the basis of the performance rubric on page 267. Further general assessment rubrics can be found in appendix B.

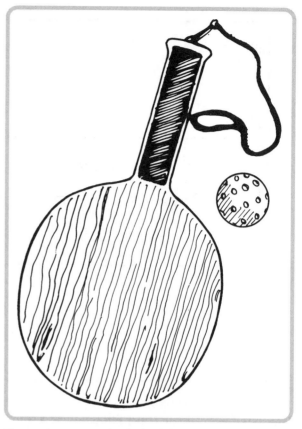

Figure 9.4—Standard pickleball paddle.

Additional Resource

Freidenberg, Mark. 1999. *The Official Pickleball Handbook*. Tacoma, WA: PB Master.

TABLE 9.1   Pickleball Student Portfolio Checklist

STUDENT NAME _____

- [ ] Is able to grip the paddle
- [ ] Can shift the paddle face and footwork from forehand to backhand
- [ ] Can direct a ball so that it passes over the net
- [ ] Can direct a ball so that it travels on a diagonal
- [ ] Can meet a bouncing ball on either the forehand or backhand side
- [ ] Can judge a ball and have the paddle meet it without a bounce
- [ ] Has learned the rules of pickleball
- [ ] Can play a doubles game of pickleball
- [ ] Can enter into competition, demonstrating good sporting behavior
- [ ] Can follow group-given directions for a tournament schedule
- [ ] Can assume responsibility for getting and returning equipment
- [ ] Will assume officiating chores when not playing

From *Complete Physical Education Plans for Grades 7–12* by Isobel Kleinman, 2001, Champaign, IL: Human Kinetics

Pickleball Lesson 1   Beginner level

Lesson Setup

Facility

One court or specified area for each group

Equipment

One pickleball for each assigned group of students
One paddle for each student

Performance Goals

Students will learn to

hold the pickleball paddle;
meet the ball on one bounce:
- On the forehand side
- On the backhand side

play safely with implements in a small space.

Cognitive Goals

Students will learn

to anticipate where the ball goes after bouncing,
safety concerns of playing in smaller places with a paddle, and
to improve their focus on the ball.

Lesson Safety

Practice areas should be separated by a minimum of 15 feet.

Warm-Up

Students will

1. Jog around the playing area
2. Learn and repeat crossover steps
3. Complete sit-ups
4. Practice pivoting mimetics
5. Complete stretches

Motivation

Mention to your students that they are beginning a unit with a funny name: pickleball. The name may be unfamiliar, but every skill they use in this game will help them become better at Ping-Pong, handball, racquetball, badminton, and tennis, because each of these games shares something in common with pickleball. Tell the class that the best thing about this game is that it's fun—even for people who are experienced with the big games. Show them how to get started.

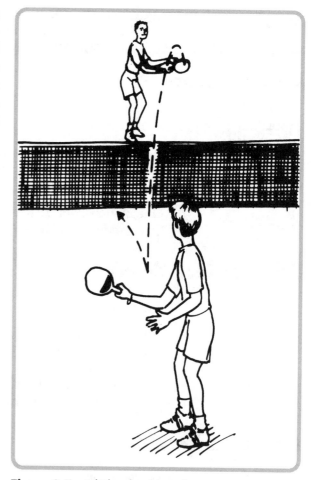

Figure 9.5—Hitting backhands.

Teaching Sequence

1. Teach and check the proper grip.
2. Set up lines of students 15 feet away from each other along a wall:
   * Explain special safety precautions for using a paddle in shared spaces.
   * Teach students what to do when their ball flies to someone else's area.
   * Teach students how to properly return balls to the person asking for them.
3. Teach, demonstrate, and have students practice hitting the ball to a wall from five feet away. Discourage full swings at this distance, but rather concentrate on students meeting the ball at its height with a firm wrist and their eyes on the ball. Then encourage a follow-through up:
   * With the forehand
   * With the backhand
4. When students have demonstrated some degree of success, have them leave the wall and go to the courts, trying to hit the ball over the net:
   * Choose a student with whom to demonstrate consecutive hits on the forehand side.
   * Have students practice.
   * Demonstrate hitting to the backhand side, as shown in figure 9.5.
   * Have students practice hitting to the backhand.

Review

Review some of the terms learned in the class and examine how students know whether they are hitting a forehand or a backhand.

Discuss on what side of the body a right-handed player would meet the ball in order to hit a forehand.

Ask students whether turning to the dominant side to swing would be considered using the forehand.

Ask them how they would explain a backhand.

Assessment

Observe for ball control.

Pickleball Lesson 2   Beginner level

Performance Goals

Students will

improve their ability to meet the ball on their backhand,
hit on a diagonal from off the court and be able to serve, and
use service rules to practice playing points.

Cognitive Goals

Students will

understand the difference between a forehand and a backhand, and
learn the rules for serving.

Lesson Safety

Encourage students to practice the same types of things at one time so they do not get in each other's way, and so they can improve focus during the lesson.

Warm-Up

Students will

1. Participate in free play—practicing on the court with equipment
2. Practice crossover steps
3. Complete sit-ups
4. Practice forehand and backhand mimetics: pivoting with a backswing, contact point, follow-through up

Motivation

All games have rules that determine the legal way to put the ball into play. Tell students that since they are doing so well at hitting the ball back and forth, they are ready to learn how to start the game. Before playing pickleball, they have to learn its rules. In this lesson, they will learn how to put the ball into play—the service.

Lesson Sequence

1. Have students practice backhand to backhand from short distances, increasing distances as they increase their number of consecutive contacts.
2. Explain the following service rules:
   - The ball must land in the diagonal service box or on its line.
   - The server must stand off the court.
   - As in volleyball, only the serving team can win a point.
   - Each person gets a turn of service until his opponents put him out.
   - Each time a team wins a point, the server must change sides and serve to the opposite diagonal.
3. Demonstrate how to make a ball go on the diagonal, and show a proper serve.
4. Have students practice serving, allowing a minimum of 10 serves per student before going on to a game.
5. If there is time, allow a game that uses the service rules students just learned.

Review

Ask the class what is the easiest way to get a ball to travel on a diagonal. Review what happens if a player doesn't get her serve in the diagonal box. Discuss why a player needs a full stroke to get the serve over the net.

Pickleball Lesson 3 — Beginner level

Lesson Setup

Facility

A specified area for each practice group to work in while waiting for a pickleball court if one is not available

Performance Goals

Students will

continue to improve their paddle skills,
follow the rules of the game, and
play games.

Cognitive Goals

Students will

review service rules, and
learn receiver's rules.

Lesson Safety

If you do not have a court for every four students but have outside practice space that will not interfere with a game, give equipment to everyone and have students practice.

If you do not have a safe place for practice,

- collect all the equipment, except for that being used on the game courts, and
- have the remaining students stand at the net and officiate while they wait for their turn to go onto the court.

Warm-Up

Students will

1. Participate in free play on court with equipment
2. Complete crossover steps, running side to side
3. Run forward and back, stopping in a knee bend
4. Practice mimetics for forehand and backhand with a follow-through

Motivation

Tell students that you haven't taught them all the rules yet, so in this lesson, they will learn the rules that the team receiving the serve must follow. And, rather than just playing out points like in the previous lesson, they will be able to play games.

Lesson Sequence

1. Teach the following rules:
   - A team's turn of service begins with whoever is in the right-hand box.
   - The receiving team may only allow the player in the right-hand box to receive serves to the right-hand box. When the serve is to the left, the teammate on the left must return serve.
   - The receiver must let the serve bounce before returning it.
   - The server must let the returned ball bounce before hitting the returned serve. Thereafter, the serving team is allowed to hit balls on a fly.
2. Answer questions about service rules.
3. Send students out to their courts for their first games.
4. Have students rotate courts after a set time so they play with a variety of people.

Review

Ask the class what side of the court a turn of service starts from.
Find out if there are any questions.

Pickleball Lesson 4 — Beginner level

Lesson Setup

Facility

A specified practice area for each group if a court is not available

Performance Goals

Students will

continue to improve their paddle skills,
volley, and
play games.

Cognitive Goals

Students will

learn that volleys do not have backswings but do have follow-throughs,
learn what the "no volley" zone is and the two-bounce rule, and
experience how different people play.

Lesson Safety

During volleying practice, students can practice in pairs opposite each other, as long as they can reach out with their paddle and be double-paddles distance from anyone to the right or left of them.

Once the games start, if there is not one court for every four students but you have outside practice space that if used will not interfere with the game, give equipment to everyone and have students practice.

If you do not have a safe place for practice,

- collect all the equipment, except for that being used on the game courts; and
- have the remaining students stand at the net and officiate while they wait their turn to go onto the court.

Warm-Up

Students will

1. Participate in free play on the court with equipment
2. Complete footwork practice:

- Crossover steps side to side
- Running forward and back
- Stopping with each change of direction with a knee bend

3. Practice full-stroke mimetics on both sides

Motivation

Ask the class if anyone knows what volleying is: Is the ball allowed to bounce in volleyball? Are there other games that students can think of that use a volley? If a player does not wait for the ball to bounce, is he speeding up or slowing down the game? The answer is speeding it up. That is why some people find volleys more intimidating than normal ground strokes. It makes everyone react more quickly, and when a player's opponents cannot react quickly enough, the volley helps him win the point.

Tell students that volleying is actually very easy to do. All they have to do is meet the ball in front of them. In this lesson they will learn how to volley, practice it a little, and then play as many five-point games as there is time for.

Lesson Sequence

1. Demonstrate the volley. Have students practice with their partner, exchanging who feeds the ball until the volley is successfully done by each 10 times.
2. Teach the rules that involve the volley:
   - That the short line is the border for the "no volley" zone
   - That the server must wait and let the return of serve bounce before volleying, and she cannot, as in tennis, rush the net on the serve
   - That the receiver, too, must wait to hit one ground stroke before volleying
3. Review the receiving rules.
4. Instruct students to first play against whomever they choose, playing a five-point game, and as soon as they are done, have them report to you so you can send them out again with new opponents. This is a good time to get a feel for how you should develop the class tournament to keep competition interesting for all skill levels. Make an effort to have winners of the minigames play other winners.

Review

Ask the class to explain the two-bounce rule.
Ask about the "no volley" zone.

Assessment

Observe each group's progress, keeping in mind the things to add to the review or to the introduction of the next lesson. Start scouting the team partnerships, with a mind to who are the strongest and weakest of teams. This will help when you develop the class tournament.

Pickleball Lesson 5   Beginner level

Lesson Setup

Equipment

Blackboard, chalk, and eraser
Round-robin tournament charts (see appendix A)

Performance Goal

Students will play their last practice games.

Cognitive Goals

Students will

learn how to survive with and without their partner on the court:
* Up and back positioning
* Right and left responsibilities
* In the event of an absence
review the "no volley" zone and two-bounce rules, and
learn to follow tournament procedure and respond to the following:
* A timer's horn
* Court assignments

Lesson Safety

Instruct the students that when they are leaving the court after completing their five-point games, they should make sure to walk well behind the baselines so they do not interfere with other people's games.

Warm-Up

Students will

1. Participate in free play on court
2. Practice mimetics for the backhand, forehand, low volley, and high volley
3. Complete footwork skills, concentrating on ending with a pivot preparatory step that has the forward leg bent at the knee as it should be for ground strokes

Motivation

Tell your students that you are setting up a class tournament. They will also be learning what to do when a partner is absent and how to get to their assigned courts without taking time from playing their games. If the class is large, tell them you will be planning a minimum of two games for everyone each day. So in order to not waste time when their game assignments change, they need to learn how the directions will be posted. The next class will begin the tournament.

Lesson Sequence

1. Bring the class to the blackboard:
   - Diagram how partners split responsibilities of the court.
   - Then put the court assignments on the board the way they would appear in the tournament schedule and send those students out to play a practice game using side-by-side doubles strategy. (See appendix A for ideas on how to handle scheduling if there are not enough courts for students to play all at once.)
2. End the first-round games with a timer's horn and bring the class back to the blackboard:
   - Show how the teams should indicate the winners.
   - Diagram the up-and-back doubles strategy.
   - Indicate the second-round game assignments as they would appear in the tournament chart and send the students back out to play the next round with their new practice opponents.
3. Bring the students back to the blackboard after suspending the second practice game. Explain what they should do when
   - they are not scheduled to play, or
   - someone's teammate is absent.
4. Review how they should report the winners.

Review

Ask them what they should check for first when they come in for the next class (the court assignments and who plays first).

Ask why they should go to the court if they are not scheduled to play.

Ask them what their call would be if they were officiating and the serving team hit the ball on a fly in the no-volley zone.

If a student's game is over but she is supposed to play the very next playing period, discuss whether she should report her score or start the next game with her new opponents. Ask if her wins should be recorded.

Assessment

This lesson clearly can be stretched into two. Use observation techniques and a sense of the students' needs for meeting new opponents, practicing, or competing and how much time is left in your unit for tournaments. It makes no sense to fly into a tournament if the class is large and cannot follow instructions well. The playing time will be eaten up by confusion if they need more time to understand what to do, time that easily could be used deciding which doubles strategy to use—up and back or side to side. Observe before deciding how fast to move on.

Teacher Homework

Make a separate round-robin tournament schedule for each ability level, with at least four teams in each of the small tournaments. Make up the tournament charts and court assignment schedules and post. Sample round-robin tournament schedules and charts can be found in appendix A.

Pickleball Lesson 6 — Beginner level

Lesson Setup

Equipment

Extra pickleballs close by in case of breakage
Blackboard, chalk, and eraser or marker
Posted tournament charts and court schedules

Performance Goals

Students will

continue to improve their paddle skills,
play round 1 of the tournament, and
exhibit good behavior during competition:
  • Playing by the rules
  • Exhibiting good sporting behavior
  • Following tournament procedure

Cognitive Goal

Students will learn to meet a challenge that requires they play at their best level.

Lesson Safety

Figure 9.6 shows a safe setup for students when one team must not play for a playing period. Those players are off the court and put to work as officials in a zone that is safe to stand in during their waiting period.
Collect all equipment not needed for each game.
Tell students, "When you leave the court, make sure to walk behind the baseline so you do not interfere with any game or run the risk of being clobbered with a paddle."

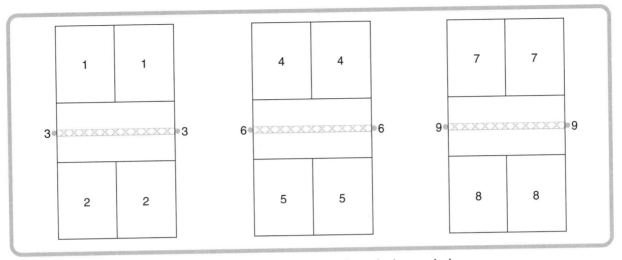

Figure 9.6—Where students would be during scheduled first playing period.

Warm-Up

Students will participate in free play on the court with equipment

Motivation

Inform students that you are there if they need a new ball, have questions about rules and how they apply, or want a strategy hint for how to beat their opponent. Tell them to enjoy their play and to make sure to report their scores and that they are playing the right team before they begin games. Announce that the clock will start immediately after warm-ups, so they should make sure to check their game schedule as soon as they come in from the locker room so they don't lose any playing time.

Lesson Sequence

1. Post the schedules on the blackboard and make them available upon entry to the gym; equipment should be out for preclass practice and warm-ups.
2. Once the warm-up period is over, collect any equipment not needed for the games.
3. Games should begin as soon as the warm-ups are over.
4. Students should make sure that their team number is circled if they win.

Review

Make sure all scores have been submitted.
Announce the day's standings.

Assessment

Observe each court and its ability to officiate, start in a timely fashion, and get good playing time. If the procedure is too complicated for students to begin without your direction, and they have only the tournament charts to guide them, then you must make changes in the next lesson.

Pickleball Lessons 7-11 — Beginner level

Lesson Setup

Equipment

Extra pickleballs close by in case of breakage
Blackboard, chalk, and eraser or marker
Updated tournament charts
The posted performance assessment rubric for beginners

Performance Goals

Students will

continue to improve their paddle skills, and
play through a tournament:
- Playing by the rules
- Exhibiting good sporting behavior
- Following tournament procedure

Cognitive Goals

Students will

learn to be self-sufficient:
- Reading the available charts
- Following their own progress by using their math skills to calculate their standings
learn to meet a challenge to play at their best levels.

Lesson Safety

Now that the class is involved in competition, be vigilant about the psychological welfare and safety of all students. Be prepared to step in if behavior becomes intimidating both physically and emotionally.

Warm-Up

Students will participate in free-play practice on the court with equipment

Motivation

Announce the standings after the current round. The scores will be entered each day and students have to add them up to see where they are in the rankings. Wish them luck.

Lesson Sequence

1. Post the schedules on the blackboard and make them available upon entry to the gym; equipment also should be out.
2. Have games begin as soon as warm-ups are over.
3. Have students make sure that their team number is circled if they win so wins can be entered on the round-robin tournament chart. (See the sample chart in appendix A, which shows how two rounds have been entered, giving students a clear image of whom they have yet to play and how they have done since the tournament started.)

Review

Make sure all scores have been submitted.
Announce who had the day's best scores.
Ask if the class has any questions.
Tell students to be prepared for a short quiz on the last day.

Assessment

During the course of the tournament, post performance and/or skills expectations. Begin assessing student performance by using the beginner performance assessment rubric on page 267, completing the process on the last day of the tournament.

Pickleball Lesson 12 — Beginner level

Lesson Setup

Equipment

A quiz for each student
Blackboard, chalk, and eraser
Tournament charts

Performance Goals

Students will

take a short quiz at the beginning of class, and
conclude their tournament.

Cognitive Goal

Students will get to measure their understanding of pickleball.

Warm-Up

Students will practice skills on the court after the quiz and before the game

Motivation

After five rounds of a tournament, tell the students that they all have gotten so much better. In this class, the first-, second-, and third-place winners of each tournament will meet and the ultimate champion will be decided. While those players are playing out their matches, the rest of the students will play their own games against teams from the other draw that they haven't played before.

Lesson Sequence

1. Post the schedules on the blackboard and make them available upon entry to the gym; equipment also should be out.
2. Games should begin as soon as the warm-ups are over:
   - The play-offs should reflect the tournament standings.
   - The games not vying for play-off spots should be student choice, or
   - They should be assigned by an even match.
3. Students should make sure that their team number is circled if they win.

Review

Leave time for a quick review of the quiz.
Announce the tournament winners and congratulate them.

Assessment

Students will be assessed based on a quiz and the performance assessment rubric (table 9.2). Further general assessment rubrics can be found in appendix B.

TABLE 9.2   Beginner Pickleball Performance Assessment Rubric

STUDENT NAME _____

	0	1	2	3	4	5
Forehand	No effort	• Uses proper grip • Uses correct mimetics on cue • Uses the correct side of the paddle • Able to meet an object in the center of the paddle five consecutive times during a self-volley	• Meets an object coming from over the net • Able to redirect a ball to a target 5 feet away after it bounces • Has proper body pivot • Able to self-volley up and down 10 times	• Moves to meet a ball after the bounce • Able to rally over the net 5 times with a partner • Meets a ball with the paddle head up • Controls a wall volley five times	• Runs and redirects a ball to a target area • Meets a ball in the center of the paddle with a firm wrist • Returns a ball with a volley • Able to rally 10 times	• Moves to cover a wide shot • Chooses correctly between a volley and a full stroke • Able to control depth or vary speed • Uses a complete swing
Backhand	No effort	• Uses correct mimetics • Uses the correct side of the paddle • Able to meet an object in the center of the paddle five consecutive times during a self-volley	• Meets an object coming from over the net • Able to redirect a ball to a target after it bounces • Has proper body pivot • Able to self-volley up and down 10 times	• Moves to meet a ball after the bounce • Meets a ball with the paddle head up • Controls a backhand wall volley five times	• Runs and redirects a ball toward a target • Returns a ball with a volley • Able to rally 10 times over the net	• Moves to cover the backhand side • Is successful whether uses a volley or a full stroke • Controls depth • Varies speed
Serve	No effort	• Uses correct mimetics • Uses a correct grip • Gets a ball over the net from a self-toss	• Occasionally able to put a ball in play • Able to direct a ball on the diagonal	• Consistently able to direct a ball diagonally • Serves reach the service box more often than not	• Serves from off the court • Performs a legal serve	• Is consistent • Is starting to vary speed or depth • Shows signs of strategic placement

Pickleball Quiz—Beginner level

NAME _____ TEACHER _____

DATE _____ CLASS PERIOD _____

True or False: Read each statement below carefully. If the statement is true, put a check under the True box in the column to the left of the statement. If the statement is false, put a check under the False box in the column to the left of the statement. If using a grid sheet, blacken in the appropriate column for each question, making sure to use the correctly numbered line for each question and its answer.

True	False	
☐	☐	1. A server must serve from off the court.
☐	☐	2. One hitter cannot allow the ball to bounce two times before hitting it back over the net.
☐	☐	3. The "no volley" zone is between the net and the short line.
☐	☐	4. If you meet the ball on the same side of your body that holds the paddle, it is called a forehand.
☐	☐	5. When the ball is served over the net and lands inside the diagonal box and passes the short line, the server loses his turn of service.
☐	☐	6. The receiving team wins a point when the serving team hits the ball out of bounds.
☐	☐	7. The first server on a team is always the person on the right-hand side of the court.
☐	☐	8. If a server goes to the net to hit the receiver's return on a fly, she is breaking the two-bounce rule.
☐	☐	9. The volley is a stroke with a backswing.
☐	☐	10. When player A loses the point serving from the left, his partner B starts his serve from the same box—the box on the left.

From *Complete Physical Education Plans for Grades 7–12* by Isobel Kleinman, 2001, Champaign, IL: Human Kinetics.

Pickleball Answer Key—Beginner level

1. T
2. T
3. T
4. T
5. F
6. F
7. T
8. T
9. F
10. F

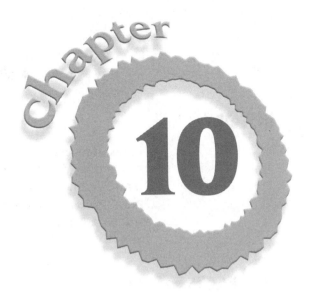

Chapter 10

Tennis

Unit Overview

1. Provide each student with a racket and a ball at each class meeting. Keep everyone engaged in some aspect of playing tennis during each lesson.

2. Follow the lesson plans, which break down the following and focus on one concept per lesson:

   - Racket skill—the grip, forehand/backhand ground strokes, the serve, and forehand/backhand volley
   - Footwork—the waiting position, pivot, knee bend, forward and back, and side-to-side movement

- Tennis terminology—fault, let, turn of service, love, set, deuce, and advantage in/out
- The rules of service, receiving, and playing out a point
- Scoring of a point, a game, a set, and a match

3. Teach the economics of tennis:

   - Cost of equipment
   - Public and private courts

Tennis

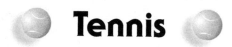

HISTORY

Tennis dates back to the Stone Age. Then, humans used clubs to hit rocks back and forth. Later, the French modernized the game of tennis. The word "tennis" comes from the French word "tenez," which means "take it" or "play." In 1913, an international conference in Paris was held and the International Lawn Tennis Federation was founded. In 1977, "lawn" was dropped from its name. Thus, today it is the International Tennis Federation.

FUN FACTS

→ Tennis disappeared from the Olympic menu after the 1924 Paris games. However, it reappeared as a full-medal sport in the 1988 Seoul games.

→ The United States Tennis Association runs more than 200 national tournaments per year.

→ In 1999, 261,535 new players began playing tennis in the United States.

→ The Women's Tennis Association prize money surpassed $45 million in 1999.

→ Total prize money from Wimbledon Championships has grown from $26,150 in 1968 to $7,595,330 in 1999.

BENEFITS OF PLAYING

1. People can burn more calories per hour playing competitive tennis than playing volleyball, swimming, canoeing, hiking, playing softball, or golfing.
2. Tennis is good for the heart!
3. Tennis can help you improve your leg strength, balance, speed, and agility.
4. Tennis is great for hand-eye coordination.
5. Tennis is fun!

TIME TO SURF!

Web Site	Web Site Address
United States Tennis Association	www.usta.com
Women's Tennis Association	http://www.wtatour.com/
International Tennis Federation	http://www.itftennis.com/fl_index.html

From *Complete Physical Education Plans for Grades 7–12* by Isobel Kleinman, 2001, Champaign, IL: Human Kinetics.

Tennis Unit Extension Project

NAME _____ CLASS _____

Equipment needed to play tennis

Item	Where you would purchase it (be specific)	Cost

Where you would play tennis

Please explain where in the community you would play tennis. Be specific.

How much does it cost to play?

Are there courts where you can play for free? What about in bad weather? Are there indoor courts available? If yes, how much does it cost to play there?

Health benefits of playing tennis

Please explain the health benefits of playing tennis. Include how much tennis you would need to play each week to gain these benefits.

Reflection question

Do you think tennis is an activity you would like to play as an adult? Why or why not? And if yes, do you think you'd rather play in a league like the USTA Adult Team Tennis league, in tournaments, or just play with friends?

From *Complete Physical Education Plans for Grades 7–12* by Isobel Kleinman, 2001, Champaign, IL: Human Kinetics.

Tennis Teaching Tips

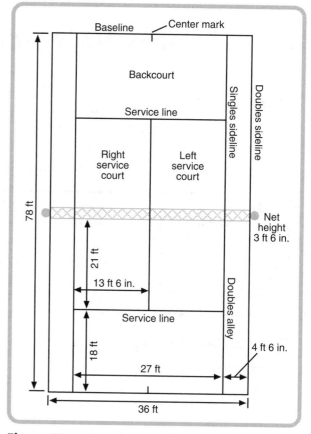

1. Allow students the opportunity for a lot of repetition.
2. Encourage students to
   - change partners,
   - change opponents, and
   - keep the ball in play.
3. Teach rules as you introduce the skill.
4. Emphasize tennis footwork and racket preparation during warm-up.
5. The fun of involvement is a priority; raise the expectations of the class after 90 percent of your students are ready to go on.
6. Each lesson includes some kind of contest.
7. There is a short tournament involving all students; it is planned as the culmination event. Students unable to participate should be involved in officiating games, scoring games, or analyzing skills. For example, they can be marking what stroke led to the most winning shots, the most unforced errors, and so forth.
8. Encourage students to practice with different classmates. If the least-skilled players stay together during their learning experience, it is likely to be frustrating for them. If you rotate practice partners in a systematic way, you will avoid that problem.
9. If advanced students are bored, have them fill in as teacher assistants, helping other students develop by feeding the ball to them and helping them keep the ball in play. Meanwhile, advanced tennis players should be encouraged to improve their consistency and accuracy.
10. Every effort should be made to assure students that improvement is what is valued, not a predisposition to be a great athlete.

Figure 10.1—Tennis court dimensions.

Unit Setup

Facility

Instructional groups should not be larger than the facilities can accommodate. Optimally, there should be no more than four students per tennis court. (This unit shows how to accommodate twice that number so that students safely work on tennis skills the entire period. But once tennis games start, having more than four students per game court is counterproductive. If students cannot play for 20 to 30 minutes without having to get off the court, the work on focusing and learning to score is lost. It is best to plan something else for the additional students and have them rotate onto the courts for games on alternate days.) The courts should be fenced in with fences a minimum of 20 feet high, so that errant balls do not require half the period to retrieve.

Equipment

One racket and ball for each student
Three balls for each pair playing over a net
Round-robin tournament schedules and charts (see appendix A)

Unit Safety

This unit equips all students in a class with rackets and balls and expects them to use them at the same time. As a result, students must develop court courtesies from the very first lesson in order for their practice and learning experiences to be safe.

Players must not run anywhere other than within their assigned practice area or court.

If a ball is errant, players must learn to ask the person whose court it is on to please throw it back.

Equipment is only to be used for contacting the tennis ball.

Balls must be picked up from the playing surface so no one trips. If it is not the student's ball, he should find out whose it is and throw it back so it reaches the person on one bounce.

Unit Timeline

There are two units of tennis in this chapter:

10 lessons to develop skill competency and basic tennis scoring and terminology, and

4 to 8 lessons for a small class tournament.

Unit Assessment

A student portfolio checklist is provided here for student use (table 10.1). Encourage students to track their progress as they master new skills. Students will conclude the unit with a quiz, and performance will be measured on the basis of the performance assessment rubric at the end of the unit. Further general assessment rubrics can be found in appendix B.

Additional Resources

American Sport Education Program. 1998. *Coaching Youth Tennis.* Champaign, IL: Human Kinetics.

Burns, Bill. 1998. *Tennis 2000: Strokes, Strategy and Psychology for a Lifetime.* Boston: Little Brown & Co.

Hoctor, Mike, Rebecca Desmond, and Ron Woods. 1995. *Coaching Tennis Successfully.* Champaign, IL: Human Kinetics.

Verdeick, Jim, and Dennis Van der Meer. *USPTR Manual for Coaches.* This book and all others by Dennis Van der Meer are out of print, but if you can find a copy, it is worth it. His approach to teaching is used by the Unites States Professional Tennis Association and is the one used in this unit.

TABLE 10.1   Tennis Student Portfolio Checklist

STUDENT NAME: _____

- ☐ Is able to grip the racket
- ☐ Can shift the racket face, footwork, and grip from forehand to backhand
- ☐ Can consecutively meet a ball on the center of the strings while self-bouncing to the ground, the air, and against a wall
- ☐ Can consecutively block a bounced forehand to a target 10 feet away
- ☐ Can consecutively block a bounced backhand to a target 10 feet away
- ☐ Understands the significance of boundaries and keeping the ball inside
- ☐ Understands how one scores in tennis games, sets, and matches
- ☐ Has learned the service toss and proper overhead service motion
- ☐ Is able to follow tennis service rules
- ☐ Is able to block a forehand or backhand volley
- ☐ Can take a full backswing and follow-through without losing control
- ☐ Can begin match play while self-directed and using the rules of tennis

From *Complete Physical Education Plans for Grades 7–12* by Isobel Kleinman, 2001, Champaign, IL: Human Kinetics

Tennis Lesson 1   Beginner level

Lesson Setup

Facility

A clear area large enough to safely accommodate the group

Equipment

One tennis ball per person
One tennis racket per person

Performance Goals

Students will

grip a tennis racket,

meet the ball on the center of the strings,
develop a firm wrist and forearm, and
get and return their own equipment.

Cognitive Goals

Students will

start developing concentration, and
learn what a tennis error is.

Lesson Safety

Practicing partners should have a minimum of 20 feet between them and
other students.
Students must learn to follow court courtesies as explained at the beginning of
this chapter.

Warm-Up

Students will

1. Jog around the playing area while carrying a tennis racket in the waiting position
2. Move from left to right, with body facing net, using crossover steps—repeat several times
3. Pivot to the right, step forward with the left foot while turning right, bring up the racket for the forehand, reverse directions and feet for a backhand, and end with the racket in the waiting position—repeat several times
4. Complete stretches

Motivation

Tennis is a great leisure-time activity and one of the few sports students will
learn in school that they'll have free and easy access to as an adult. Tell
students that there are many local community tennis courts available to
them without cost. The other advantage of playing tennis is that one doesn't
need a whole bunch of players to get together for a game. All that's needed
is one other person, and if a student can't find that, she can practice by
herself, she can go to a wall, or, if her family belongs to a tennis club or is
willing to get her private lessons, she will have access to a ball machine or a
tennis pro for a workout. The United States Tennis Association (USTA) runs
many local leagues at every skill level, so there are many opportunities for
all kinds of people to compete. Of course, if students haven't watched
Wimbledon, the U.S. Open, the French Open, or any other tennis tournament, they might not already know that the greats in this game, just like any
other game, make a lot of money. There is a very profitable competitive
tour for them.

Lesson Sequence

1. Before beginning any use of the tennis racket, teach court courtesy and safety rules.
2. Teach, demonstrate, and check the proper tennis grip for the forehand.
3. Teach, demonstrate, and allow practice of using the racket (with a forehand grip) to bounce the ball to the ground as shown in figure 10.2:
   - Give the students a few minutes to do this.
   - Ask if anyone can keep it under control 10 times.
4. Call students back in:
   - Demonstrate bouncing the ball to the ground using the center of the racket strings to meet the ball while keeping a forehand grip, then, without changing the grip, use the other side (upper side of the strings) to do the same in the air.
   - Ask if anyone is able to control the ball on this side of the strings 10 times.
5. After students practice and are able to control the ball off the racket, tapping 10 times to the ground and 10 times to the air, bring them to the wall (figure 10.3):
   - Demonstrate the same controlled bounces, now directed at the wall.
   - Have students begin from one arm's length and racket distance away, using their forehand side.

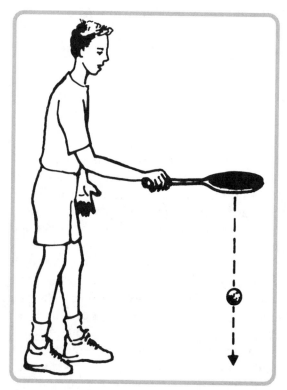

Figure 10.2—Self-bounce for racket control.

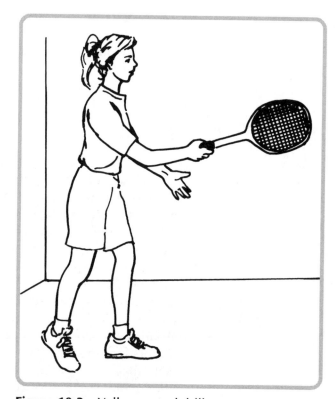

Figure 10.3—Volley control drill.

- Encourage the same moderation of just meeting and blocking the ball with a firm wrist—no swing at all. Aim to control 10 times, but don't let students stay on this for more than a few minutes:

  It is difficult if they do not stay close to the wall and use a simple block.

  If they try to swing, there will be lots of wild balls and frustration.

6. With a student, demonstrate the following, as shown in figure 10.4: Place a ball on the ground five feet from the student, then stand five feet from the ball, too. Using the same type of block, with a slight upward follow-through, meet the ball so it travels slightly upward and forward and drops to the target (the ball) on the ground. Ask your partner, on the ball's rise, to block the ball back, making sure not to drop the racket head and not to hit it down, but to block it with a slight upward follow-through. Show the class how the two of you can reach out with your racket, get the strings behind the ball, and block it back after it bounces off the ground:

  - Demonstrate consecutive hits, counting each tap as you go.
  - Use a volley to block the ball when your practice partner hits the ball further than the target on the ground.
  - Allow the students to set up and practice the game.

7. Encourage consecutive contacts with a slight upward follow-through after each bounce, meeting the ball on the rise. If the partner loses control and hits the ball a little long, encourage using the volley to meet it and hit it back so the ball stays in play. Make it into a contest:

  - Who can get to 10 first?
  - Who can get the highest number of consecutive taps without an error?

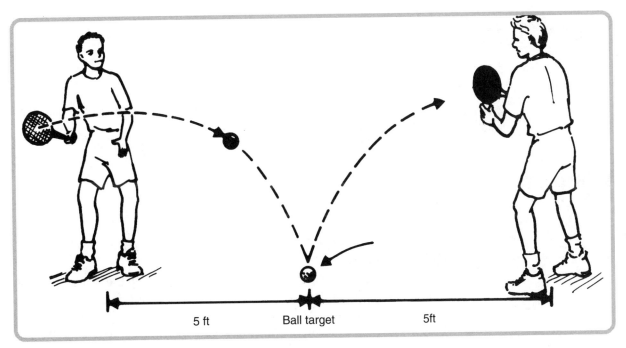

Figure 10.4—Racket/ball control with a partner.

5 ft   Ball target   5ft

Review

Ask if anyone can show the class a proper grip.

Ask what part of the racket should meet the ball, and whether the player's eyes should see it meet.

Discuss which is better—a limp, dangling wrist and racket or a firm wrist and forearm with the racket head up.

Review where a right-handed player meets the ball for a forehand—on the right or on the left—and where he meets a backhand.

Discuss whether it's legal to allow the ball to bounce twice before hitting it.

Assessment

Observe each group's ball control. If 90 percent of the class can control the ball in this close control drill for 10 consecutive taps, then the group is ready to move on to the next lesson. If not, repeat all aspects of this lesson, leaving the most time for the partner work.

Tennis Lesson 2 — Beginner level

Performance Goals

Students will

exercise proper footwork and waiting position, and
address the ball for backhand and forehand.

Cognitive Goals

Students will learn

what a waiting position is and why to use it,
how to adjust to balls on the left and right and terminology for the forehand and backhand, and
the value of getting physically consistent when meeting the ball.

Warm-Up

Students will

1. Practice the wall volley, as taught in lesson 1 (arm and racket length distance from the wall)
2. Jog around the playing area with the tennis racket held in the waiting position
3. Complete footwork drilling, moving from left to right using crossover steps
4. Practice mimetics for the forehand:
   - From the waiting position, pivot to the forehand side—do this three times
   - Do the same as above but add the step forward while turning to the right—do this three times

- Focus on the same as above but allow the secondary arm to let go of the racket throat so the racket head appears ready to meet the "imaginary" ball—do this three times
- Now with all of the above together, follow through at the end of the above sequence so that the racket head rises upward and the strings face the line of direction—repeat five or more times

5. Practice mimetics for the backhand—break down the learning pattern as above:
   - Pivot left, while rotating the grip back a quarter turn
   - Allow the racket to follow the body's natural turn
   - With a firm wrist and forearm, follow through slightly up, with the strings facing the same line of direction—repeat five or more times

Motivation

In order to play tennis on a whole court, everyone must learn to get in position so that they can swing and hit the ball over and over again and know that when they hit it, the ball will stay in bounds. Tell students that while they improve their consistency at a close distance, they are developing the building blocks to becoming fine and steady tennis players. One of those building blocks, a very important one, is footwork and preparation.

Lesson Sequence

1. Begin with a demonstration of the previous day's drill, focusing on
   - the footwork,
   - the waiting position, and
   - the pivot as well as the racket control.
2. Have students practice while coaching:
   - Move the feet
   - Pivot to meet the ball on the forehand or backhand side
   - Return to the waiting position after each contact
3. Stop the class and bring the students together to show them the volley:
   - Demonstrate how to keep the rally going with a partner when the partner misses the target of the ball on the ground and hits the ball too high and/or hard (figure 10.5).
4. Reinforce goals by sending students back to practice again, asking the following questions:
   - Who is able to meet the ball with a firm wrist on the forehand or backhand side?
   - Who is returning to the waiting position after every contact?
   - Who can meet the ball and keep it under control for 10 times? Or more? Or the most?
5. Rotate partners, instructing students to
   - tell you who gets to 10 hits with no error, and
   - move those feet so they get the strings behind the ball.
6. Rotate partners again and set a new goal of consistency and preparation.

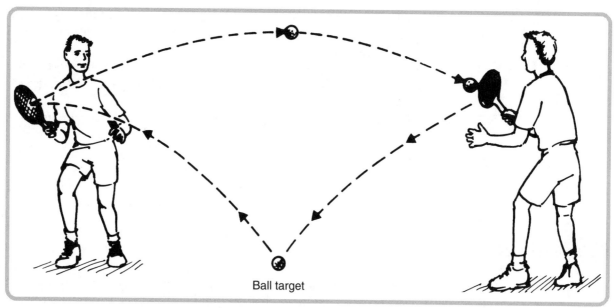

Figure 10.5—Using the volley to keep the ball in play.

Review

Ask who knows why good footwork is so important.
Ask why consistency is so important.
Discuss which feels better—hitting with a limp, dangling wrist and racket or with a firm wrist and forearm with the racket head up.
Ask why an upward follow-through is important.

Tennis Lesson 3 — Beginner level

Lesson Setup

Facility

A minimum of one tennis court for every eight students.

Equipment

Three tennis balls for every group of two students

Performance Goals

Students will

return to the waiting position after every contact with the ball,
meet the ball on the forehand or backhand side with a follow-through, and
hit the ball over the net.

Cognitive Goals

Students will

learn to deal with the obstacle of the net, and
improve their concentration during a lesson.

Lesson Safety

For this drill, three couples, or a maximum of four, can work over the net at a time. They can only do this because the drill is close to the net, the target being only five feet from the net, and each partner is trying to hit the ball straight. If there is a lack of control, have the students continue on the first drill until they can maintain control over the net, since the crowded conditions require control for safety.

Warm-Up

Students will

1. Practice a wall volley, at racket length distance from the wall
2. Jog around the playing area with the tennis racket in the waiting position
3. Complete footwork drills
4. Practice tennis mimetics:
   - Practice forehand mimetics from the waiting position, pivoting right and stepping forward for the forehand, wrist firm, arm firm, follow-through up, and returning to the waiting position—do it 10 times
   - Practice backhand mimetics—do it 10 times

Motivation

Tell your students that, believe it or not, they have begun the building blocks of solid tennis play by adding a few things at a time. In this lesson, they will try to not only keep mastering control of the racket and the ball, but they also will learn to deal with the fact that the net is in the way.

Lesson Sequence

1. After warm-ups, begin with the racket/ball control drill (see figure 10.4):
   - Ask students to count the consecutive taps when hitting the ball back and forth between each other.
   - Give them a goal:
        In the previous class, they were aiming for 10; ask them to see if they can do better.
        Let them know the highest score of a previous class and ask if they can beat it.

2. Demonstrate a drill very similar to the one they have been doing. This time their target is approximately 5 feet from the other side of a net, and their practice partner is 10 feet from the other side of the net and 5 feet from where the target is and where the ball is supposed to land (figure 10.6):

- Place a ball five feet from the net on each side of the court (two balls are needed) so they become a target.
- Line up five feet from the target. Align players to that when holding their rackets on the forehand side both rackets are string to string.
- Begin rallying over the net, demonstrating how to block the ball as it rises from the bounce, so you're hitting it back with little or no swing, and it lands near the ball on the other side, bouncing up so your partner can easily meet it with a forehand and return it. Rally forehand to forehand over the net, making sure to use the same controlled and steady swing, meeting the ball and following through (with no major backswing and no speed).

3. Send students out to practice over the net, allowing as many as four couples to share a net. After five minutes of practice, do the following:

- Ask who has gotten five hits without an error. Allow more practice. Then ask who got 10 or more contacts.
- Allow some more time, encouraging students to count on every hit.
- Rotate the partners, reemphasizing the return to the waiting position after each contact.

4. Repeat the same procedure for the backhand side:

- Ask who got 10 contacts or more.
- Rotate the partners again.

5. Discuss why to return to the waiting position after every contact.

Review

Ask the class why it is important to return to the waiting position after each contact.

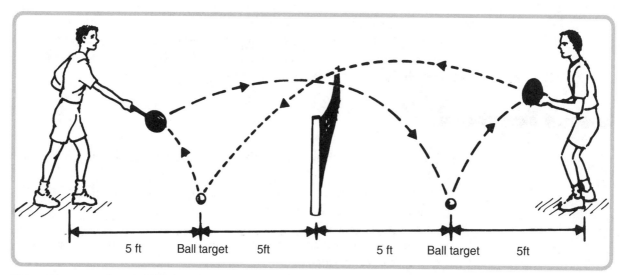

Figure 10.6—Control drill over the net.

Ask who can show a proper follow-through, and why it should go up.
Review what direction the strings should be facing.
Discuss what happens if they face the sky, or if they face the ground.

Tennis Lesson 4   Beginner level

Lesson Setup

Facility

This lesson requires a service box area for every two students. If the class is too large to accommodate one couple per service box, no more than two couples should be assigned.

Performance Goals

Students will

play a modified game using real tennis scoring, and
play the whole game within the defined boundary of the service box.

Cognitive Goals

Students will learn

how the turn of service is determined;
that a full game is served by one person until it is over;
tennis scoring—love, 15, 30, 40, game, deuce, and advantage in/out; and
to be concerned for boundaries—that when someone hits the ball out, his opponent wins a point.

Warm-Up

Students will

1. Practice a wall volley at racket-length distance from the wall
2. Practice mimetics for the forehand and backhand, using footwork before the pivot turn
3. Use the short over-the-net control drill learned in the last lesson as a warm-up

Motivation

Scoring in tennis is like a foreign language. This is probably because the game developed in France. If someone calls out "40-love," it would make no sense until you knew what it meant. Tell the class that "40-love" means the server is about to win and the receiver needs three points in a row just to tie the game.

Talk about what scores mean and using this "special language" during the day's games.

Lesson Sequence

1. Gather the students together and go over the following:
   - Scoring terminology—love, 15, 30, 40, game
   - How a tie is handled—deuce, advantage
   - Discuss these rules:

     A point is won by someone, no matter who the server.

     A server's score is always called out first.

     One person serves until the game is over.

     A ball landing on any part of the line is good.

2. Assign each couple to play a control game in which the ball's bounce is confined to the service box (figure 10.7):
   - Have them play point out, rallying back and forth until someone misses or the ball lands outside a boundary.
   - Use tennis scoring, making sure that when one tennis game is over, the server changes.
   - Allow as many games as there is time for.

3. If there is a couple waiting, have them wait by the box, helping to keep score for the people they watch. They should get to use the court and be ready to switch the minute one game is over.

4. Circulate, answering any questions about scoring that arise.

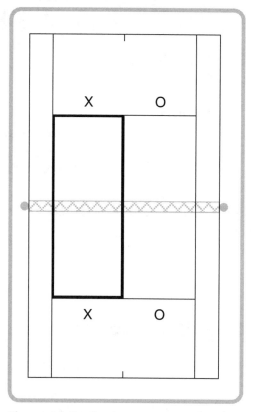

Figure 10.7—Students can practice the scoring used in tennis while completing control drills using two service boxes.

Review

Ask the class who is winning if the score is deuce.

If the score is 15-40, review whether it is the receiver or the server who is about to win.

Discuss if love is a winning score in tennis.

Ask students, if their opponent hits the ball and it lands half on the line and half off, whether it is good.

Tennis Lesson 5   Beginner level

Lesson Setup

Facility

This lesson requires a service box area for every two students. If there are not enough service box courts for each couple, create another space for those waiting:

- Use volleyball standards with dropped nets and alternative courts set up on a handball court or basketball court where they can play.
- Define space behind the baseline where the extra students can practice or even play without interfering with the game.

Performance Goals

Students will

play a modified game using real tennis scoring, aiming to complete a set; and change sides of the court after every odd game.

Cognitive Goals

Students will

learn that a game is like a word in a sentence, a set is like a sentence in a story, and a match is like the story;
understand what a *set* and a *match* are; and
learn why players change sides of the court and when they do it.

Warm-Up

Students will

1. Complete a short control drill over the net or in any space available
2. Practice mimetics for the forehand, backhand, and volley on the forehand and backhand side, using footwork before pivoting to one side or the other

Motivation

Discuss with the class that tennis has an unusual scoring system, but it was designed that way to make the game fair to all players. It gives each player an equal chance regardless of playing style (e.g., big server vs. a baseliner) and weather conditions (e.g., wind and sun). The scoring system allows players equal opportunities to serve and to play on each side of the court. You might think of playing a match like writing a story. Each game is like a word in a sentence. In order to complete the sentence, you need to win six games and be ahead by at least two games (thus you have to do more than just win your serve each time). If you get ahead 6 games to 5, you still need to win another game to win the set 7-5. However, if the set is tied at 6 games all, the modern game calls for a tiebreaker, where the winner is the first person to win 7 points and be ahead by 2 points (and there are specific rules for alternating the serve and side). Then once the first sentence is complete, you still need a second sentence to complete the story. In other words, you need to win two sets to win a match. But, for now, students will concentrate on having enough time so they can play enough games to complete a set.

Lesson Sequence

1. Teach why and when opponents switch sides of the court.
2. Explain that the game is still being played within the service box boundaries.
3. Review scoring and turn-of-service rules, and assign courts.
4. Have students play a set, using the service box as a court and using all the rules learned to date.
5. If there are not enough courts, either
   - set up a modified game plan, having students with no court play rallying games in another practice area, or
   - have students rotate off the service box court after two games (each player has served a game) and encourage them to remember their game scores so when they regain a court they can continue their sets.

Review

Ask if the class has any questions.
Review why it is important to change sides after every odd game.
Discuss how a player can win a set.
Ask which students were winning their set when the class was stopped. Ask if they were ahead by two games.

Tennis Lesson 6 — Beginner level

Performance Goals

Students will

take a proper backswing,
work on strokes from baseline to baseline, and
cover a larger portion of the court.

Cognitive Goals

Students will

learn the value of a backswing;
adjust to different power and timing from baseline to baseline; and
learn to keep three balls safely on them, though using only one at a time.

Lesson Safety

Under no circumstances should more than two couples be rallying with their own balls on one court at a time.

Warm-Up

Students will

1. Complete a short control drill over the net or in any space available
2. Practice mimetics of a full backswing while taking a pivot step—backhand and forehand—followed by a full follow-through; practice until the mimetic stroke is smooth and fluid, 10 times
3. Add footwork to the process, taking a backswing while moving right or left, 10 times

Motivation

Tell students not to underestimate how well they are doing. They are about to start something that's not too easy to do—play the whole length of the court (half the width). Tell them you think they'll be able to do it, although many players with more practice sometimes have difficulty doing this. Many experienced tennis players cannot hit a ball over and over again, straight ahead. But tell students you are making this change now because you think the class is ready and it is time to add to their tennis tools. Once they take a complete swing, they can generate shots that go from baseline to baseline. Then they will be ready to play the whole court instead of service box to service box.

Lesson Sequence

1. Teach students the appropriate way to gather their tennis balls and hold them so they are not interfering with their playing space.
2. Assign students court space to practice full strokes, as shown in figure 10.8.
3. Rotate whom they are hitting with every five minutes.

Review

Ask students what makes full-court swings different from the shorter game they played before.

Ask when they should take their backswing.
Discuss whether the backswing should be low.
Review the follow-through.

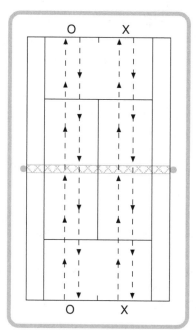

Figure 10.8—Full-court strokes.

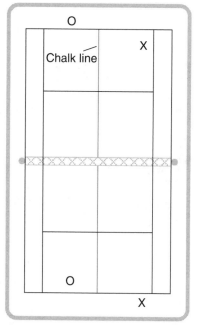

Figure 10.9—Playing singles in half a court.

Tennis Lesson 7   Beginner level

Lesson Setup

Facility

This lesson requires half the width of a court for every two players (figure 10.9).

Extra students must use the wall or practice volleying on the field.

Performance Goals

Students will play the full-length court using most tennis rules, with the following modifications:

A service modification allows a regular drop-and-hit method of putting the ball into play.

The serve will not be directed to the diagonal box.

Their games must be played in half the width of the court.

Cognitive Goals

Students will learn

the boundaries for the whole court, and
the following service rules:
- The ball must be put into play from off the court.
- The serve must land in the service box or on its lines, without touching the net.
- The server is allowed a second serve if the first does not enter the box.
- A serve that touches the net is called a *let*.
- A *double fault* results in a point for the opponent.

Warm-Up

Students will

1. Complete a short control drill over the net or in any space available
2. Practice mimetics of a full backswing with a pivot step for backhand and forehand

Motivation

One of the most frustrating parts of tennis, for new and old players, is that opponents can win games without ever doing anything at all. Tell students to imagine being able to play a great game once the ball gets put into play, but always losing their own service game because they cannot make the ball land in the correct service box. In this class, students will be using almost all the service rules of an official game while sticking to the skills they already have mastered on the short court. Invite them to use whatever method they choose for getting the ball over the net into play, because they have to make sure they can get the ball in the service box from off the court.

Lesson Sequence

1. Teach the service rules to be used:
   - The server must serve from off the court, behind the baseline.
   - The ball must land in the service box or on the line, or it is a fault.
   - The ball cannot touch the net—when it is a let and when it is a fault.
   - Double faults lead to the opponent's point.
   - Servers get two turns to serve before losing a point if they are not able to get the serve in the diagonal service box.
2. Teach students the courtesy of returning all the balls to the server, so the server always has two and an uninterrupted turn of service.
3. Plan for equitable court time for all players. If you have more players than courts, substitutes must be given some job: calling the faults, keeping score, or practicing against a close-by wall. (All court space is now being used since games are full court.)

Review

Congratulate the class, and tell students they have done some great work playing a game in half the space used during normal singles play.

Ask if there are any questions.

Review what the score would be if a player cannot get the ball in the service box once or twice.

Discuss what happens if the serve touches the net and goes in the box, and if it doesn't.

Ask students why they want at least two balls in their pockets when they serve.

Assessment

This lesson has developed the students' abilities to control the ball. If the class is not in control, stay on lesson 6 or 7. Playing a game in half the width of the court can be rewarding. It allows players more hits and a better opportunity to improve their skills, focus, and concentration—but if students are not up to it, don't do it.

Tennis Lesson 8 — Beginner level

Lesson Setup

Equipment

Take every ball available and divide them up so each student has the maximum number of balls possible.

Performance Goal

Students will learn and practice an overhead serve.

Cognitive Goals

Students will learn

the service toss, point of contact, and follow-through for an overhead serve;

that the server must serve on a diagonal;

the value of doing a minimum of 30 repetitions when practicing an overhead serve;

the concept of a *second serve*; and

the serving rules that requiring serving to alternate boxes.

Lesson Safety

Students must remain on the same side of the court until all the practice balls have been used. When the whole group is finished hitting its serves, it should go and collect the balls and begin all over.

Tennis

Warm-Up

Students will practice serving and tossing mimetics

Motivation

Tell students that you don't know whether this lesson can be the beginning of building a new tennis star, but tennis players such as Pete Sampras, Andre Agassi, Patrick Rafter, Mark Philippoussis, Venus and Serena Williams, Martina Hingis, Irina Spirlea, Stefi Graff, and Lindsey Davenport get a huge competitive advantage from a big first serve. Report that this is how they started.

Lesson Sequence

1. Teach students that the serve must go to the diagonal box.
2. Teach the serve with no racket:
   - Begin with the entire service motion.
   - Then give them each a ball to practice the toss.
   - Combine the toss and backswing.
   - Combine the toss, backswing, and swinging up to catch the ball at its height , as in figure 10.10, continuing with the follow-through after grabbing the ball out of the air.
   - Have them use the whole service motion, hitting the ball with the palm of the hand and following through with the swinging arm across the body.

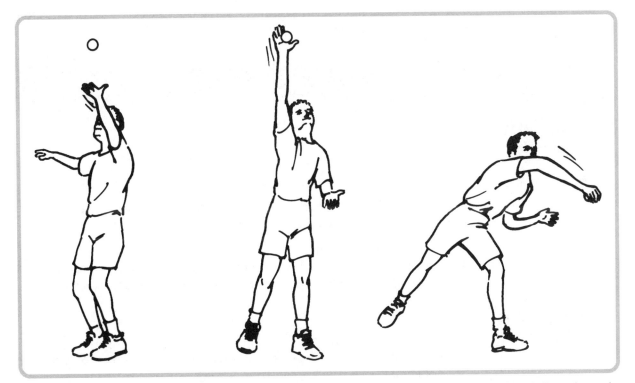

Figure 10.10—Using the service motion to catch a ball at the height of the toss and the follow-through.

3. Add the racket, showing the importance of wrist position on contact with the ball.
4. Demonstrate the full serve and the box it must go to.
5. Have students use each of their balls, one ball at a time, to serve over the net. Set up the class as in figure 10.11.
6. After all balls have been hit, change sides, collect balls, and try again for 30 or more serves.

Review

Remind students that a good serve requires a good toss.
Ask them where the toss should be in relation to the front toe.
Review the optimum height for the toss.
Discuss whether players should swing around to meet the ball or swing up to hit it.
Ask students what the racket does after it hits the ball.
Review where the follow-through should go.

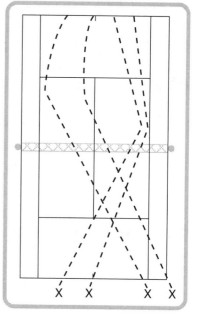

Figure 10.11—Service practice.

Assessment

Observe individual students for common errors to correct as a class or individual errors to correct privately.

Tennis Lesson 9   Beginner level

Lesson Setup

Facility

If the class is too large to accommodate four players to a tennis court, a separate practice area must be arranged, with

a wall to practice rallying;
areas for practicing volleying with a partner (concrete floor not needed); and
a marked-off zone, set up with a net and target area for practicing tennis serves.

Equipment

A can or set of three balls with the same markings per game
Practice balls for students who are not involved in doubles games (only if there are not enough courts)
A blackboard, chart, or magnetic board

Performance Goal

Students will play doubles.

Cognitive Goals

Students will

learn the rules for doubles:
- The order of service
- The order of return of service
- The different boundaries and how they affect ground strokes and serves

learn the team concept in tennis doubles, and

be reminded about court courtesy in relationship to balls:
- Learning how to identify their own balls
- Learning to clear the court and return the balls of others

Lesson Safety

If there are not enough courts to accommodate everyone, students should not be left to simply watch for the period. Whatever practice and exercise they do must be done off the tennis court. A second space is necessary so students do not endanger themselves or the people playing on the tennis court.

Warm-Up

Students will

1. Jog once around the facility
2. Complete a short control drill
3. Practice mimetics: serving and tossing motion followed by five practice serves

Motivation

Announce that up until now the students have been playing singles, but in this class, they will play with a teammate.

Lesson Sequence

1. Teach the order of service rules for doubles. See that in figure 10.12, the X team won the first serve. Player X1 has to serve first, while his partner must wait until one of his opponents serves the second game. Then he serves in the third game. Go over the following:

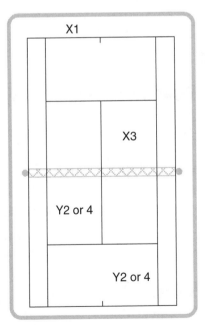

Figure 10.12—Doubles play serving order.

- The order of receiving the serve for doubles
- Any prior questions on service

2. Assign evenly matched opponents to one court to play a doubles game.
3. If there are remaining students, they can
    - practice service, toss, motion, ball contact, and follow-through;
    - practice the volley with each other; or
    - volley in fours.

Review

Discuss with the class if it's possible for one receiver to return service attempts to either box.

Ask if the return of serve has to land in any specific area on the court.

After the serve is received and returned, review whether the person closest to the ball can hit it legally.

Ask if the person closest to the incoming serve can hit the ball.

Tennis Lesson 10   Beginner level

Lesson Setup

Facility

A second marked-off area outside the tennis court compound for students not scheduled for a game

Equipment

A magnetic or chalk board

Performance Goal

Students will have doubles play.

Cognitive Goals

Students will learn general doubles positioning:

Up and back
Right and left

Warm-Up

Students will

1. Jog once around the facility
2. Complete a short control drill close enough to the net to generate volleys
3. Complete mimetics:

- Practice the volley, including how to
    step into the volley, and
    keep the wrist and forearm firm on the imaginary contact with the
        ball
- Practice the serve and toss motion. Allow five practice serves

Motivation

Review the doubles service rules and boundary lines again, and tell students to learn how to divide up the court so they can enjoy playing with a teammate.

Lesson Sequence

1. Teach doubles court positions and transitions that should occur when one partner has to
   - move wide for a shot (use a visual aid or students to demonstrate the shift of players—one to get the ball, the other to cover the middle of the court), or
   - cover a short ball.
2. If there are remaining students, they can use the alternate space that is off the tennis courts for:
   - Practicing the service, toss motion, ball contact, and follow-through
   - Volleying to each other
   - Rallying against a wall

Review

Ask students what they should do if a ball goes over their partner's head.
Review, if their partner goes out wide, whether they should stay put, or move with their partner so they can cover the middle.
Collect tournament partners' names before students leave class.

Assessment

Observe individual students for common errors to correct as a class or individual errors to correct privately.

Teacher Homework

Set up a tournament that allows players to compete on their own ability level. For example, see table 10.2, which sets up a round robin among the advanced players on one set of courts over the days, and the more intermediate players on a second set of courts, and the beginners on a third set of courts. For more examples of round-robin tournament charts and schedules, see appendix A.

All students should have the experience of a game. Everyone should have an equal opportunity to have a court to themselves. If the court space does not accommodate all players at once, then do lessons twice, rotating who plays and who practices.

TABLE 10.2 Arranging Successful Competition for Students With Different Skills

Group A: Three teams, with trouble maintaining a full-court rally (teams 8, 9, and 11)

Group B: Four teams, which control the ball with no pace (teams 2, 4, 5, and 10)

Group C: Four teams, with fast coverage and shots (teams 1, 3, 6, and 7)

DAY	GROUP A (USING SHORT-COURT RULES)	GROUP B	GROUP C
1	8 plays 9, and 11 practices (at wall or between each other)	2 plays 5 4 plays 10	1 plays 7 3 plays 6
2	11 plays 8, and 9 practices	2 plays 10 5 plays 4	1 plays 6 3 plays 7
3	11 plays 9, and 8 practices	2 plays 4 10 plays 5	6 plays 7 1 plays 3

Tennis Lessons 11-15 — Beginner level

Lesson Setup

Equipment

A posted team roster, tournament schedule, and team standings sheets (see appendix A)

A posted performance assessment rubric for the beginner level

Performance Goal

Students will play doubles.

Cognitive Goal

Students will use the team concept and follow applicable rules.

Warm-Up

Students will

1. Jog once around the facility
2. Complete stretches

Motivation

Announce that it's time to start a little competition. Students can see how well they learned and how they have to adjust when playing different people. Tell the class that you will assign courts and opponents. They should play as many games as they can in the period. Instruct them to tell you the number of games they win before they leave.

Lesson Sequence

Begin the tournament. Students without a court should be given an alternate—but challenging—activity related to tennis.

Review

Tell students to be prepared for a quiz on the next rainy day.
Ask if they have any questions.
Instruct them to give you their scores.

Assessment

Observations are based on the performance assessment rubric (table 10.3, next page). Further general assessment rubrics can be found in appendix B. There also will be a quiz (see page 312).

Tennis Lesson 1   Intermediate level

Lesson Setup

Facility

One tennis court for every four students

Equipment

One tennis ball and one racket for each student

Performance Goals

Students will

  review the grip, meet the ball on the center of the strings, and maintain a firm wrist and forearm; and
  do progressive warm-ups of their strokes—start close to each other and back up to the baseline after a few minutes of success at close range.

TABLE 10.3 Beginner Tennis Performance Assessment Rubric

STUDENT NAME _____

	0	1	2	3	4	5
Forehand	No effort	• Uses proper grip • Uses correct mimetics • Uses the correct side of the racket • Able to meet an object in the center of the racket five consecutive times during a self-volley	• Meets an object coming from over the net • Able to redirect a ball to a target five feet away after it bounces • Uses proper body pivot • Able to self-volley up and down 10 times	• Moves to meet a ball after the bounce • Able to rally over the net 10 times with a partner at 30 feet distance • Meets a ball with the racket head up • Controls the forehand wall volley three times	• Runs four steps or more and still redirects a ball to a target area • Meets the ball in front • Returns the ball with a volley • Able to rally 10 times over the net up to 60 feet distance	• Moves to cover a wide shot • Chooses correctly between a volley and a full stroke • Able to control depth or vary speed • Backswing and follow-through are complete
Backhand	No effort	• Changes grip • Uses correct mimetics • Uses the correct side of the racket • Able to meet an object in the center of the racket three consecutive times during a self-volley	• Meets an object coming from over the net • Able to redirect a ball to a target five feet away after it bounces • Uses proper body pivot • Able to self-volley up or down 10 times	• Moves to meet a ball after the bounce • Able to rally over the net 10 times with a partner at 30 feet distance • Meets a ball with the racket head up • Controls the backhand wall volley three times	• Runs four steps or more and still redirects a ball toward a target • Meets the ball in front • Returns the ball with a volley • Able to rally 10 times over the net up to 60 feet of distance	• Moves easily to cover the back-hand side • Is equally profi-cient with a volley and a full stroke • Able to control depth • Able to vary speed • Backswing and follow-through are complete
Serve	No effort	• Uses correct mimetics • Uses a correct grip • Gets a ball over the net from a self-toss	• Occasionally able to put a ball in play • Able to direct the ball on the diagonal	• Consistently able to direct the ball diagonally • Serves reach the service box more often than not	• Serves from off the court • Puts the ball in play legally more often than not	• Is consistent • Is starting to vary speed or depth • Shows sign of strategic place-ment

Cognitive Goals

Students will

review the reasons for a low-to-high swing—reduce errors and get topspin;
remember that every ball they send out is a point for the other side;
learn to value steady play; and
learn to be responsible for getting and returning their own equipment.

Lesson Safety

Each couple should practice on half the width of a full court.
Each couple on the court should be rallying from the same general position in relation to the net.

Warm-Up

Students will

1. Jog around the playing area
2. Practice mimetics for the backhand, forehand, serve, and volley:
   - First do the movement pattern of the stroke alone
   - Then add the footwork
   - Repeat 10 times for each, making sure that
     the racket head is positioned properly at the backswing, contact point, and follow-through;
     the motion is smooth and unforced; and
     the motion is ended by returning to the waiting position

Motivation

Tell students that they will take just a few days for practice and then will be playing their own tournament. Suggest they make the practice count.

Lesson Sequence

1. Review the grip, preparation (footwork and racket-head positioning), and follow-through.
2. Review and demonstrate the beginning of the control drill and allow practice:
   - Encourage consecutive hits
   - If practice partners' shots go beyond the target, attempt to keep the ball in play with a volley.
   - Keeping the ball in play
3. Make the control drill into a contest, asking the following:
   - Who can get to 10 first?
   - Who can get the highest number of consecutive taps without an error?
4. Progressively move students back until they reach the baseline.

Review

If a player's ball is going into the net, review with the class what the problem could be and how it should be fixed.

Ask why it is important to be able to keep the ball on the court.

Discuss at what time players should take their backswing.

Ask if it's better to drop the racket head for a low ball or to bend their knees so they can get under the ball.

Assessment

It is important to gauge the progress of the class. When students as a whole are having little or no trouble controlling a short rally and can maintain that rally for 10 strokes, they are ready to move back. If that is not true, do not move them back. If the class progress is slow, spend more time on this lesson. If there is a good number of students ready to move on after one lesson, while others are not, group them together on their own court and permit that court to gradually move back to the baseline.

Tennis Lesson 2 — Intermediate level

Performance Goals

Students will

practice the serve (more than 30 serves per student),
practice volleying at the net, and
get and return their own equipment.

Cognitive Goals

Students will

review service rules,
learn to meet the ball out in front with a firm wrist for volleys, and
seek steadiness.

Warm-Up

Students will

1. Jog around the playing area with the tennis racket in the waiting position
2. Practice mimetics—a full swing and its footwork:
   • The footwork and preparation for a *volley*
   • The *service motion*:
      Make a smooth service motion without hitting the ball (using the racket)
      Toss with the weight shift and the racket backswing
      Swing to a full extension to reach the imaginary ball at the height of the toss
      Complete the follow-through, allowing the shoulder to turn and the weight to come over the front foot
      Do the whole serve, from the imaginary toss and backswing to the follow-through so it becomes one smooth, flowing motion.

Motivation

Announce that doubles play will begin in the next day's lesson. Suggest that students think about who they want as partners and that they practice with them today. They have learned all the necessary skills—being able to put the ball into play with a serve, being able to return the serve using little or no backswing, meeting the ball during a rally and sending it back over the net, and being able to volley the ball while up at the net. By the end of this lesson, they will have practiced all the things necessary to enjoy their game.

Lesson Sequence

1. Review, demonstrate, and have students practice the serve, breaking it down with mimetics first.
2. Have students divide up all the balls and bring them to one side of the tennis courts:
   - Have them serve all the balls to the closest diagonal service box (as seen in figure 10.11).
   - When all balls have been served, have the group retrieve them.
   - On the other side of the net, have them set up and serve all the balls again.
   - They should do this until everyone has had 30 or more serves.
3. Review and demonstrate the essential features of a good volley (no backswing, in waiting position with the racket head up front, a firm wrist, and eyes on the ball):
   - Have students practice volleying to each other's forehand.
   - Then switch to backhand.
   - Then see if they can move from a forehand to a backhand volley.

Review

Ask the class to demonstrate the waiting position for a net player preparing to volley at the net.

Ask for a demonstration of the service motion.

If a player goes for a big first serve and misses, review what she should do on the second serve when she plays a game and why.

Discuss from what side of the court one must serve first.

If the ball touches the line dividing the service boxes, review whether it is good.

Ask if any server can continue to serve from her favorite side of the court.

Teacher Homework

Create doubles teams based on students' abilities.

Tennis Lesson 3 — Intermediate level

Lesson Setup

Equipment

A can of balls for each court
A blank round-robin roster sheet
A clipboard and pen or pencil

Performance Goal

Students will play a doubles practice game with their tournament teammate by their side.

Cognitive Goals

Students will review the following:

- Scoring for a game, set, and match
- The rules for receiving serve
- Court courtesy
- How to identify their balls from those of other courts
- Clearing their court of balls before each point and properly returning balls that are not theirs

Warm-Up

Students will

1. Complete a control drill for volley and short game
2. Practice a rally from the baseline
3. Complete five practice serves

Motivation

Explain to the class that playing with a teammate leads to new concerns—how to divide up the responsibility of the court, who should serve first, who should receive in the deuce box or the ad box.

Also, once students get into a game, they want to make sure that they use the same balls and that they return balls that land up on their court to the balls' owners. Go over how to begin game play and what is expected on a public court.

Lesson Sequence

1. Explain about cans of balls:
   - Each court comes out with its own can of balls.
   - Each can has its own identifying marks (such as Penn 3 or Wilson 2).
   - It is proper to
     - clear the court of balls lying around, for safety reasons; and
     - return balls that are not one's own by sending them back to their owners so they get there on one bounce.
2. Review the receiving rules.
3. Announce tournament partners, and send teams to the courts to begin doubles play.

Review

Ask if the class has any questions.
Go over common problems that you may have witnessed

Assessment

Observe for the following:

Ball control
Common group problems that should be addressed to the class
Individual hints that should be shared privately

Tennis Lesson 4   Intermediate level

Lesson Setup

Equipment

A portable blackboard, magnetic board, or variety of charts and diagrams

Performance Goal

Students will play doubles.

Cognitive Goals

Students will

learn what strategies there are for doubles and their rationale:
- Hitting the ball down the middle unless one has an opening
- Doubles is a game of angles
- Avoid hitting to the other team's net person
- Poaching—the net player moves over to cut off a ball going to his partner and volleys the ball back onto the other court
learn some general ideas for responding to a returning shot down the middle that splits both players:
- The forehand takes the shot.
- The person who just played the ball is the one most natural to play the shot down the middle.

Warm-Up

Students will

1. Complete a control drill for volley and short game
2. Practice a rally from the baseline
3. Complete five practice serves

Motivation

Confusion is the worst enemy of one's opponent. It prevents the other team from playing well together. Ask students how they can try to confuse their opponent and how their team can decide not to be confused.

Lesson Sequence

1. Explain strategies:
   - Sometimes being steady and letting the opponent err is the way to win.
   - Going out and winning the game means placing opponents at a disadvantage or in a state of confusion:

     Doubles strategies that create confusion include hitting the ball down the middle.

     Strategies that place opponents at a disadvantage are poaching, using wide angles, and hitting the ball to the open spaces.

     Strategies that avoid puting one's own team at a disadvantage include
     - Not hitting the ball to the other team's net person,
     - Letting the forehand take the shot down the middle, and
     - Covering one's own zone on the court.
2. Assign students to their own courts and have them begin doubles play.

Review

Ask students how many hit a shot down the middle.
Ask how many anticipated the shot and prevented it from becoming a winner.
Discuss whether anyone poached.

Teacher Homework

Create a master schedule of doubles games and post it.

Tennis Lesson 5   Intermediate level

Lesson Setup

Equipment

A round-robin team roster and game schedule (see appendix A)
A pen or pencil

Performance Goals

Students will

play doubles in a competitive situation, and
rotate sides after every odd game is over.

Cognitive Goals

Students will learn

how to deal with their own eagerness when playing in games that count, and to consider planning strategies before beginning a match, such as
- who serves first, and
- what side of the court they should try to take.

Warm-Up

Students will

1. Complete a control drill for a volley and short game
2. Practice a rally from the baseline
3. Complete five practice serves

Motivation

Announce that the class should be ready for the games to start counting. Tell students that if they run into problems, you will be nearby and they should just call out. But they should remember that real tennis tournaments, except for Davis Cup competitions, do not allow coaches to speak with or advise players or interfere with play, so for the most part, they will have to learn to solve their problems themselves.

Lesson Sequence

1. Assign courts and opponents.
2. Go over how to determine who serves first, both which team and which player.
3. Teach that the team not serving first gets their choice of sides. Teach students to pay attention to the sun's location when making this decision.

Review

Ask the class if anyone had points in which both partners went for the same ball.
Ask if anyone had points in which no one thought the ball was theirs.
Find out who won.

Tennis Lesson 6 — Intermediate level

Performance Goal

Students will play doubles in a competitive situation.

Cognitive Goal

Students will learn more match strategy:

When to consider hitting the ball up
Who goes for a ball too deep for the net person to reach

Warm-Up

Students will

1. Complete a control drill for volley and short game.
2. Practice a rally from the baseline
3. Complete five practice serves

Motivation

Tell students that going down the middle takes away the opponent's angles so that it is harder for him to win the point, but it allows him to anticipate exactly what they are going to do if they do it all the time. Another strategy will be covered: lobbing. Show students how they can get the ball up without varying their stroke.

Wish students good luck outsmarting their opponents, and announce the standings after one full round of competition.

Lesson Sequence

1. Show students how to use the same stroke but get the ball up and explain strategy.
2. Assign courts and opponents.

Review

Ask if anyone tried to hit a ball over the net person's head.
Ask if anyone had points in which no one thought the ball was theirs.
Collect the game scores.

Tennis Lesson 7 — Intermediate level

Performance Goal

Students will play doubles in a competitive situation.

Cognitive Goal

Students will learn good behavior on the court when there is a disagreement in the score and line calls.

Warm-Up

Students will

1. Complete a control drill for volley and short game
2. Practice a rally from the baseline
3. Complete five practice serves
4. Complete stretches

Motivation

Tell the class that the worst repetitive behavior on the tennis court usually occurs when one team thinks the other gave a bad line call. Discuss whose ultimate responsibility line calls are and ways to resolve disagreements when they arise. Announce the standings after two rounds of the tournament.

Lesson Sequence

1. Explain the following:
   • Calls are the responsibility of the person on whose side the ball lands.
   • When there is a question, one should look for a mark on the surface.
   • If a player thinks a call is wrong, she should call for a line judge.
2. Assign courts and opponents.

Review

Ask the class if disagreements were resolved by finding the mark on the court surface.
Collect the game scores.

Tennis Lessons 8-10 — Intermediate level

Performance Goal

Students will play doubles in a competitive situation.

Cognitive Goals

Students will understand and value

the warm-up before beginning competition,
good sporting behavior during play, and
court courtesy.

Warm-Up

Students will

1. Complete a control drill for volley and short game
2. Practice a rally from the baseline

3. Complete five practice serves
4. Complete stretches

Motivation

Announce the standings.

Lesson Sequence

After the warm-ups and announcements, students will go to their assigned courts and play their doubles matches.

Review

Collect the game scores.
Ask if anyone has any questions.
Tell students that they should be prepared for a short quiz on the next rainy day.

Assessment

Observe performance standards (on page 311), which should be posted for students to see.
There will be a 10-minute written quiz (see page 313).

Tennis Lessons 11-12 — Intermediate level

Performance Goal

Students will play their last match, attempting to complete a real match, two of three sets in two class periods, against opponents most evenly matched with them.

Cognitive Goals

Students will

be reminded of what a tennis match consists of, and
learn to enjoy competition that is equal and challenging.

Warm-Up

Students will

1. Complete a control drill for volley and short game.
2. Practice a rally from the baseline
3. Complete five practice serves
4. Complete stretches

Motivation

Announce the standings before giving students their opponents.

Lesson Sequence

Assign courts and opponents whose success in the six rounds have been comparable.

Review

Collect the game scores.

Ask if there are any questions.

Ask students what type of play they enjoyed most—the kind in which it was easy to win, or the games in which they had to work for each point.

Ask if they knew that the USTA creates local tournaments that schedule teams of players on one's own playing level to compete against each other. Teams that are successful, whether beginners or advanced, have play-offs and go to sectional, regional, and national tournaments.

Assessment

Students can be assessed with the quiz on page 313 and by using the performance assessment rubric in table 10.4. Further general assessment rubrics can be found in appendix B.

TABLE 10.4 Intermediate Tennis Performance Assessment Rubric

STUDENT NAME _____

	0	1	2	3	4	5
Forehand and backhand	No effort	• Has proper body pivot • Has proper grip and mechanics • Able to rally inside the service box five times	• Returns a ground stroke • Able to volley during a game if the ball is not hit too hard	• Moves up to four steps away for the ball • Controls a baseline rally up to three times • Able to return serve	• Volleys are directed • Ground strokes are directed	• Able to control depth or vary speed • Uses complete backswing and follow-through
Serve	No effort	• Uses correct mechanics • Toss is above the head • Able to direct the ball on a diagonal	• Occasionally able to put the ball in play • Serves from the correct place on the court	• Usually puts the ball in play • First serve reaches the service box one of four tries	• Makes sure the first serve goes in • Serves deep into the service box • Sometimes the serve is a weapon	• Is consistent • Serves with power and depth • Shows signs of strategic placement
Court position and team work	No effort	• On the court promptly • Goes to the correct position for the serve	• Shifts in the direction of the ball • Covers most shots on own side of court if shots are in front	• Covers own alley • Volleys shots down the middle if they are close • Backs up balls over partner's head	• Will move to poach • Takes the ball in the air when it is overhead • Switches sides to keep the court covered	• Puts the ball away when shifting to poach • Comes to net at every opportunity • Recovers quickly if drawn off the court

Tennis Quiz—Beginner level

NAME _____ TEACHER _____

DATE _____ CLASS PERIOD _____

True or False: Read each statement below carefully. If the statement is true, put a check under the True box in the column to the left of the statement. If the statement is false, put a check under the False box in the column to the left of the statement. If using a grid sheet, blacken in the appropriate column for each question, making sure to use the correctly numbered line for each question and its answer.

True False

☐ ☐ 1. A ball allowed to bounce twice before it is returned has been put into play legally.

☐ ☐ 2. A ball landing on the line is out.

☐ ☐ 3. When meeting the ball, the racket should be gripped firmly and placed so the ball lands on the center of the strings.

☐ ☐ 4. The server begins each new game from the right side of the court.

☐ ☐ 5. It is a fault when the ball is served over the net and lands inside the diagonal service box.

☐ ☐ 6. The server is the player in the lead if the score is 30-40.

☐ ☐ 7. "Deuce" means that no one is leading and both teams need two more points to win.

☐ ☐ 8. Having "love" in tennis is like having nothing at all.

☐ ☐ 9. The volley is a stroke that requires a big backswing.

☐ ☐ 10. During an overhead serve, the toss and backswing should be done at the same time.

☐ ☐ 11. You are preparing to meet a ball on your right side when you pivot by stepping forward with your left foot.

☐ ☐ 12. If your strings face the ground, the ball will go up in the air.

☐ ☐ 13. The server serves an entire game until it is over.

☐ ☐ 14. A tennis game can be over in four points, if only one team wins all the points.

☐ ☐ 15. If the game score is 4 to 2, the set is over because six games were played and one player is ahead by two games.

From *Complete Physical Education Plans for Grades 7–12* by Isobel Kleinman, 2001, Champaign, IL: Human Kinetics.

Tennis Quiz—Intermediate level

NAME _____ TEACHER _____

DATE _____ CLASS PERIOD _____

True or False: Read each statement below carefully. If the statement is true, put a check under the True box in the column to the left of the statement. If the statement is false, put a check under the False box in the column to the left of the statement. If using a grid sheet, blacken in the appropriate column for each question, making sure to use the correctly numbered line for each question and its answer.

True **False**

☐ ☐ 1. The server who serves the first game of a doubles match does not serve again until the third game of the match is completed.

☐ ☐ 2. All games start with the server serving from the left side of the court.

☐ ☐ 3. The game score is 40-30. The serving team has five games to one game. The serving team can win the set if it wins one more point.

☐ ☐ 4. A receiver who begins play in the deuce box must receive only the serves directed to the box that's on the right side of the court.

☐ ☐ 5. The most confusing shot in doubles play is the shot that splits the teammates and goes down the middle.

☐ ☐ 6. A volley is a skill that does not allow the ball to bounce and requires the person to meet the ball with no backswing.

☐ ☐ 7. "Deuce" means that no one is leading and both teams need two more points to win.

☐ ☐ 8. A shot that lands 1/16 on the line and 15/16 off the line is still good.

☐ ☐ 9. If you want to put a hard-hitting ball on the court the most often, brush the ball from low to high as you swing.

☐ ☐ 10. During an overhead serve, the toss should be over and behind your head instead of over and in front of your head.

☐ ☐ 11. Poaching is when the net person runs over to cut off a ball meant for her partner.

☐ ☐ 12. To hit a lob, your racket strings should face the sky while you follow through.

☐ ☐ 13. Any player can hit any ball in tennis as long as the serve has been returned by the proper receiver.

☐ ☐ 14. A score of "ad-in" means that the server is about to win the game and the receiver needs three points in a row to win it instead.

☐ ☐ 15. It is discourteous to run onto someone's court to get your ball.

From *Complete Physical Education Plans for Grades 7–12* by Isobel Kleinman, 2001, Champaign, IL: Human Kinetics.

Tennis Answer Key—Beginner level

1. F. The rules require that the ball be returned on one bounce or less.
2. F. The line or any part of it is considered good.
3. T. While the ball can be hit without a firm wrist and off center, this is the best way to meet the ball.
4. T. All games start from the right side of the slash mark.
5. F. The serve must pass over the net and land inside or on the lines of the diagonal service box.
6. F. Since the server's score is always said first, a score of 30-40 means the receiving team leads.
7. T. Deuce is another word for a tied score and means a player only needs two more points to win.
8. T. Love means zero in tennis.
9. F. The volley will be ruined if a backswing is taken.
10. T. The backswing and toss should occur at the same time.
11. T. The left foot should be the forwardmost foot when hitting a ball on the right side.
12. F. Strings that face down to the ground cause the ball to go down to the ground.
13. T. The server must complete the service game he starts.
14. T. 15, 30, 40, game.
15. F. A set requires that one team win at least six games and be ahead by two.

Tennis Answer Key—Intermediate level

1. F. Each of four doubles players must serve a complete game before anyone can serve again. The first server won't serve again until the fifth game.
2. F. Each game starts from the right.
3. T. If the serving team wins, it will have six games.
4. T. Players cannot switch sides for return of serve once the game begins. The deuce box is the "0,2,4,6" box on the right side of the court.
5. T. Partners hesitate to take a shot they think their teammate is going after.
6. T
7. T. When the score is tied, either team needs two points to win.
8. T. Any fraction of the ball touching a line means that the ball is good.
9. T. The topspin of the ball will help it drop in the court.
10. F. The toss should be above and slightly in front of the head.
11. T.
12. T. The balls will go in the direction the strings face, which is up.
13. T. Court coverage is only predetermined for the service return. After that, any one can play the ball wherever they want.
14. T. To win, the receiving team will need to gain a point for deuce and then two more points for game.
15. T. It interrupts their game.

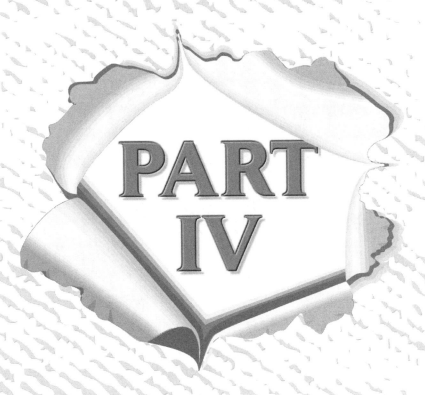

PART IV

Team Sports Unit Plans

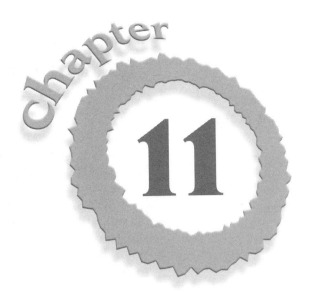

Chapter 11

Basketball

Unit Overview

1. Give a short history of basketball and its evolution.

2. Introduce a skill and then have it used in some type of game situation:
   - A pass—chest, bounce, one arm
   - A catch
   - A dribble—right hand, left hand, the strategy
   - A shot—inside: layup, outside, jumper

3. Teach rules when they are relevant to the skill being taught:
   - Illegal dribble—discontinued dribble, traveling, palming.
   - What happens if the ball goes outside the boundaries and how to put it back in.
   - What happens during a tie ball, or if the feet keep moving with the ball in hand.
   - Scoring.
   - Three-second rule.
   - Fouls when covering driving to the basket or defending against the opposition.

4. Teach court positions—center, guard, forward.

5. Prior to games, teach guarding and the rules against blocking and holding.

6. Teach defensive strategies—shifting, boxing out, double teaming, pressing.

7. Teach systems of defense—zone (2-1-2, 1-3-1, 2-2-1) or person to person.

8. During the tournaments, focus on offensive strategies and skills—cutting or making a quick change of direction, passing and going, pivots and turns, feint screens, picks.

9. As students progress, combine skills:
   - In catching: run to catch, run to catch and shoot, turn to catch
   - In jumping: turn to jump and shoot, jump to shoot

10. Each lesson should include some kind of contest and emphasize the point of the lesson.

Basketball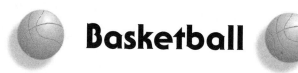

HISTORY

Dr. James A. Naismith invented basketball in 1891 in Springfield, Massachusetts. In the beginning, a peach basket was used as the hoop. A year later, Senda Berenson Abbott adapted Naismith's rules for women at Smith College. By 1932, things changed drastically for basketball when eight national federations founded the International Basketball Federation in Switzerland. Fourteen years later the National Basketball Association began. Then, in 1997, women began their own professional league, the Women's National Basketball Association.

FUN FACTS

→ In 1962, Wilt Chamberlain scored 100 points in a single game.

→ Basketball is played by more than 400 million people.

→ Today, there are 208 national federations for basketball.

→ Men at the University of California–Los Angeles won the National College Athletic Association (NCAA) Championship for seven consecutive years from 1967 to 1973.

→ In 1982, Lorri Bauman from Drake College scored the most points in a women's NCAA Division I game, with 50 points.

BENEFITS OF PLAYING

1. You get a great workout.
2. You learn about the importance of teamwork.
3. You condition your leg muscles.
4. You can play inside or outside.
5. It's a lot of fun!

TIME TO SURF!

Web Site	Web Site Address
International Basketball Federation	http://www.fiba.com/
National Basketball Association	http://www.nba.com
Women's National Basketball Association	http://www.wnba.com

From *Complete Physical Education Plans for Grades 7–12* by Isobel Kleinman, 2001, Champaign, IL: Human Kinetics.

Basketball Unit Extension Project

NAME _____ CLASS _____

Equipment needed to play basketball

Item	Where you would purchase it (be specific)	Cost

Where you would play basketball

Please explain where in the community you would play basketball. Be specific.

Health benefits of playing basketball

Please explain the health benefits of playing basketball. Include how much basketball you would need to play each week to gain these benefits.

Reflection question

Do you think basketball is an activity you would like to play as an adult? Why or why not? And if you believe you'd like to play basketball, would you rather play in an organized recreation league, in pick-up games at a park, or in your own driveway?

Bonus question

Attend an adult recreation league basketball game and write a brief paper on what you liked and didn't like about the way the game was played. Add whether or not you'd like to participate in this league as an adult (include why or why not).

From *Complete Physical Education Plans for Grades 7–12* by Isobel Kleinman, 2001, Champaign, IL: Human Kinetics.

Basketball Teaching Tips

1. If students do not have sufficient noncompetitive practice time to learn and improve skills, so that 90 percent of the class is ready to move on, don't add the performance pressure of competition.

2. Students will come to you with a wide range of abilities, with many feeling that they are "no good" and no match for classmates with prior basketball playing experience. Size differences in the close quarters of a basketball court can be intimidating. As a result, consideration should be given to developing and encouraging the least experienced athletes to make realistic goals and meet them. It goes without saying that teachers must be vigilant that everyone has equal playing time.

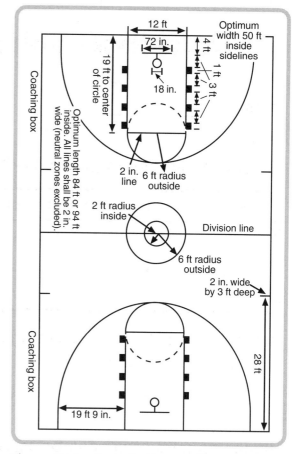

Figure 11.1—Basketball court dimensions.

3. The nonaggressive player and nonathletic player must not be overrun by the others on the team:
   - Teach everyone that they can score and under what circumstances.
   - Once the game starts, disallow the dribble until each team gets the idea of passing to the open person.
   - Coach the player who assumes point-guard responsibilities that his role is to set up the team, not just himself.
   - Make sure that personal fouls are called.

4. Every effort should be made for each student to have a location to play at each day:
   - Every student should be on a team and every team should have a court to play on.
   - If substitution is necessary because the class is too large, make it a rule that no one is out for more than five or so minutes.

5. Develop a short tournament.

6. Everyone likes to shoot a basketball, but surprisingly, not everyone likes to play the game. Too often, if their skills are not up to those of their classmates, they are made to feel bad. This problem can be avoided if teams are divided equally and the more experienced players don't make fools of the least experienced players. With teacher guidance, students who do not feel quick enough or accurate enough to make a team contribution will learn

that they can contribute, and the teammates who scorned them can learn to appreciate their effort and growth. Showing everyone that they can score is a good starting point.

7. If students are unable to participate fully in class activities, remember that they can be involved by coaching, officiating, keeping score, or conducting a research project.

Unit Setup

Facility

A full basketball court or a half-court to accommodate every two teams
Full and half-court playing areas should be marked with the basketball key, three-point shooting zones, and side and end boundary lines
Practice baskets, some of which aren't flush to a wall

Equipment

A minimum of one ball for every two students—practice and game balls
Stopwatch or wristwatch with a second hand
Scrimmage vests
Whistles for student officials
Clipboards and pencils for student scorers
Tournament charts and team standings lists (see appendix A)
Blackboard and chalk or markers

Unit Timeline

There are units for grades 7-8, 9-10, and 11-12. Each is broken down to include

four lessons to develop basic skills enough to enjoy a low-level game,
two lessons to work with new team groups in a cooperative learning environment,
six to 12 lessons for a class round-robin tournament, and
two lessons for quiz and assessment during a culminating activity.

Unit Assessment

The day-by-day assessment of whether the lessons are in tune with the class is dependent on the observation skills of the teacher. There is no need to teach all the new skills planned. Allowing a pleasurable development of essential skills, along with an understanding of how they relate to the game, is the most essential aspect of this unit. Teachers have to gauge their own emotional climate and decide whether to move on or slow down. Whatever is decided in terms of lessons, students should see the relevance of their skills acquisition in terms of how it helps them enjoy the game.

Students can keep their own record by updating the student portfolio checklist (table 11.1).
The assessment can be done objectively.

Quizzes appear for each grade level.

A detailed performance assessment rubric concludes the unit for each grade level. General assessment rubrics can be found in appendix B..

TABLE 11.1   Basketball Student Portfolio Checklist

STUDENT NAME _____

☐ Can pass and catch the ball
☐ Can dribble with either hand
☐ Can shoot and score
☐ Can play a game while following the rules of basketball
☐ Can jump to catch and can rebound
☐ Can follow a dribble by passing or shooting without having to stop the motion
☐ Can guard an opponent of equal ability
☐ Knows common violations and the procedure for returning the ball to play
☐ Knows what causes fouls to be called, their penalties, and procedures
☐ Has learned offensive strategies
☐ Knows responsibilities of guards, forwards, and centers
☐ Exhibits responsibility and good sporting behavior during competition

From *Complete Physical Education Plans for Grades 7–12* by Isobel Kleinman, 2001, Champaign, IL: Human Kinetics

Additional Resources

Goldstein, Sidney, and Dale Brown. 1994. *The Basketball Coaches Bible: A Comprehensive and Systematic Guide to Coaching.* Philadelphia: Golden Aura Publishers.

Krause, Jerry, Don Meyer, and Jerry Meyer. 1999. *Basketball Skills and Drills* (2nd ed.). Champaign, IL: Human Kinetics.

Marcus, Howard. 1991. *Basketball Basics: Drills, Techniques and Strategies for Coaches.* Chicago: NTC/Contemporary Publishing.

William, Joe. 1993. *Youth League Basketball: Coaching and Playing.* Indianapolis: Masters Publishing.

Basketball Lesson 1 — Beginner level

Lesson Setup

Facility

Clean, unobstructed wall
Baskets for every four students

Equipment

One ball for every four students
A stopwatch or wristwatch with a second hand

Performance Goals

Students will

be able to pass and catch a basketball, and
learn the lay-up shot.

Cognitive Goals

Students will learn

a brief history of basketball and its evolution,
what constitutes a good pass,
the effect that spin has on the flight of the ball, and
why lay-up shots are desirable.

Lesson Safety

Practice drill teams should be separated by a minimum of six feet.
Groups need their own baskets.

Warm-Up

Students will

1. Jog around the playing area
2. Complete push-ups and sit-ups
3. Practice full-motion mimetic of the chest pass
4. Practice mimetic for the lay-up shot:
   • Start with wrist action
   • Add arm motion, bringing ball up from waist to shoulder height to release of ball
   • Add the footwork—catch step, step-hop, and release

Motivation

Basketball is an American invention, developed in Springfield, Massachusetts. It is the only national sport that has worldwide popularity and is still dominated by the United States. Through the 1960s, the powers that made up the rules and set standards did not allow women more than two dribbles. They did not allow women to play whole court, rationalizing that they were not strong enough. Things have changed so much that now the games for men and women are almost the same. But there are still a few differences: ball size, for one. Now it's time to take up the game that everyone loves.

Lesson Sequence

1. Teach and demonstrate the chest pass and desired target:
   - Have students pass five times back and forth between partners from six feet away.
   - Increase the distance between them until they are comfortable at 12 feet.
   - When it looks like students are passing easily, have a contest (i.e., ask who can pass and catch 10 passes first).
2. Teach the bounce pass, discussing
   - the advantages and disadvantages of the bounce pass,
   - the distance from the target that the pass should hit the floor, and
   - an emphasis on the follow-through for a solid pass.
3. Demonstrate how spin affects the flight and speed of the ball.
4. Teach the lay-up shot and how many points a successful shot is worth to a team:
   - Review step-hop footwork and proper arm position as students learned in the warm-up.
   - Demonstrate where the ball should touch the basket for it to drop in. Figure 11.2 shows the easiest shot for a right-handed shooter.
   - Give students 15-second trials and ask them to identify their highest score.
   - Have the highest scorer demonstrate the technique for getting the most shots in 15 seconds.
   - Repeat the trials.
   - Have a lay-up contest—who can score the most in 15 seconds.

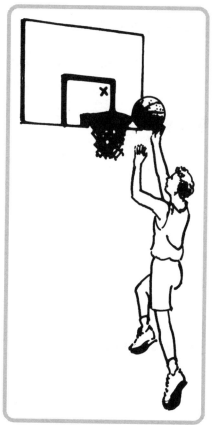

Figure 11.2—Lay-up shot on the right side of the basket.

Review

Ask students where the best place is for a teammate to catch a pass.

Review why they want passes that are quick and short.

Ask at what point in the throwing motion spin is imparted.

Discuss whether a ball thrown with underspin will go farther than one thrown without it.

Ask if a ball thrown without underspin will bounce back off the basket or drop down into the basketball hoop.

Review how one gets underspin on the ball.

Assessment

Observe each group's progress to determine how much of the lesson needs repetition.

Basketball Lesson 2   Beginner level

Performance Goals

Students will be able to

dribble, and
follow up the dribble with a pass.

Cognitive Goals

Students will learn

what constitutes a good dribble and its uses; and
why it is important for players not to look at the ball when they dribble, because it enables them to
- see the open person and pass on the move, and
- see the basket on approach and shoot from the dribble.

Lesson Safety

Practice drill teams should be separated by a minimum of six feet.
Groups need their own baskets.
Before getting students into the "dribble maze", make sure that all players have basic control of their dribble and warn the class that looking where they are going is more important than getting there quickly.

Warm-Up

Students will

1. Practice on-court with available basketballs during a free play period
2. Complete pogo spring jumps (like bounces generated by ankle flexions), sit-ups, push-ups, and stretches
3. Practice mimetics for the chest pass and layup

Motivation

Ask the class if anyone knows why the dribble is used in a basketball game. Which would be faster, a game that moves the ball ahead by passing or one in which it is brought down the court by dribbling? In this lesson, students should learn to dribble without being oblivious to what is happening around them. They will learn how to dribble so that they don't have to watch the ball. If they don't need to look at the ball when they are dribbling now, then once games start, they will be able to see the basket as they get closer to it and see if their teammates are open to get their passes.

Lesson Sequence

1. Teach and demonstrate the dribble.
2. Practice for familiarity:
   - Students should meet the ball at waist height and slightly in front of them.
   - Gradually have the students pick up their pace, making sure they continue to meet the ball at waist height.
   - Encourage students to look where they are going, not at the ball.
   - Introduce obstacles so that they have to look where they are going.
   - Gradually set up a drill pattern, which starts simply until it progresses to the dribble maze. Begin with students all going in the same direction (figure 11.3a). Change to a shuttle formation so students are dribbling from different directions at the same time (figure 11.3b). That way, they have to look where they are going instead of at the ball. Warn students to proceed carefully. (This drill works wonders for teaching students to keep their eye off the ball, for stopping their feet while they're continuing to bounce the ball to avoid a discontinued dribble violation, and, if you stop the group only for small hints, for increasing their stamina.) When students are doing well with two directions, add a third by having some students dribble perpendicular to the rest of the class (figure 11.3c).
3. Have students start using their weak hands for dribbling.
4. Teach a sequence to combine the dribble with throwing skills:
   - Students dribble to a zone and pass.
   - Students dribble to a basket and shoot.
5. Set up contests, using the dribble prior to each pass or shot.

Review

Ask students where their hand should meet the ball.
Ask them what their eyes should be looking at.
Review whether it's better to have a stiff wrist (to push the ball) or a loose wrist (to slap at the ball).
Ask if the ball should be pushed out to the side or in front and why.
Discuss the reasons for dribbling.

Assessment

Observe each dribbling skill to determine the best ways to improve it.

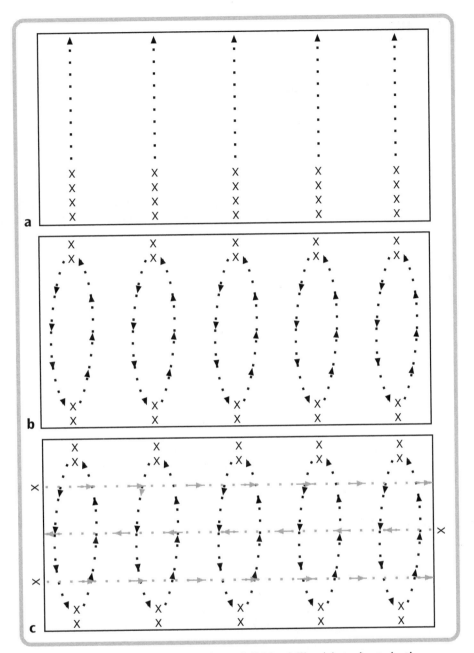

Figure 11.3—Three formations for a dribble drill—*(a)* students in the same direction; *(b)* dribble progression facing each other; *(c)* dribble maze.

Basketball Lesson 3   Beginner level

Performance Goals

Students will be able to

dribble and shoot, and
shoot from outside the basketball key.

Cognitive Goals

Students will learn

dribbling violations for palming, discontinued dribble, and traveling; what the basketball key is; and what an outside shot is.

Lesson Safety

Each practice team should have its own basket and a clear lane to basket from the opposite side of the gym. Special care should be given in instructing students not to interfere with the ball carrier's path to the basket.

Warm-Up

Students will

1. Practice free play on the basketball court
2. Practice footwork mimetics for the lay-up approach and shot

Motivation

Some young players get the ball, dribble all around, and lose the game for their team because they cannot win unless they score. They are so busy trying to get away from everyone that they use the dribble to do everything but get the ball to the basket. Let's discuss how to legally score points for your team from the dribble.

Lesson Sequence

1. Teach and demonstrate the legal step-hop for a layup shot on the right foot and the left foot.
2. Using every basket in the gym,
   • divide the class by the number of baskets so that each group is equal in size; and
   • one at a time, have students practice repeated lay-up shooting when inside the basketball key at 10-second intervals.
3. Have students practice using the dribble as an approach to the basket for the layup, beginning from the foul line, as shown in figure 11.4.

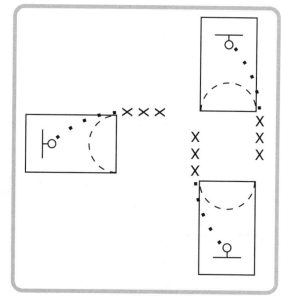

Figure 11.4—Dribbling from foul line for a layup.

330

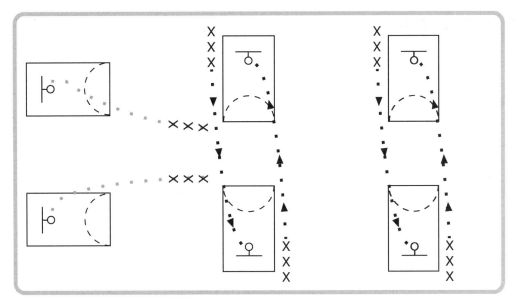

Figure 11.5—Gym with six baskets and keys.

4. Discuss dribbling violations and teach students how to detect them.
5. Set up a contest using every basket in the gym. Line up groups 50 feet from their basket, so they are traveling the same distance, dribbling, as every other group. Make sure that students wait their turns without interfering with the approaching ball carrier who is coming to take a shot (figure 11.5). Have students follow this sequence:
   • Dribble to the basket and shoot; do not come back until you sink a shot.
   • Dribble to the basket and shoot. If it does not go in, dribble to the next basket and try again—and so on.
   • Dribble to the basket and take one shot. If it goes in, your team gets two points. Come back, and let the next person go; keep the line going in turn until the whistle is blown. Then see which group scored the most points in the time allotted.
6. If there is time, teach students how to shoot from outside the key.

Review

Ask if anyone can explain their understanding of palming, traveling, and the discontinued dribble.

Basketball Lesson 4   Beginner level

Performance Goals

Students will

shoot from outside the key, and
improve their lay-up shots.

Cognitive Goals

Students will learn to aim and follow through while shooting outside shots.

Warm-Up

Students will

1. Practice the dribble
2. Practice shooting
3. Practice mimetics of footwork for the lay-up approach and shot

Motivation

If everyone on defense knew that a player would only shoot from the easiest location, what would they do? They would keep all their defense inside the key. How to keep the offense moving? Make them open up by learning to guard people outside the key. Why would they do that? Because people outside the key are scoring. Players need to learn how to score from farther away. Spend some time teaching students how to find their special place on the court, a place where they reach the basket easily and have enough control to score.

Lesson Sequence

1. Teach and demonstrate the outside shot.
2. Allow every ball you have to be used for practicing the outside shot the way basketball teams do, with some people under the basket returning the balls to shooters—no waiting turns, just getting the ball and shooting. Do not go ahead until everyone has taken at least 20 shots.
3. Have students make up the number of groups equal to the number of baskets:
   - Line them up on the opposite side of the gym from the basket they use.
   - Repeat dribbling and shooting drills they have learned to date.
4. Stop the class and reinstruct them to dribble to the position where they take their outside shots and then shoot:
   - Allow several trials, dribbling and shooting automatically once in position.
   - Vary it by having them follow up a miss with a layup.
5. Once groups are comfortable with the sequence, have them keep score for all their members as a team total in the amount of time allotted.

Review

Ask how many people scored one basket for their teams, and two, and three. Discuss how many points each shot is.

Ask students if anyone got in their way. Explain that in the next lesson things will be different and someone will get in their way.

Basketball Lesson 5   Beginner level

Lesson Setup

Equipment

Scrimmage vests

Performance Goals

Students will

improve their shooting, and
learn guarding techniques.

Cognitive Goals

Students will learn what denying a shot is, how to deny a shot, and why they should deny opponents' easy shots.

Warm-Up

Students will

1. Complete free play
2. Complete footwork drills—backpedaling, side to side, jumping up and coming straight down

Motivation

If players could shoot as well as the students have been shooting in practice, the typical game score for a seventh- or eighth-grade class would be about 80 points in a period. That is unusual. In this lesson, the players should try scoring with opposition. Someone will be trying to stop them from being successful. But the goal is not to prevent someone from taking a shot. It is to make the shooter take a difficult shot so that she misses, allowing the defense to get the ball.

Lesson Sequence

1. Teach and demonstrate body position, focus, and footwork for guarding an opponent.
2. Drill defensive positioning—moving between opponent and basket so one's back is to the basket:
   • Have students try without the ball.
   • Have them try with the ball.

3. Teach a keep-away game:
  • Create two teams for each basket (three to five players on a team).
  • Assign the *pinny* team to be the first shooters and the white team to be the first defenders. Shooters get two minutes to score as many points as possible. If nonshooters get the ball, they must try to use up the clock without shooting. Then switch the group that shoots, allowing those players the same two minutes to be shooters. Which scored the most when on offense?
  • Repeat, suggesting coaching hints derived from what was seen, making sure to give equal time on offense to both teams.

Review

Discuss what was different today when students shot the ball.

Basketball Lesson 6   Beginner level

Lesson Setup

Facility

Half-court areas marked with basketball key, three-point shooting range, sidelines, and endlines
Baskets that are not flush to the wall

Equipment

Practice and game balls
Scrimmage vests

Performance Goal

Students will play a game.

Cognitive Goal

Students will learn the rules of a half-court game (or a full-court game if the class has that option).

Warm-Up

Students will

1. Complete free play
2. Complete footwork drills—backpedaling, side to side, jumping up and coming straight down

3. Practice mimetics to rehearse jump to catch, as in figure 11.6—lay-up approach and shooting motion

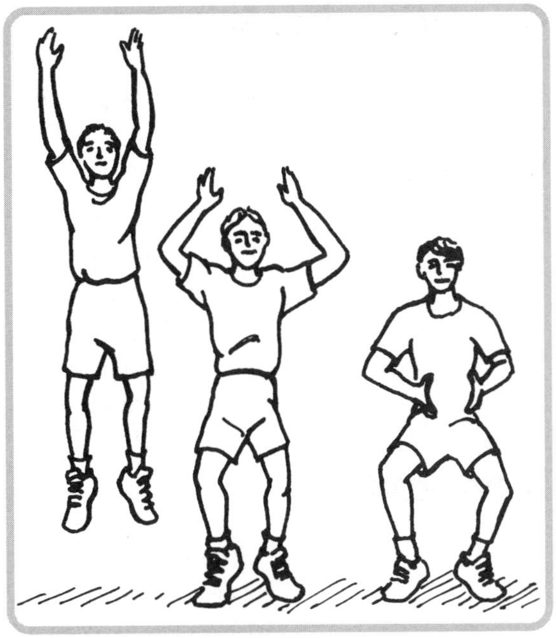

Motivation

You should announce tournament teams in the next lesson. But for now, teach the rules to be used in class (if you are playing half-court) and have students play the game in the same practice groups they've been working with.

Figure 11.6—Teaching rebounding mechanics without using equipment.

Lesson Sequence

1. Teach half-court basketball rules, pointing out the following:
   • The boundaries
   • When teams must bring the ball back, where, and why
2. Assign equally skilled teams to a court to play each other.
3. Have them play games. Use a halftime to answer any questions you haven't already answered or to share a class problem and its solution.

Review

Ask students why they have to bring the ball back in half-court basketball.

Discuss what skill needs to be used the least if teams are already near the basket they will be shooting for, and why.

Teacher Homework

Make up teams so that each is equal. Account for skill, gender, height, and speed.

Basketball Lesson 7   Beginner level

Performance Goal

Students will play games.

Cognitive Goals

Students will learn the tournament teams and play games with them.

Warm-Up

Students will

1. Complete free play followed by stretches
2. Complete footwork drills—backpedaling, side to side, jumping up and coming straight down
3. Practice mimetics: jumping to catch, lay-up approach, shooting motion

Motivation

Come to this lesson with the teams created, making them as even as possible. Explain to the class that you've tried to make every team with someone tall on it, with someone who dribbles fairly well, with a good shooter or two or three. You have had days to watch all the students and have really thought about how to divide them up. In short, they should learn how to take advantage of the skills that each player possesses so together they can win.

Announce the teams so that they can meet and start their practice games. Instruct them at first to play a half-court game without using the dribble.

Lesson Sequence

1. Announce teams and assign courts. Consider asking students to make up team names and use those names for keeping track of tournament standings.
2. Go over tournament procedure; the team getting the ball must wear a pinny.
3. Have teams begin with a no-dribble game. No-dribbling games force all players to look at their teammates to move the ball, since players can't move when they have possession of the ball. It prevents the ball handlers from hogging and dribbling endlessly. The shy, reticent player becomes needed and begins to feel a part of the team as soon as the second pass comes to him. And, it gets the players moving once they get rid of the ball.
4. Go from court to court, officiating or coaching.
5. Consider suspending the no-dribble game halfway through the period.

Review

Have the players pick a captain and co-captain. Once a team agrees, record the names.
Ask students if the dribble slows down a game or speeds it up.

Teacher Homework

Make and post the game schedule and tournament chart. Tournament charts and schedules can be found in appendix A.

Basketball Lesson 8　　　　　　　　　　Beginner level

Lesson Setup

Equipment

A team chart with captains' names, team numbers, record
A posted round-robing schedule (see appendix A)

Performance Goal

Students will play games while improving their skills.

Cognitive Goals

Students will

learn the strategy of "pass and go,"
begin to work as a team unit, and
learn what it means to be evasive and why it is important.

Warm-Up

Students will begin instant activity and free play

Motivation

On a crowded court, or against a very good opponent, it is difficult to get open. In this lesson, students will play the first round of the tournament, and they will need to get free so they can score. There is a simple trick that makes a player's opponents watch the ball instead of the player, so that she can get free. It is called "pass and go." It is not very hard, it's just that when the ball is passed, most people want to look at it. If a guard is covering a passer, where will the guard's attention be focused when the ball is passed? Here's what she can do.

Lesson Sequence

1. Have teams line up in shuttle formation, as shown in figure 11.7. Demonstrate the pass-and-go drill:
   • Remind students that they must pass before they go so they avoid traveling.
   • Repeat the drill, using different passes and correcting traveling violations.
2. After traveling violations are under control, assign the courts and begin round 1.
3. Go from court to court, officiating or coaching.

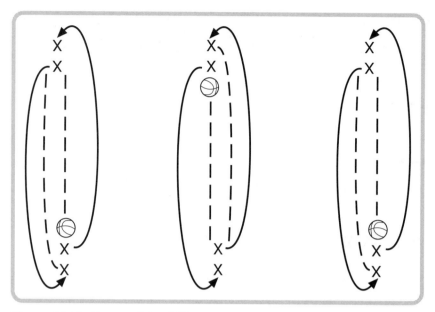

Figure 11.7—Pass and Go drill.

Review

Discuss general problems the class is having.
Collect scores and congratulate all students for their good efforts.

Basketball Lesson 9   Beginner level

Performance Goals

Students will

play round 2 with more attention to safety, and
play games while improving their skills and learning to work with others.

Cognitive Goals

Students will

learn to compete as a team, and
learn about personal fouls.

Warm-Up

Students will

1. Complete free play
2. Complete footwork drills, jumping, and mimetic drills

Motivation

At some point you may have told the players that their job, when they don't have the ball, is to make their opponents take shots that are not easy. This is done so players can rebound the misses. Sometimes players try to stop opponents from getting where they are going—and it usually works. But it is illegal. And because one usually has to physically hold someone or get in his path in order to stop him, it is dangerous. To prevent danger, basketball rules call those kinds of activities "fouls." Review what fouls are and how to avoid causing them.

Lesson Sequence

1. Gather the students together:
   • Go over fouls for charging; blocking; pushing, tripping, and holding; and a loose ball.
   • Explain that fouls are treated more harshly than violations and why.
2. Begin round 2.
3. Go from court to court, officiating or coaching.

Review

Ask students what the difference is between a foul and a violation.
Ask them the difference between a charge and a block.
Discuss general problems the class is having.
Collect scores and congratulate all students for their good efforts.

Basketball Lesson 10   Beginner level

Performance Goals

Students will

play round 3 of the tournament, and
implement penalties for personal fouls while playing their games.

Cognitive Goal

Students will learn the appropriate penalties for fouls.

Warm-Up

Students will

1. Complete free play
2. Perform sit-ups, push-ups, and stretches

Motivation

The previous lesson covered fouls and how dangerous they are. This lesson is about the penalties. People who play basketball cannot keep endangering the safety of others without some sort of penalty. Now it's time to start acknowledging penalties and awarding the victim his due.

Lesson Sequence

1. Have students gather around, and go over the penalties for
   - when the shooter is fouled,
   - when any other player is fouled,
   - when a team has exceeded the foul limit (you can set your own since the playing time is so short), and
   - when a person is responsible for excessive fouling.
2. Begin round 3.
3. Go from court to court, officiating or coaching.

Review

Ask whether anyone has fouled while shooting or pushed while dribbling.

Review how many people went to the foul line and took shots.

Collect scores and congratulate all students for their good efforts.

Basketball Lesson 11   Beginner level

Performance Goals

Students will

play round 4 of the tournament, and
try to incorporate "boxing out" in their game.

Cognitive Goal

Students will learn the concept of "boxing out."

Warm-Up

Students will

1. Complete free play
2. Practice shooting

Motivation

Although fouls exist, that doesn't mean that a player has to give up a position. In fact, because of fouls, if a player has position and is not violating any rules, she may keep that position. That is part of the concept of "boxing out." When a team knows that it is easier to rebound inside the basketball key, the players try to get there first and use their bodies to prevent their opponents' good positions to get the rebound. Have students spend a little time at the beginning of the period practicing taking foul shots while their teammates run in to box out. Ask each member of the team to take five foul shots before play begins.

Lesson Sequence

1. Stop the natural warm-up and demonstrate boxing out, using a group of three to demonstrate at a basket, as shown in figure 11.8:
   • Each person takes turns shooting a sequence of foul shots.
   • Nonshooters move into the key in anticipation of the ball hitting the basket. They take a wide stance and on the hit, jump to rebound.
2. Send students back to where they were practicing, making sure groups are of equal size, and allow practice of shooting and boxing out.
3. Have players stretch as a group.
4. Begin round 4 of the tournament.
5. Go from court to court, officiating or coaching.

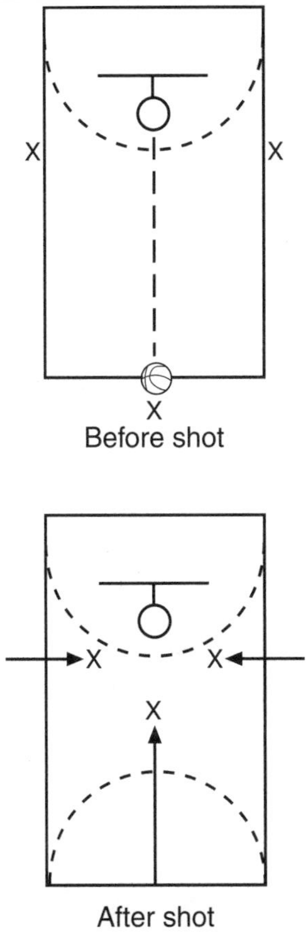

Review

Announce the standings, which players also can see posted.
Collect scores and congratulate all students for their good efforts.

Figure 11.8—Combining practice of boxing out and foul shooting.

Basketball Lesson 12 — Beginner level

Performance Goal

Students will play round 5.

Cognitive Goal

Students will learn the concept of setting up a screen.

Warm-Up

Students will complete free play

Motivation

Before announcing the scores and standings, bring up another idea that might help players score more. Talk about how when players look up to shoot, they may have someone bigger in the way trying to block them. To get the opponent to keep his distance so he cannot reach the player or the ball, explain about setting up a screen.

After that, announce the standings. Let the teams know what they need to do in order to change their standings.

Lesson Sequence

1. Demonstrate the advantage of a screen.
2. Begin round 5 of the tournament.
3. Go from court to court, officiating or coaching.

Review

Collect scores and congratulate all students for their good efforts, announcing their places. Announce the kinds of things that appear on the beginner's performance assessment rubric (on page 347).

Basketball Lesson 13   Beginner level

Lesson Setup

Equipment

A posted chart of the beginner's basketball performance assessement rubric (on page 347)

Performance Goal

Students will play round 6.

Cognitive Goal

Students will continue to learn what important personal goals they should have reached during the unit.

Warm-Up

Students will complete free play

Motivation

Round 5 of the round-robin tournament is over. Announce the standings at this time and mention how many games there are to go. Let the players know what a particular team must do to change its standings.

Tell the students that as they continue their rounds, you will be starting to grade their efforts. Go over what you will be looking for, and leave a list of those items posted so they can look it over at their leisure. Let them know that if they get out there and do their best, they should have no problem getting the full skills credit. Tell them that you are grading on how they assume a job for their team, not on whether they are a great scorer, dribbler, or rebounder.

Lesson Sequence

1. Go over the beginner's goals that appear on the basketball performance assessment rubric:
   - On offense, players should get "open," be able to catch a ball sent by a teammate, and shoot if open and close enough to hit the basket.
   - On defense, players should stay between their person and the basket when opponents have the ball.
2. Begin round 6 of the tournament.
3. Go from court to court, officiating or coaching.

Review

Collect scores and congratulate all students for their good efforts.

Assessment

Begin observing for minimum skills standards.

Basketball Lesson 14   Beginner level

Performance Goal

Students will play round 7.

Cognitive Goals

Students will

try to compete with thoughts on what they should be doing for their team and reaching the highest level on the performance assessment rubric, and
use a halftime to try to adapt their playing to their opponents.

Warm-Up

Students will complete free play

Motivation

Round 6 of the round-robin tournament is over. Announce the standings at this time and mention how many games there are to go. Let the players know what a particular team must do in order to change its standings.

Tell students that you'll start their games right away. In this lesson, you'll be stopping the players halfway through the playing period, not only to give them a breather, but to give them an opportunity to assess what they need to be doing to shut down the other team's scoring. You will be roaming around during halftime to give your perspective if the players want it. Tell them you'll be there to offer coaching hints and officiating during the games.

Lesson Sequence

1. Begin round 7 of the tournament.
2. Go from court to court, officiating or coaching.
3. Stop the game halfway through the time period for a two-minute rest or coaching time-out.

Review

Collect scores and congratulate all students for their good efforts.

Assessment

Observe skills for grading purposes following the performance assessment rubric.

Basketball Lesson 15 — Beginner level

Performance Goal

Students will play round 8.

Cognitive Goal

Students will continue to compete, using a halftime to try to adjust and turn things around.

Warm-Up

Students will complete free play

Motivation

Round 7 of the round-robin tournament is over. Announce the standings at this time and mention how many games there are to go. Let the players know what a particular team must do in order to change its standings.

Tell students that this is the last day of the tournament. In the next class there will be a short quiz, and then they will complete what play-offs they need to determine a class winner. Alternatively, you can let them make up their own teams for the final day of the unit. Ask students to raise their hands if they're in favor of facing their closest competitor for the final basketball game, playing with friends of their choice, or a battle of the sexes.

Lesson Sequence

1. Begin round 8 of the tournament or an announced playoff game.
2. Go from court to court, officiating or coaching.
3. Stop the game halfway through for a two-minute rest or coaching time-out.

Review

Collect scores and congratulate all students for their good efforts.
Remind them to bring a pencil for the quiz and about their change of clothing.

Assessment

Observe and record skills standards.

Basketball Lesson 16   Beginner level

Lesson Setup

Equipment

One quiz for each student
Extra pens and pencils

Performance Goals

Students will

complete a quiz on basketball,
play a game of basketball with teams of their choice, and
have a minimum of 20 minutes of activity.

Cognitive Goal

Students will demonstrate their knowledge of rules and basic concepts via a short quiz (on page 386).

Warm-Up

Students will complete sit-ups, push-ups, and stretches

Motivation

Extend congratulations to the first-place, second-place, and third-place winners. This is the last day of basketball. Tell the students to get with their teams and you will give them their court assignments.

Lesson Sequence

1. After warm-ups, ask if students have any questions about the rules or strategies before handing out papers.
2. Direct students to take their quizzes.
3. Assign courts.

Review

Recognize students who performed with excellence and explain why you thought so.
Indicate the students who made the most dramatic improvement, and congratulate all students for their good efforts.

Assessment

Complete the grading for the skills portion of the physical education grade in basketball. A quiz is available to test student knowledge of the sport, as well as the performance assessment rubric in table 11.2. For further general assessment rubrics, see appendix B.

TABLE 11.2 Beginner Basketball Performance Assessment Rubric

STUDENT NAME _____

	0	1	2	3
Shooting	No effort	• Has proper body mechanics • Has intentional aiming focus • Meets backboard	• Shoots when open • Has frequent success inside key • Developing outside shot	• Frequent success from inside and outside key • Follows up outside shot
Passing	No effort	• Has proper body mechanics • Is accurate to 10 feet • Has proper follow-through	• Pass arrives accurately • Passes to someone on the move • Varies passes: bounce, chest	• Passes to open person • Passes on the run • Pass arrives with speed
Dribbling	No effort	• Uses proper fundamentals • Begins dribble when moving	• Makes effort to keep eyes off ball • Switches hands or stop to defend the ball • Dribbles only to gain ground	• Rarely breaks dribble rules • Is developing both hands • Uses dribble offensively
Defense	No effort	• Attempts to stay between hoop and opponent • Uses hands to block ball	• Anticipates change of direction • Attempts rebounds • Jumps to block shots	• Goes to person or position on change of possession • Does not allow open shots
Teamwork and sporting behavior	No effort	• Gets to court on time • Gets along with teammates • Hogs ball or blames others	• Tries to play within rules • Does not hog ball • Makes effort to improve weaknesses	• Leads team constructively • Plays within the rules • Is the go-to person

---

Basketball Lesson 1 — Intermediate level

Lesson Setup

Facility

A large area of cleared floor space
One basket for every four players

Equipment

One basketball for every four students
Stopwatch or wristwatch with a second hand

Performance Goal

Students will review skills for lay-up shooting, the pivot turn, and the dribble.

Cognitive Goals

Students will

review the rules of the dribble, and
learn the purpose of the dribble.

Lesson Safety

During the lay-up drill, have only one ball at each basket at a time.
Basketball generally takes place in a crowded court space. This lesson should train students to be aware of where they are going. Be especially cautious to keep encouraging that dribblers look where they are going as you create the dribble maze. If you are unsure, see Basketball Lesson 2 in the Beginner section where the dribble maze is introduced.
Once the dribble to lay-up shot drill is used, limit basketballs to the number of baskets and have groups line up equally behind each ball.

Warm-Up

Students will

1. Run to a two-step stop
2. Pivot on the left foot, pivot on the right foot
3. Practice mimetic for a lay-up shot: arm and step-hop footwork

Motivation

The main reason some people grow to hate playing basketball is that they get hurt. Sometimes the hurt is not always physical—it could be the "know-it-all" teammate who hogs the ball and makes a person feel like she cannot make a contribution. Anyone who thinks she cannot make a contribution to her team has not taken the time to understand the game and learn the fundamentals. In this lesson, students should learn that everyone is capable of getting the ball in the basket. Start with the lay-up shot and discuss where players have to place the ball.

Lesson Sequence

1. Teach and demonstrate the desired target for the lay-up shot:
   - Have students take two or three shots each.
   - Demonstrate the effect of spin.
   - Ask students how many baskets they can sink in 10 seconds. Let each person at each basket have a 10-second trial.
   - Have the most successful shooter demonstrate his successful technique to the class.
   - Try again, giving everyone a few more 10-second turns.
2. Review the essentials of the dribble:
   - Set up a dribble drill, creating new reminders as they go. Tell players to
     meet the ball at their waist,
     push the ball out in front of them,
     use their weaker hands, and
     look where they are going.
   - As you improve their attention, add obstacles until you have the full-blown dribble maze drill:
     Have half the class moving in the opposite direction.
     Stop the class and ask the extra-good dribblers to begin their dribbling from the side, so they are moving perpendicularly to the main lines.
   - Set up a drill that uses the dribble for one of its purposes—for example, have students dribble one lap around the gym, shooting a lay-up shot when they get to a basket.

Review

Ask students, if they want a ball to drop in the basket, whether they should heave it or let it roll off their fingers.

Review why it is important to be able to dribble without looking at the ball.

Ask players whether they and their teams can score when they are dribbling the ball.

Discuss the purpose of the dribble.

Assessment

Observe each group's ball control, making sure it is ready to move on to the next aspect of the lesson or even the next lesson. There is no rush; do not move on until 90 percent of the class look like they are making good progress.

Basketball Lesson 2 — Intermediate level

Performance Goal

Students will review outside shooting.

Cognitive Goals

Students will

learn the essentials of successful outside shooting, and
understand the purpose of the dribble.

Lesson Safety

Use every ball for the outside shooting practice. Set up one or two people to retrieve balls and feed them back to shooters, trying to avoid anyone running under the basket and getting bopped in the head with a ball. Once the scoring drills begin, have one group per basket.

Warm-Up

Students will

1. Run to a two-step stop, run to a stop and then pivot, reversing direction to run more
2. Practice outside shot mimetics—feet on the ground with arm action only:
   • Same arm action while leaving the ground
   • Same arm action once in the air
3. Practice mimetic for a lay-up shot: arm and step-hop footwork

Motivation

Some short players can't get fast break opportunities. Without fast break opportunities they rarely can get inside the basketball key without looking up to shoot and find towers of arms over their head blocking their shots. These players will love to learn the outside shot. It is the outside shot that will give them their most scoring opportunities in a heated game.

The outside shot has other advantages: up to three points if in the zone, keeping defense true so it doesn't clog up the basketball key, and making everyone a potential scorer. Instruct the class to work on it now.

Lesson Sequence

1. Teach and demonstrate the outside shot and how it will be practiced as a group:

- Identify the basketball key
- How to focus and aim
- Demonstrate the effect of spin
- Each student finds their "spot":
    Use every ball, feeding balls to shooters so they continue to get the range.
    Have other students dribble and pass the balls to the shooters. The shooters catch and immediately shoot, as shown in figure 11.9a.
    Move everyone to another place on the gym floor and have each student try dribbling to their spot, following it up with an immediate outside shot (figure 11.9 b and c).
2. Allow the number of teams as there are baskets and set up a competition:
    - Dribbling to the lay-up shot, one shot, team scores or not, returning to the line and keeping score
    - Dribbling to one outside shot and shooting; if a score, great, either way returning to the line afterward

Review

Ask the class which spin is helpful in shooting: the flat, top, or underspin.
Discuss whether the ball will fall short if a player uses too much underspin.
Ask players how many scored more than three baskets.
Review how many scored by dribbling straight to their outside spots and getting it in from there.
Find out how many were surprised that the ball dropped in for them.

Assessment

Observe each group's ball handling to determine how much review and repetition is necessary.

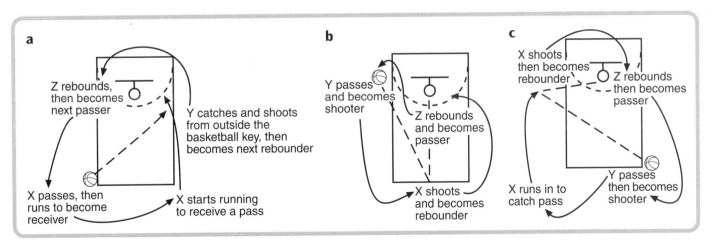

Figure 11.9—Shooting from a pass.

Basketball Lesson 3 — Intermediate level

Performance Goals

Students will

review how to successfully rebound, and
learn how to shoot foul shots.

Cognitive Goals

Students will learn

what causes fouls and why foul shots are awarded, and
the significance of a basketball key:
  • Where most points get scored
  • Timing their entrance into the key for rebounding offensive shots
  • The three-second rule

Warm-Up

Students will

1. Complete free play
2. Practice pass-and-go drill and dribble drill while in attendance lines,
3. Practice mimetic for rebounding and a lay-up shot: arm and step-hop footwork

Motivation

If everyone realized a missed shot might still result in their team scoring, would they consider scoring more often? It is true—but how? Rebounding is an art. On offense, it gives one's team a second or third or fourth chance to score, and on defense it prevents extra scoring chances. Of course, it is easiest for the tallest players, but good timing, good court position, jumping ability, and grabbing the ball securely are equally important. While not everyone will be the designated rebounder, there are many occasions for everyone to rebound. Discuss how to do it and how to have the sensibility to be assured of when it is a good time to take that outside shot.

Lesson Sequence

1. Teach and demonstrate rebounding by jumping to catch the ball while it's in the air:
   • Have students line up at a wall first, as shown in figure 11.10:
     One person throws to a wall target with underspin.

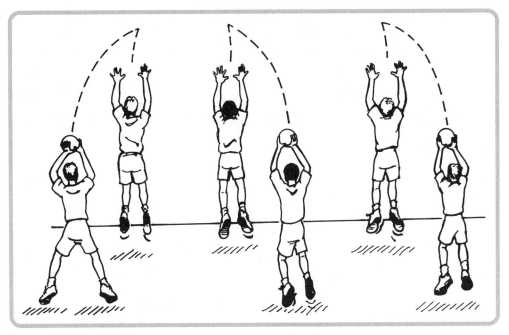

Figure 11.10—Learning to time jump for rebounding using a wall.

The rebounder jumps when the ball hits the wall, reaches up, and catches the ball, landing with the ball pulled down and feet spread apart.
- Repeat a few times, encouraging the reach and pulling the ball into the body.
2. Bring the group to the basketball key:
   - Teach them the three-second rule.
   - Go over the drill for practicing slipping into the key and rebounding the foul shot.
   - Have every student take three foul shots while the others rebound and lay up.
3. Line up the group somewhere else in the gym, have them dribble to the point where they like to take their outside shots, assume it will miss, rebound the miss, and follow up with a layup:
   - Set up a little competition:
       Give teams three minutes to score as much as they can, beginning with an outside shot.
       If the shot goes in, they get two points and return to the line.
       If not, follow up the miss with one layup; if that shot goes in, they get two points and return to the line.
       Each team keeps its own score.
   - Get the scores and allow the enthusiasm to build.
   - Remind the group that something is missing: defense.

Review

Ask students if they scored more points on the outside shot or on the follow-up layup.

Discuss whether it is better to take an inside shot or an outside one during a
   game, and why.

Review what a player should wait for if he is going to take an outside shot.

Basketball Lesson 4   Intermediate level

Lesson Setup

Equipment

Scrimmage vests for half the students
Whistles for student officials

Performance Goal

Students will play half-court basketball games using the "bringing back the ball"
rules.

Cognitive Goal

Students will review half-court basketball "bringing it back" rules and general
strategies.

Warm-Up

Students will

1. Complete free play
2. Practice mimetics
3. Complete calisthenics and stretches
4. Practice pass-and-go drills and dribble drills while in attendance lines

Motivation

Ask the students if the basketball games on television are full-court or half-court.
Discuss how they could duplicate the full-court experience if they only had two
baskets but wanted two games to go on. Go over the rules for half-court, the way
players can open the court, and how the three-second rule discussed in the
previous lesson would apply to a half-court game.

Lesson Sequence

1. Bring the group to a half-court basketball area and discuss boundary lines,
and half-court rules and the reason for them.
2. Go from court to court, officiating the three-second and "bringing it back" rules.

TABLE 11.3 Teacher Worksheet for Making Up Four Basketball Teams

	TEAM 1	TEAM 2	TEAM 3	TEAM 4
Tall—potential rebounding				
Good outside shooter				
Good ball handler				
Fast				
Lagging skills				

Review

Comment on how the students have played well and mention anything that they should pay attention to.

Tell them that in the next lesson they will learn who their tournament team players are. You will be dividing the class up so that each team has a natural at dribbling, someone who has rebounding advantages, and someone who is a good shooter.

Teacher Homework

Make up teams that are as equal as possible. The worksheet in table 11.3 will help.

Basketball Lesson 5   Intermediate level

Performance Goals

Students will

emphasize pass-and-go skills;
play a no-dribble, pass-and-go half-court basketball game; and
learn their round-robin tournament teams and play with them.

Cognitive Goals

Students will

review the purpose of the dribble,
learn the advantage of pass and go, and
learn the typical rules that poorly executed pass-and-go skills might incur:
• Traveling
• Holding the ball too long (five-second rule)

Warm-Up

Students will

1. Complete free play
2. Practice mimetics
3. Complete calisthenics and stretches
4. Complete pass-and-go drills and dribble drills while in attendance lines

Motivation

In this lesson, students will try to stop that automatic dribble reflex. The reason is twofold: first, when a player is playing a half-court game she is already at her own end, so her job is to get open for scoring. Second, unless there is an open lane and the ball handler is going to the basket or threatening to go, dribbling in half-court is overdribbling.

Lesson Sequence

1. Review and practice the pass and go, warning about traveling and the need for accurate passes.
2. Read off the tournament teams. Consider asking students to make up team names and use those names for keeping track of tournament standings.
3. Direct students to the court for no-dribble practice games.
4. Travel from game to game, reinforcing all no-dribble rules for the day and reminding students to go (as in pass and go) after they pass.

Review

Ask the students if they realize that they have a lot more scoring opportunities during half-court if they rely on the pass instead of the dribble.

Basketball Lesson 6 — Intermediate level

Performance Goal

Students will play a half-court basketball game with tournament teams.

Cognitive Goals

Students will learn

the job of the center and choose one,
the appropriate time to shoot (when open and close enough to hit the rim), and
that each player can make a team contribution.

Students will pick their own leaders (captains and co-captains).

Warm-Up

Students will

1. Complete free play
2. Practice mimetics
3. Complete calisthenics and stretches
4. Practice dribbling before the game

Motivation

Basketball is one of the few games in which one has to master offense and defense. Because it can get confusing and things can happen quickly, the necessary jobs are broken down. People become specialists at some things. Tell students how their team can take advantage of the missed shots and about the rules that are in place that will make that more of a challenge. How can a team take advantage of a missed shot? By rebounding. The rule? Three seconds. Discuss with the class the best rebounders in the national league, why, and what their job is. Talk about the center.

Lesson Sequence

1. Teach students about the center and how a team can and should take advantage of its center.
2. Direct players to the court for a practice game—dribbling allowed.
3. Travel from game to game, reinforcing
   - the three-second rule,
   - teammates waiting to take an outside shot until the center can slip into the key, and
   - the center learning to sense when teammates are shooting.

Review

Ask students where the most points got scored this class.
Find out how many rebounds their center cashed in on.
Request that students tell you who their team captains and co-captains are before they leave class.

Basketball Lesson 7 — Intermediate level

Performance Goal

Students will play a half-court basketball game with tournament teams.

Cognitive Goals

Students will

learn the job of the guard and assign teammates to the job,
be encouraged to shoot when open and close enough to hit the rim, and
continue to learn that they can make a team contribution.

Warm-Up

Students will

1. Complete free play
2. Practice mimetics
3. Complete calisthenics and stretches
4. Practice dribbling before the game

Motivation

Ask students how many like to dribble. Discuss whether there is such a thing as dribbling too much and how to tell when someone dribbles too much.

In a full-court game, the person with the best dribbling skills usually brings the ball down the court. Ask the class what position that person plays and why one person usually is doing that. Also review what the others are supposed to be doing.

In this lesson, the games will continue and the teams will be tuned up by assigning two people to another job: the job of the guards. Discuss that job and then have the students play with guards.

Lesson Sequence

1. Teach students about the guard:
   • Necessary skills—the dribble, passing on the move, outside shooting, fearless layups
   • Jobs—bringing the ball down, taking out, setting up plays
   • Fast break
2. Direct students to the court for a practice game.
3. Travel from game to game,
   • reinforcing all rules;
   • reminding guards to get the ball for takeouts; and
   • coaching guards to look for open teammates, force a play, and shoot from outside when the center is inside the key, nothing is developing, and they are open.

Review

Ask players to think about whether their guard set them up or hogged the ball. Tell the class that tomorrow is the last practice before beginning the tournaments.

Basketball Lesson 8 — Intermediate level

Performance Goal

Students will play a last practice game before the tournament.

Cognitive Goals

Students will

learn the job of the forward and assign teammates to the job,
be encouraged to shoot when open and close enough to hit the rim, and
learn that every team member has a job or role to play, and is responsible for
taking a job on the team.

Warm-Up

Students will

1. Complete free play
2. Practice mimetics
3. Complete calisthenics and stretches
4. Practice dribbling to shoot before the game

Motivation

There are five people on a basketball team. Two are guards who try to set up the plays and one is a center whose job it is to rebound the missed shots. Who remains? The forwards. In this lesson students will learn the role of a forward.

Lesson Sequence

1. Teach students about the forward:
   • Necessary skills—getting open, shooting, rebounding
   • Jobs—setting screens or picks, boxing out, rebounding
2. Direct students to the court for a practice game.
3. Travel from game to game,
   • reinforcing all rules,
   • reminding forwards to get open and take advantage of shooting opportunities, and
   • coaching guards to feed the ball to their forwards.

Review

Ask students how they feel about breaking down the court offensive responsibilities.

Review whose primary job it is to shoot and to score, to set up plays, and to rebound.

Let students know that the tournament will start in the next class. You will post their game schedules and the captains' names; they will follow the tournament schedule, with a new game and opponent everyday.

Teacher Homework

Create tournament charts. Sample charts can be found in appendix A.

Basketball Lesson 9   Intermediate level

Lesson Setup

Equipment

Post tournament schedules and standings (see Appendix A)

Performance Goal

Students will play round 1 in a half-court basketball tournament.

Cognitive Goals

Students will

learn the value of taking a halftime rest to reorganize,
be encouraged to do their own jobs the best they can, and
be reminded of the value of defense.

Warm-Up

Students will

1. Complete free play
2. Practice mimetics—jump to block, catch, rebound

Motivation

So far, you haven't said one word to the class about defense. Now that the students are in a tournament, it's time to discuss not letting their opponents run up the score on them. Cutting off the scoring legally is essential to getting a win. Before the players start their games, make sure they know their defensive responsibilities—who they cover or where they cover.

Lesson Sequence

1. Direct students to the court for the round 1 game.
2. Stop games halfway through playing time and ask the teams to solve the following:
   - Is their defense breaking down?
   - Are they giving up the ball to the other team without scoring, and why?
3. Allow teams some time to talk (two to three minutes) and then resume games.
4. Travel from game to game, officiating the rules.

Review

Tell students that their games looked great, but, unfortunately, there is always a loser even when everyone plays the best they can. Take this time to draw the players' attention to things you saw on the courts that if changed can help a team be more successful.

Ask the winning captains to see you on their way out so that you can record their wins for the tournament.

Basketball Lesson 10   Intermediate level

Performance Goals

Students will

play round 2 in a half-court basketball tournament, and
improve their learned skills.

Cognitive Goals

Students will

look over 2-1-2 zone defense and decide if it would be valuable to use,
take a halftime to rest and reorganize, and
be encouraged to do their own jobs the best that they can.

Warm-Up

Students will

1. Complete free play
2. Practice mimetics
3. Perform stretches

Motivation

Some very good teams are slower than others. As a result, they do not keep up their person-to-person coverage well and a player slips away. Leaving someone unguarded is dangerous. But students have another option, and this is a good time for them to lean it. They might want to take the old approach of "going where the fish are"—if they know where the ball carrier's team is going, they can get there first and be ready to block them when they and the ball arrive. If the defensive players are there, waiting for the other team, they can make shooting opportunities more difficult and be in position, ready and waiting for the rebound. Such a defense is called the zone defense. Show the class this defense before they play the next round. It might be the right thing for their team to do.

Lesson Sequence

1. Demonstrate the 2-1-2 zone defense by using players on the court:
   - Show where each player usually sets up.
   - Show how a team shifts as a whole in the direction of the ball.
   - You also might want to show, on the blackboard, the big hole in defense that occurs if someone does not stay in the team configuration.
2. Direct students to the court for the round 2 game.
3. Stop games halfway through playing time and ask the teams to solve the following:
   - Should they stick to person-to-person coverage or convert to zone defense?
   - Are their passes quick and getting to the player on the run?
4. Allow teams some time to talk (two to three minutes) and then resume games.
5. Travel from game to game, officiating the rules.

Review

Review the advantage of the zone defense.
Ask students which zone they learned in this lesson.
Ask who guards the top of the key by the foul line, who is in the middle of the key, and where are the forwards.
Request the winning captains to stand.

Basketball Lesson 11   Intermediate level

Performance Goal

Students will play round 3.

Cognitive Goal

Students will review the importance of boxing out and the use of screens.

362

Warm-Up

Students will

1. Complete free play
2. Practice footwork, shifting in the direction of the ball, keeping the same space between classmates
3. Perform stretches

Motivation

Before beginning this lesson's games, show students how they can use their bodies to prevent their opponents from blocking their teammates' shots, or, in other words, screening them from the block. Equally, they can use their bodies to prevent their opponents from getting into the key to get a rebound, called boxing out. Show this to the class. The screen is very useful when a team's shooters are constantly being denied. Boxing out gives a player command of the rebounds, giving her second shooting opportunities or taking opponents' repeated tries to score away from them.

Lesson Sequence

1. Demonstrate the screen and boxing out.
2. Direct students to the court for the round 3 game.
3. Stop the games halfway through playing time and ask the teams to solve the following:
   - Should they stick to person-to-person coverage or convert to zone defense?
   - Are their passes quick and getting to the player on the run?
4. Allow teams some time to talk (one minute) and then resume games.
5. Travel from game to game, officiating the rules.

Review

Ask if anyone screened for his teammate.
Request the winning team captains to stand.

Basketball Lesson 12   Intermediate level

Performance Goal

Students will play round 4.

Cognitive Goal

Students will learn what performance goals will be graded.

Warm-Up

Students will

1. Complete free play
2. Practice mimetics
3. Perform stretches

Motivation

Before starting this lesson's games, tell the class what you're looking for in the levels of accomplishment on the performance rubric (on page 369).

On offense, players should be able to score and move so they are able to receive a pass.

On defense, players should stay between their opponents and the baskets, and jump to block or rebound.

Mention to students that they are in round 4. Announce what the standings are after three rounds.

Lesson Sequence

1. Direct students to the court for the round 4 game.
2. Stop games halfway through playing time.
3. Allow teams some time to talk (one minute) and then resume games.
4. Travel from game to game, officiating the rules.

Review

Review what students will be graded on and why. Let them know the rubric will be posted so they can look at it at their leisure.

Ask students what they think you're looking for on offense and why—scoring, being able to receive a pass? Also ask about offense jumping to block or catch (a rebound) and positioning.

Request the winning captains to report you.

Basketball Lesson 13   Intermediate level

Lesson Setup

Equipment

A posted chart of the intermediate performance assessment rubric

Performance Goal

Students will play round 5 in a half-court basketball tournament.

Cognitive Goal

Students will review what skills will be graded.

Warm-Up

Students will

1. Complete free play
2. Practice mimetics
3. Perform stretches

Motivation

Announce that from now until the unit is over, you will be recording student achievement in class based on the performance rubric. Tell students to make sure on offense that they try to shoot when open and that they continue moving so their guard is able to pass them the ball. On defense, instruct them to stay between their opponent and the basket and make sure they jump to block or rebound. Assure them that if they get out there and do their best, they will have no problem getting the full skills credit. Say that you are grading on how they assume the job for their team, not on whether they are great scorers, dribblers, or rebounders.

Mention to students that they are in round 5. Announce what the standings are after four rounds.

Lesson Sequence

1. Direct students to the court for the round 5 game.
2. Stop games halfway through playing time.
3. Allow teams some time to talk (one minute) and then resume games.
4. Travel from game to game, officiating the rules and observing for skills.
5. Record skills checkoff after class.

Review

Take time to especially compliment a student for being the best guard in the class. Explain why.

Ask the winning captains to stand.

Assessment

Record student skills grades based on the learning standards reached on the intermediate basketball performance assessment rubric.

Basketball Lesson 14   Intermediate level

Performance Goal

Students will play round 6.

Cognitive Goal

Students will learn about the quiz coming up and have an opportunity to ask questions before it does.

Warm-Up

Students will

1. Complete free play
2. Complete calisthenics and stretches

Motivation

Mention to students that they are in round 6. Announce what the standings are after five rounds. Mention that this is the last of the round-robin tournament games. In the next class, students will have a short quiz (on page 387) and spend the remainder of the period playing whatever playoffs are necessary. Before beginning the games, ask if anyone has any questions about the rules, the positions, the strategies, or the penalties.

Lesson Sequence

1. Direct students to the court for the round 6 game.
2. Stop games halfway through playing time and allow teams some time to talk (one minute) and then resume games.
3. Travel from game to game, officiating the rules and observing for skills breakdown.
4. Record skills checkoff after class.

Review

Take time to especially compliment a student for the most improvement since the beginning of the unit.

Ask the class if the games raised any questions that they did not think of before they started playing.

Request the winning captains to stand so you can credit their teams with their tournament points.

Remind students that the next class will have a short quiz.

Assessment

Finish assessing the performance levels of each student.

Teacher Homework

Make sure that you have enough quizzes for all the students.

Basketball Lesson 15   Intermediate level

Lesson Setup

Equipment

Intermediate-level quizzes for every student (page 387)
Pens and pencils

Performance Goals

Students will

take a basketball quiz, and
play the last basketball game of the unit.

Cognitive Goal

Students will turn what they have been doing into written form by taking a quiz.

Warm-Up

Students will

1. Complete free play
2. Complete calisthenics and stretches

Motivation

Pass out the quizzes and tell students to do the best that they can. Ask if there are any questions before students begin the quiz. Games will resume after they are finished.

Lesson Sequence

1. Distribute quizzes after answering any questions. Have students sit on the floor to take the quiz. Collect quizzes when everyone is done.
2. Direct students to the court for their last basketball game.
3. Travel from game to game, officiating the rules and observing for skills breakdown.
4. Record skills checkoff after class.

Review

Continue compliments on whatever seems worthy.
Ask the winning captains to stand.

Assessment

Finish the performance assessment and grade the quizzes. Use the performance assessment rubric in table 11.4. Further general assessment rubrics can be found in appendix B.

Basketball Lesson 1 — Advanced level

Lesson Setup

Facility

A large area of cleared floor space
One basket for every four players

Equipment

One basketball for every two players
Stopwatch or wristwatch with a second hand

Performance Goals

Students will review basketball skills:

Passing and dribbling
Lay-up shooting
Outside shooting
Rebounding

TABLE 11.4 Intermediate Basketball Performance Assessment Rubric

STUDENT NAME _____

	0	1	2	3
Offensive skills	No effort	• Passes to an open player • Succeeds at an inside shot • Catches passes	• Scores when open • Passes or catches on the go • Developing a specialty	• Usually scores • Able to dodge opponent • Creates opportunities
Defensive skills	No effort	• Finds zone or opponent • Uses hands • Has legal contact with ball	• Stays between hoop and opponent • Able to break up plays legally	• Blocks a shot in the air • Rebounds if not guarding shooter
Court transition	No effort	• Is not confused by change of possession • Does not shoot at wrong basket or pass to opponent	• Has good anticipation of role change • Gets into new position quickly • Avoids fouls during exchange • Gets open on offensive side	• Leads directional change with dribble or leading passes • Creates legal changeovers
Team strategy	No effort	• Starting to learn position • Developing specific skills	• Fulfills team plan smoothly • Plays both offense and defense	• Has excellent skills to meet team role
Sporting behavior	No effort	• Tries to win regardless of rules • Blames others	• Tries to develop and improve • Works well with team • Violations are unintentional	• Plays within rules • Is a team leader • Helps others

Cognitive Goals

Students will

review the rules for and purpose of the dribble, and
begin learning to use all skills in a full basketball court.

Lesson Safety

During the 10-second lay-up drill, have students only use one ball at each basket. Basketball generally takes place in a crowded court space. This lesson should train students to be aware of where they are going. Be especially careful of reminding students that they must look up during the dribble maze.

Before the dribble to lay-up shot drill begins, collect extra basketballs so there is only one for each basket and have equal groups line up behind each ball.

Warm-Up

Students will

1. Complete free play
2. Practice mimetics for jump to rebound, jump to catch, and jump to block
3. Run the gym perimeter until the whistle blows, then using a two-step stop, pivot on front foot, to left and right without dragging foot
4. Practice mimetics for the lay-up shot:
   • Practice arm motion and release
   • Practice step-hop footwork
5. Perform stretches

Motivation

The students have played half-court basketball in class for years. You taught them the dribble but discouraged its use in a half-court game because there was no need to bring the ball down the court as there is in a full-court game. Players could dribble, but they didn't have to. Dribbling was taught as a way to go to the basket if a lane was open. And it would be necessary one day.

In this lesson, tell the students that you will make every effort to give them multiple opportunities to play a full-court game. Being able to dribble on the run, pass from the dribble, and avoid opponents who are pressing will be more necessary, especially if one has a slow team. Take some time for players to get the feel of the basketball again and tune up their skills. It may seem like a waste of time for those students who have played basketball all year, but others in the class have not had the same opportunities. Suggest that for every drill players use, if they are feeling comfortable with one hand, then they should use the other.

Lesson Sequence

1. Demonstrate the 10-second lay-up shot drill:
   • Divide the class so that every basket is being used.
   • Give everyone in class at least two trials.
2. Review the essentials of the dribble and do the dribble maze.
3. Set up the drill using the dribble to take
   • a lay-up shot, and
   • an outside shot.
4. Set up a three-person drill, as shown in figure 11.11, so students can move the ball up to shoot with no dribble.

Review

Review with students that the person dribbling should meet the ball in front and no higher than her waist.

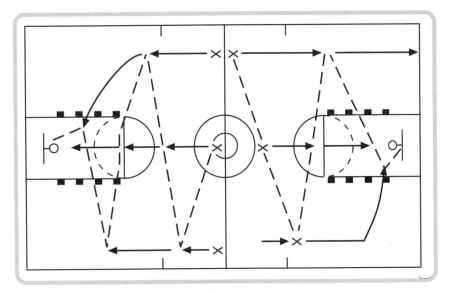

Figure 11.11—Advancing the ball with a pass.

Mention that the person dribbling should keep her eyes on what is going on around her.

Remind students that bouncing the ball takes more time than passing the ball.

Discuss how players can use their bodies to protect themselves:

- If they are right-handed and are dribbling, and their opponent is on their right
- If they have stopped to pass and their opponents are in front of them

Assessment

This lesson is chock-full of different skills, and you must observe to see if students need more time. If their performance is awkward they can benefit from an extra day. Make sure you do not move on until they are ready.

Basketball Lesson 2   Advanced level

Lesson Setup

Facility

One full-court for every 10 players, or
The opportunity to play on a full-court for half of the period and a half-court the other part of the period

Equipment

Scrimmage vests for half the class
Whistles for student officials

Performance Goal

Students will improve the skills of dribbling, shooting, and passing.

Cognitive Goals

Students will

review the difficulty of making the transition from offense to defense on a full court, and

learn what a *press* is.

Warm-Up

Students will

1. Complete free play
2. Practice dribbling, dribbling and passing, and the pass and go drill while in attendance line
3. Practice mimetics: jumping to rebound
4. Perform stretches

Motivation

Explain that the half-court game that students have played for the past few years is the game they want to play once they get to the other team's half of the court. What changes in full-court basketball from half-court is getting from one end to the other. Go over some of the problems that occur at midcourt, give students some solutions, and then start them in a game. Also look at the difference in mentality between offense and defense.

Lesson Sequence

1. Discuss the following:
   - The options for a pass rather than a dribble
   - The need for a team to set up before the ball arrives
   - The dangers of sluggish defense arriving after the ball and after the offense
2. Have groups get in fives and assign a court for full-court play.

Review

Ask players how many dribbled as soon as they got the ball.

Ask how many caused their opponents to lose the ball before they could shoot.

Start a discussion about separating the teams into guards, forwards, and centers.

Basketball Lesson 3 — Advanced level

Lesson Setup

Facility

One full-court for every 10 players, or
One full-court and the rest half-courts for every 10 players

Performance Goals

Students will

improve their transitions from offense to defense, and
play full-court games for all or part of the period.

Cognitive Goals

Students will

review positions and their roles during offense and defense, and
concentrate on transitions to defense.

Warm-Up

Students will

1. Complete free play
2. Practice footwork: backpedal, side to side, squaring shoulders, change of direction
3. Practice mimetics: jumping to block and rebound
4. Perform stretches

Motivation

The first thing that happens in unskilled games is that fouls occur more frequently. Everyone wants the same ball and as soon as someone gets it, unskilled players crash into the ball carrier. The tendency not to go back for defense is the biggest, most obvious flaw. Talk to the class about defensive responsibilities and how to avoid that tendency.

Lesson Sequence

1. Discuss the following:
   - The positions in a zone defense and when to take them
   - When to pick up an opponent if playing person to person and not pressing
   - The difference between charging and blocking fouls

2. Have groups get in fives and assign two teams to full-court play. If there are more than two teams, arrange for each team to play on a half-court and change courts to full so that they have equal playing time on the big court.

Review

Ask if anyone can describe the feeling of trying to shoot against a zone defense and what happens.

Find out how many players couldn't find their person to cover when the other team got the ball. Ask if they have any suggestions to make.

Let students know that you will be coming up with the tournament teams for the next lesson. They can continue practicing as a team, working to resolve team problems.

Teacher Homework

Make up teams that are equal in ability and player assets.

Basketball Lesson 4 — Advanced level

Performance Goal

Students will play full-court games for all or part of the period.

Cognitive Goals

Students will

learn the new tournament teams,
review offensive roles and their strategies, and
divide up positions among their new teammates.

Warm-Up

Students will

1. Complete free play
2. Practice footwork: backpedaling, side to side, squaring shoulders, change of direction
3. Practice mimetics: jumping to block, rebound, and shoot
4. Perform stretches

Motivation

This is the time students find out their class tournament teammates. It is a good time for them to get a sense of where each will fit in best and to start to get some sense of team organization. Mention to the students that most of them are not complete strangers to the game of basketball. Some of them may play on outside teams, and to fit that team's needs, they play one position. But if they are a forward on their outside team and here their experience and speed make them the most likely candidate to play a guard—should they continue to play forward here? Or, if here they are the tallest on the team, should they play center, even though their outside team has someone else play that position?

Lesson Sequence

1. Announce the teams. Consider asking students to make up team names and use those names for keeping track of tournament standings.
2. Discuss the following:
   - The overall skills needs of a point guard, the other guard, and strategies
   - The scoring success a team has if its center is successful
   - The role of the forward on getting open, setting screens, and rebounding
3. Give students time to get scrimmage vests and decide who will play what position.
4. Have them play full-court games.
5. Stop the game after about 10 minutes to consider position changes.
6. Continue the games.

Review

Ask if everyone is clear on their offensive responsibilities.
Review who tends to bring the ball down the most often and what skill that person needs.
Ask whose rebounding skills are a gold mine when it comes to cashing in on missed shots from teammates.
Discuss which positions have to think, "Get open and score, get open inside and score, score, score."

Basketball Lesson 5   Advanced level

Performance Goal

Students will play basketball games, in a full-court when possible.

Cognitive Goals

Students will

review all fouls on and off the ball,
review the penalties for fouling a shooter and a nonshooter, and
choose captains and co-captains.

Warm-Up

Students will

1. Complete free play with all equipment available
2. Dribble using the weak hand while in teams
3. Perform stretches

Motivation

Basketball has more players in a concentrated area than any other game that students play. Physical contact is almost the rule, rather than the exception. It is illegal, because it results in injuries and is the primary reason some students dread the game. Have the players take a look at their responsibilities on the court with an eye to penalizing body contact and learning how to demand skill from the play, rather than purely survival techniques.

Lesson Sequence

1. Instruct the teams to pick captains and co-captains before starting anything.
2. Discuss the following:
   - The types of fouls, how to recognize them, and their consequences
     Personal fouls and fouling out
     Team fouls
   - How many free shots are awarded
   - The procedure for foul shots
3. Have students play full-court games.
4. Stop the games after about 10 minutes to redirect teams on offense or defense.
5. Continue the games.

Review

Ask students if the occasion ever arose in which there were five team fouls and the other team was awarded one-to-one free throws, the shooter got two free throws, or a team increased its score because it was given free throws.
Ask the winning captains to report to you before they leave.

Teacher Homework

Make up the tournament schedule. See appendix A for examples of round-robin tournament charts and schedules.

Basketball Lesson 6 — Advanced level

Performance Goal

Students will play practice basketball games, in a full-court when possible.

Cognitive Goal

Students will identify how to set a *pick* and its purpose.

Warm-Up

Students will

1. Complete free play
2. Shoot and rebound foul shots with each team at a basket
3. Perform stretches

Motivation

Announce that the tournament will start in the next lesson and that you will take very little time to interfere with the students' games. It is time they use what they learned for their own gain. Tell them you will be available for advice and will officiate for part of the time in each of the games. Mention that they should find the tournament fairly easy to follow. They will meet one team a class. Their win/loss/tie records will be recorded next to their team or captain/co-captains' names. This class is the last practice game, so discuss how to use a pick so they can practice using it.

Lesson Sequence

1. Discuss and demonstrate *picks*.
2. Play full-court games.
3. Stop the games after about 10 minutes to redirect teams on offense or defense.
4. Continue the games.

Review

Ask if any team benefited from a pick.
Review what a pick is and why one would want to use it.

Teacher Homework

Prepare and post the team standings charts. Round-robin tournament schedules and charts can be found in appendix A.

Basketball Lesson 7   Advanced level

Lesson Setup

Equipment

Post tournament schedules and charts
One game ball for each game

Performance Goal

Students will play round 1 of their tournament.

Cognitive Goals

Students will learn the following:

How to follow the tournament chart and assume responsibility for arriving on
the correct court, choosing the ball, and getting scrimmage vests or pinnies
How to play with good sporting behavior

Warm-Up

Students will

1. Complete free play
2. Jump to practice blocking, rebounding, and shooting
3. Perform stretches

Motivation

Announce that round 1 is about to start. Ask the captains to direct their teams to their
courts and choose with the opposite team for who gets the ball first. Whoever gets first
possession has to wear the pinnies. The other team can choose the side of the court.

Lesson Sequence

1. Answer questions and then begin round 1.
2. Have students play full-court games, officiating for equal time on each court.
3. Stop the game at halftime and allow reorganization and change of basket.
4. Continue games until one minute before dismissal.

Review

Check if anyone has any questions.
Ask the winning captains to stand and report their scores.

Assessment

Observe each group. Use the observations to provide students with private suggestions and coaching hints.

Basketball Lessons 8-11   Advanced level

Lesson Setup

Equipment

A posted advanced performance assessment rubric (on page 385)

Performance Goal

Students will complete rounds 2, 3, 4, and 5.

Cognitive Goals

Students will assume responsibility

for daily expectations,
for seeking out or trying to make strategic adjustments to new opponents, and
for playing hard but exercising good judgment and sporting behavior.

Warm-Up

Students will

1. Complete free play
2. Complete calisthenics
3. Perform stretches

Motivation

Announce the round number and, after so many rounds, what teams are in the lead. Mention how many games there are to go in the tournament, and wish the students good luck.

Lesson Sequence

1. Answer questions and then begin the next round.
2. Have students play full-court games, officiating for equal time on each court.
3. Stop the games at halftime and allow reorganization and change of basket.
4. Continue games until one minute before dismissal.

Review

Check if anyone in class has any questions.

Tell students you are grading them based on the advanced performance rubric, which is posted. If they are interested, they can take a look or ask you the next time class meets.

Ask the winning captains to stand and report their scores.

Extend compliments to any deserving students.

Assessment

Begin observing for the performance standards spelled out in the advanced performance basketball rubric on page 385.

Basketball Lesson 12 — Advanced level

Performance Goal

Students will play round 6 while being graded.

Cognitive Goal

Students will hear what the performance-level standards are for each rating.

Warm-Up

Students will

1. Complete free play
2. Complete calisthenics
3. Perform stretches

Motivation

Tell students that they are coming close to the conclusion of the basketball unit, which means they soon will be getting a quiz. Inform them also that you are going to come up with a grade for them, breaking it down into how they play their positions on offense and how they assume defensive responsibilities. You will assess their efforts to do the right thing, even if their shooting or timing is slightly off on the day you watch. Tell the class that they can review what you're looking for by checking out the posting on the blackboard.

Announce the round number and, after so many rounds, what teams are in the lead. Mention how many games there are to go in the tournament.

Lesson Sequence

1. Answer questions and then begin the next round.
2. Have students play full-court games, officiating for equal time on each court.
3. Stop the game at halftime and allow reorganization and change of basket.
4. Continue games until one minute before dismissal.

Review

Check if anyone in class has any questions.
Ask the winning captains to stand and report their scores.
Extend compliments to any deserving students.

Assessment

Use the performance assessment rubric to grade or grade by team responsibility:

Guards—bringing the ball down, feeding the team, using shooting options occasionally
Center—getting into the key on offense and putting the ball right up again
Forwards—getting down before the ball, getting open, and taking open outside shots when the team is in position to rebound
Defense—positioning, preparing to jump to block and rebound

Basketball Lesson 13   Advanced level

Performance Goal

Students will play round 7.

Cognitive Goal

Students will learn to react to the pressure of competition with good sporting behavior.

Warm-Up

Students will

1. Complete free play
2. Complete calisthenics
3. Perform stretches

Motivation

Inform students that you will continue grading them. If they have been trying to do what they learned all through the unit, they should just get out there and do their best and have no problem getting the full skills credit. Let them know that you basically are grading on how they assume the jobs for their teams, not on whether they are great scorers, dribblers, or rebounders.

Announce that they are in round 7 and, after six rounds, what teams are in the lead. Mention how many games there are to go in the tournament.

Lesson Sequence

1. Answer questions and then begin round 7.
2. Have students play full-court games, officiating for equal time on each court.
3. Stop the game at halftime and allow reorganization and change of basket.
4. Continue games until one minute before dismissal.

Review

Check if anyone in class has any questions.
Ask the winning captains to stand and report their scores.
Extend compliments to any deserving students.

Assessment

Continue assessing based on the performance assessment rubric or on team responsibility:

Guards—bringing the ball down, feeding the team, using shooting options occasionally

Center—getting into the key on offense and putting the ball right up again

Forwards—getting down before the ball, getting open, taking open outside shots when the team is in a position to rebound

Defense—positioning, preparing to jump to block and rebound

Basketball Lesson 14   Advanced level

Performance Goal

Students will play round 8, the last competitive round of the tournament.

Cognitive Goal

Students will enjoy their last tournament game and learn how much they have improved.

Warm-Up

Students will

1. Complete free play
2. Complete calisthenics
3. Perform stretches

Motivation

Tell students that you have watched all of them and they have done a great job. Let them know that whether they win or lose the tournament, you are impressed with how each team learned to work together, how each player took up her responsibilities, and how some players have made amazing improvements. Tell them to enjoy their last tournament game. The next lesson will have a short quiz and then one last playing opportunity before concluding the unit.

Announce that they are in round 8 and, after seven rounds, what teams are in the lead.

Lesson Sequence

1. Answer questions and then begin round 8.
2. Have students play full-court games, officiating for equal time on each court.
3. Stop the game at halftime and allow reorganization and change of basket.
4. Continue games until one minute before dismissal.

Review

Ask the winning captains to stand and report their scores.
Extend compliments to any deserving students.
Remind students that the next class marks the end of the basketball unit—they will be taking a short quiz and then playing.
Ask them to bring something to write with.

Assessment

Finish assessing based on the performance assessment rubric or on team responsibility:

Guards—bringing the ball down, feeding the team, using shooting options occasionally
Center—getting into the key on offense and putting the ball right up again
Forwards—getting down before the ball, getting open, taking open outside shots when the team is in position to rebound
Defense—positioning, preparing to jump to block and rebound

Basketball Lesson 15 — Advanced level

Lesson Setup

Equipment

One quiz for each student
Pens and pencils

Performance Goal

Students will

Take a quiz
Play tournament games

Cognitive Goal

Students will measure how well they understand the game of basketball.

Warm-Up

Students will

1. Complete calisthenics
2. Perform stretches

Motivation

Let students know that if they sit down and get right to their tests, they will have at least 20 minutes to play their last games.

Lesson Sequence

1. Distribute quizzes as students enter class and collect them when they are done.
2. Allow students to decide how they want to play the last day of basketball and either
   • assign courts to play-off teams if play-off games are necessary, or
   • have students play pickup games.
3. Continue games until one minute before dismissal time.

Review

Announce the final standings of the tournament.
Announce the most improved player, the most improved team, and the most valuable players—and why. Find reasons to compliment the students.

Assessment

Do a cognitive assessment via the quiz. Finish assessing student performance with the aid of the performance assessment rubric in table 11.5. Further general assessment rubrics can be found in appendix B.

Teacher Homework

Grade the quizzes.

TABLE 11.5 Advanced Basketball Performance Assessment Rubric

STUDENT NAME _____

	0	1	2	3	4	5
Skills	No effort	• Finds ways to move ball legally • Selects appropriate times to shoot • Has stamina to play offense and defense • Is responsible for a position	• Makes fast and accurate passes • Jumps to rebound, catch, shoot, or block • Runs to get open on offense and to close in on defense • Stays between opponent and basket	• Shots from outside are not forced and are sometimes successful • Catches while on the go • Will not let opponent take an unguarded shot	• Is a scoring threat • Will get open • Has good defense with rare fouls • Anticipates team cuts and can pass to person cutting to inside	• Drives to basket to score • Feeds open person for score • Has developed an outside shot for score • Causes turnovers
Position and transition	No effort	• Concentrates on the play • Does not play expected position • Does not drop back for defense as necessary	• Tries to assume assigned position • Does not cause unforced turnovers • Attempts to get to the defensive position • Has stamina on both ends	• Changes direction as needed • Moves to cover defensive position • Plays offensive role • Plays person to person without unnecessary fouls	• Gets open on offense • Anticipates transition and tries to get there early • Executes full-court press • Switches from person to person or zone defense	• Creates turnovers • Slows down the ball on transition or gets to position ahead of it • Has skills to keep possession when double-teamed
Teamwork and attitude	No effort	• Blames others • Needs supervision to stay on task • Interferes with the other team • Tries to take over	• Gets to court on time • Warms up with team • Plays within the rules	• Works well with teammates • Plays within the rules • Takes responsibility for position	• Consistently tries to play at personal best • Recognizes good teammate effort and success • Exhibits good sporting behavior	• Inspires team • Backs up, not takes over, for teammates • Has reliable, consistent leadership • Assists individual team members to personally improve

Basketball Quiz—Beginner level

NAME _____   TEACHER _____

DATE _____   CLASS PERIOD _____

True or False: Read each statement below carefully. If the statement is true, put a check under the True box in the column to the left of the statement. If the statement is false, put a check under the False box in the column to the left of the statement. If using a grid sheet, blacken in the appropriate column for each question, making sure to use the correctly numbered line for each question and its answer.

True	False	
☐	☐	1. If you dribble to a stop in two steps, you are allowed to move the front foot as often as you like as long as you keep the back foot stationary.
☐	☐	2. A person who is hit by his opponent while he is shooting the basketball gets two foul shots if his shot misses the basket and one foul shot if it goes in.
☐	☐	3. A lay-up shot is worth two points.
☐	☐	4. When a team makes a mistake that is not a personal foul, the other team takes the ball "out."
☐	☐	5. If you want to rebound the basketball, you need to get near the basket and jump when the ball hits the basket.
☐	☐	6. Meeting the dribble at shoulder height is good technique.
☐	☐	7. To play the pass-and-go strategy correctly, you should pass the ball and stay.
☐	☐	8. When guarding an opponent, keep your eyes on the basket.
☐	☐	9. It is bad sporting behavior to stop an opponent's pass or shot from getting where she wants it to go.
☐	☐	10. For the best control of the ball, the fingers of your hands should be spread out on the ball.

From *Complete Physical Education Plans for Grades 7–12* by Isobel Kleinman, 2001, Champaign, IL: Human Kinetics.

Basketball Quiz—Intermediate level

NAME _____ TEACHER _____

DATE _____ CLASS PERIOD _____

Multiple Choice: Read each question and each answer carefully. Be sure to choose the best answer that fits the statement preceding it. When you have made your choice, put the appropriate letter on the line to the left of the numbered question.

_____1. What makes the job of the center difficult is
    a. dribbling
    b. blocking an outside shot
    c. timing his entrance into the basketball key on the offensive side of the court
    d. taking the ball out

_____2. A good guard
    a. uses the dribble to slow down the game so the team can get organized
    b. feeds the ball to the open forwards
    c. takes advantage of an open lane to the basket by driving in for a lay-up shot
    d. all of the above

_____3. The foul shot
    a. is the most practiced outside shot in basketball
    b. must be taken with the feet stationary
    c. is taken when a shooter is fouled in the act of shooting
    d. all of the above

_____4. The forward's important offensive role is
    a. dribbling the ball around the court
    b. boxing out opponents
    c. rebounding
    d. shooting and scoring

_____5. The three seconds in the key rule applies to
    a. all players in the key
    b. only defensive players in the key
    c. offensive players when they are in the key and in possession of the ball
    d. all of the above

_____6. The three-second count ends when
    a. someone shoots
    b. a defensive player gets the ball
    c. players from both teams have the ball at the same time
    d. all of the above

_____7. The best kind of spin to use when shooting is
    a. underspin
    b. no spin
    c. topspin
    d. all of the above

_____8. A defense making you responsible for opponents in your area of the court is
    a. a 2-1-2 zone defense
    b. a person-to-person defense
    c. double-teaming their best shooter
    d. all of the above

_____9. The best way to play a zone defense is
    a. to chase the ball as it is coming down the court
    b. to go to your zone as soon as the other team gets the ball
    c. to follow the ball carrier entering your zone, even when he leaves your zone
    d. all of the above

_____10. The advantage of a screen is
    a. it protects the shooter from being blocked
    b. it prevents the dribbler from losing the ball
    c. it enables the center to get into the key for a rebound
    d. all of the above

From *Complete Physical Education Plans for Grades 7–12* by Isobel Kleinman, 2001, Champaign, IL: Human Kinetics.

Basketball Quiz—Advanced level

NAME _____ TEACHER _____

DATE _____ CLASS PERIOD _____

True or False: Read each statement below carefully. If the statement is true, put a check under the True box in the column to the left of the statement. If the statement is false, put a check under the False box in the column to the left of the statement. If using a grid sheet, blacken in the appropriate column for each question, making sure to use the correctly numbered line for each question and its answer.

True   **False**

☐   ☐   1. The three-second rule limits the time the defensive player may stay in the basketball key.

☐   ☐   2. Once the ball is in the air, it is free, no team is in possession, and everyone can remain in the key to block or to rebound or to shoot.

☐   ☐   3. If your shot is hitting the basket and coming right back to you, you are probably using too much underspin.

☐   ☐   4. A player who fouls too much is ejected from a basketball game.

☐   ☐   5. You decide to dribble to the basket to take a lay-up shot because the lane is clear. Suddenly, smack! A defender runs into you, and you're correctly charged with a charging foul.

☐   ☐   6. When one team is responsible for six team fouls during the course of a playing period, opponents are awarded a foul shot; if successful, they are awarded another foul shot.

☐   ☐   7. Letting the tips of your fingers touch the ball as it rolls out of your hands imparts underspin.

☐   ☐   8. When the ball changes possession, the forwards and centers should change sides of the court as quickly as possible.

☐   ☐   9. If the center is playing his role for the team, he will be taking lots of outside shots.

☐   ☐   10. The point guard can speed up the game by dribbling.

From *Complete Physical Education Plans for Grades 7–12* by Isobel Kleinman, 2001, Champaign, IL: Human Kinetics.

Basketball Answer Key—Beginner level

1. T. The pivot turn is perfectly legal.
2. T. That is the procedure for taking foul shots after being fouled while shooting.
3. T. A lay-up shot is a regular field goal.
4. T. Violations are followed by opposing teams going out of bounds and putting the ball back in play with a pass.
5. T. Both those things are a necessity: position and jumping.
6. F. Good dribbling technique requires that you meet the ball at the waist.
7. F. The pass-and-go strategy requires that you change your place on the court immediately after passing the ball.
8. F. If you watch the basket when you are guarding, you won't be able to stay with your person.
9. F. It is good team play and the proper goal of any team player on defense—to stop the score and try to get the ball.
10. T. Spreading the hand on the ball yields better ball control.

Basketball Answer Key—Intermediate level

1. C.
2. D
3. D
4. D
5. C
6. D
7. A
8. A
9. B
10. A

Basketball Answer Key—Advanced level

1. F. The three-second rule only applies to the offense when they are in possession of the ball.

2. T

3. F. Underspin will make the ball drop, not come straight back at you.

4. T. A limit is set to how many fouls a player can have in one game. Class, interschool, club, and professional limits may vary.

5. F. The person who entered your lane is charged with a blocking foul.

6. T. Teams line up for a foul shot; the referee instructs that the shooter has "1 and 1."

7. T

8. T. The faster they move, the more options on offense and the less likely opponents can score easily on defense.

9. F. The center should be positioning himself to rebound everyone else's outside shots.

10. F. The game is slowed down by the dribble.

Football

Unit Overview

1. Lessons provide repetition to enhance skills and teach rules and strategies.

2. Teach throwing (grip, stance, arm motion, follow-through) and catching (hand position, eye contact, footwork) from a stationary position and the applicable rules (completed pass, pass interference).

3. Teach football patterns, how to throw ahead of the player, and how to catch on the move (hook, square right and left, post, etc.).

4. Teach offensive options—quarterback sneak, handoff—as well as pass plays and applicable rules.

5. Teach defensive skills—how to legally use flags, break up pass plays, block, and stop the ball-carrying runner.

6. Teach football terminology: line of scrimmage, downs, fumble, rushing the quarterback, dead/downed ball

7. Introduce the strategies appropriate to the skill when the skill is being practiced.

8. Once the games are ready to begin, introduce whatever rules were not introduced during skills lessons. The following should be included: onsides/offsides, how to keep possession, the boundaries, scoring

9. Teach the common penalties for rules violations so students can assist in the games of others or monitor their own games:
   - Holding—offensive/defensive—10 yards
   - Pass interference—an automatic completed pass
   - Unnecessary roughness—disqualification
   - Illegal belts—15 yards and loss of down (disqualification)
   - Flag guarding—10 yards
   - Offsides—10 yards

10. Teach fundamental game strategies for offense and for defense.

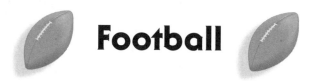

Football

HISTORY

Football began when ancient Greeks played harpaston, in which they tried to move a ball across a goal line. England adapted harpaston into a more modern version of football, which it later split into two sports: rugby and football (American soccer). Then, in 1869, the first intercollegiate football game was played, when Rutgers and Princeton played each other. Twenty-six years later, the first professional game was played. Finally, in 1922, the National Football League began.

FUN FACTS

→ John W. Heisman legalized the forward pass in 1906.

→ The San Francisco 49ers made the "Shotgun" formation popular in 1960.

→ Super Bowl I was won by the Green Bay Packers in 1967.

→ The University of Michigan's football stadium holds more than 100,000 fans.

→ Today's Super Bowl reaches an estimated 750 million viewers around the world.

BENEFITS OF PLAYING

1. Playing football involves a lot of teamwork.
2. There are many different positions that you can play.
3. Depending on the position, football can give you a good workout.
4. You can play many types of football—touch, flag, and tackle.
5. Football is a lot of fun!

TIME TO SURF!

Web Site	Web Site Address
National Football League	http://www.nfl.com
Canadian Football League	http://www.cfl.ca/
National Collegiate Athletic Association	http://www.ncaafootball.net/

From *Complete Physical Education Plans for Grades 7–12* by Isobel Kleinman, 2001, Champaign, IL: Human Kinetics.

Football Unit Extension Project

NAME _____ CLASS _____

Equipment needed to play flag/touch football

Item	Where you would purchase it (be specific)	Cost

Where you would play flag/touch football

Please explain where in the community you would play flag/touch football. Be specific.

Health benefit of playing flag/touch football

Please explain the health benefits of playing flag/touch football. Include how much badminton you would need to play each week to gain these benefits.

Reflection question

Do you think flag or touch football is an activity you would like to play as an adult? Why or why not? If you would like to play, would you rather play in an organized game in a recreation league or just in pick-up games at the park or in your backyard? Why?

From *Complete Physical Education Plans for Grades 7–12* by Isobel Kleinman, 2001, Champaign, IL: Human Kinetics.

Football Teaching Tips

1. Allow sufficient noncompetitive practice time with equipment for students to learn and improve skills without additional performance pressure.
2. Use as much football footwork, specific skill, and terminology as possible during the warm-up phase of the lesson.
3. After several lessons, when you have a feel for the depth of skill of the class, divide it up into equal teams, no more than five or six players per team. Do it on the basis of skill, gender, speed, and prior experience. Encourage working together as a unit. Promote leadership, feelings of belonging, and feelings of being needed.
4. Develop a short tournament that involves all students. Assign each to a team. Give the jobs of officiating, marking the ball, or keeping score to those unable to participate in the regular program.
5. Students clearly will have different amounts of experience with football. Advanced football athletes should be encouraged to help others and to improve their own skills while following class instructions. Those with prior experience should be looking to improve consistency, accuracy, distance, time, and speed.
6. Every effort should be made to assure students that improvement is what is valued, not a predisposition to be a great football player or great athlete.
7. If students are unable to fully participate in class activities, remember that they can be involved by coaching, officiating, keeping score, or conducting a research project.

Unit Setup

Facility

A large space, unencumbered by obstruction, permitting movement 30 yards forward and 10 yards right and left, without running into a wall, a person, or temporary obstructions

Clearly set boundaries for each simultaneous game

Equipment

One football for every two students

One belt for every student and a set of matching flags for every teammate

Two complete sets of flags of different colors for teams to identify themselves

A visual aid and writing implements

Paper for each student

Round-robin tournament schedules and charts (see appendix A)

Cones

Unit Timeline

There are three units in this chapter, one for each experience level. There are 12 to 16 lessons for the beginner groups:

6 lessons to develop skill competency in fundamentals and the basic game concept

6 to 10 lessons to compete so they can use the fundamentals in a challenging way

There are 11 lessons in this chapter for students at an intermediate level of play:

4 lessons to review skills, terminology, rules, and elementary football strategy
1 lesson to organize teams for the tournament
6 lessons for a small class tournament

There are 8 lessons for advanced groups that have mastered the basics of the game and its rules:

1 lesson for review, organization, and warming up skills previously learned
1 lesson to meet new teammates and set up starting strategies and responsibilities
6 lessons for a small class tournament

Unit Assessment

A student portfolio checklist is provided here for student use (table 12.1). Encourage students to track their progress as they master new skills. Students will conclude the unit with a written test. Their performance will be assessed on the basis of the performance rubric included at the end of their unit.

Additional Resources

American Football Coaches Association. 1995. *Football Coaching Strategies*. Champaign, IL: Human Kinetics.

American Sports Education Program. 1996. *Coaching Youth Football*. Champaign, IL.: Human Kinetics.

Flores, Tom, and Bob O'Connor. 1993. *Coaching Football*. Indianapolis, IN: Masters Press.

TABLE 12.1 Football Student Portfolio Checklist

STUDENT NAME _____

- ☐ Is able to throw a football to a person 10 yards away
- ☐ Is able to catch a football thrown from 10 yards away
- ☐ Can run one football pattern of the following: hook, square out, square in
- ☐ Understands the goal of the team in possession of the ball
- ☐ Understands the goal of the team without the ball
- ☐ Understands basic football terminology
- ☐ Understands what offensive contribution can be made by offensive players without the ball
- ☐ Knows how and can attempt to disrupt the successful play of opponents
- ☐ Is able to follow basic flag football rules
- ☐ Is able to exhibit good sporting behavior
- ☐ Can play without endangering the safety of others

From *Complete Physical Education Plans for Grades 7–12* by Isobel Kleinman, 2001, Champaign, IL: Human Kinetics

Football Lesson 1   Beginner level

Lesson Setup

Facility

Large, clear space for the entire class to move freely in

Equipment

One football for every two students

Performance Goal

Students will learn how to hold, throw, and catch a football.

Cognitive Goals

Students will learn

how to handle the peculiar shape of a football,
how to throw with reduced wind resistance,
how to direct it where they want it to go, and
what a completed pass is and why it is important.

Lesson Safety

Have practice groups separated by a minimum of five yards per group with a ball.
Throwing and running should take place in the same line of direction.

Warm-Up

Students will

1. Jog around the playing area
2. Practice football throwing mimetics: grip, wrist snap, elbow-level and arm follow-through, shoulder rotation, stepping forward
3. Practice football catching mimetics: lining up behind the path of the ball, the hand position, watching the ball into hands, pulling the ball into body
4. Perform stretches, with particular attention to the shoulder joint

Motivation

American football is different from international games that are called football. What we call soccer is the international game of football. Ask your students how many of them play international football/soccer. Suggest they see if they can learn to enjoy American football. Some people who watch it on TV may think it is just a brutal game of contact. But actually, in this class they are going to play with no contact at all. You will teach them how to stop players with no contact. But first, they'll begin learning how to throw and catch a football. It is different than throwing anything else because of its shape.

Lesson Sequence

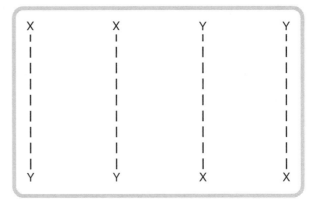

Figure 12.1—Separate partners by five yards to practice throwing and catching.

1. Demonstrate a proper football throw. Emphasize stepping forward and the follow-through.
2. Have students get a partner and practice throwing back and forth, as shown in figure 12.1. Emphasize a spiral and reaching the partner "in the numbers." Begin at close distances, separating partners as students seem proficient in their throws at close distances.
3. Emphasize the catch:
   - Teach the rules about completed passes.
   - Teach that to progress to the end zone and score using passes, those passes must be caught.
4. Make a practice contest so students do not get bored while developing skills. Change the goals of the contest to maintain interest. Some examples:
   - Who can catch 10 passes first?
   - If you run 10 yards from the thrower before turning to catch the pass are you still able to catch it?
   - If you move forward each time your partner and you have a completed pass, which partnership can move the farthest down the field after four throws? (See figure 12.2, which shows the progress of four different groups attempting four passes.)
   - Which group can get to the opposite side of the field first?

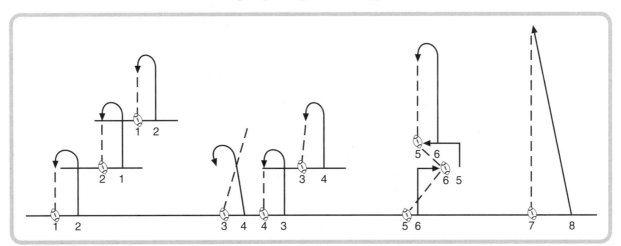

Figure 12.2—Advancing the ball by passing.

Review

Ask students how their fingers should be lined up on the ball.
Ask who can show the class a proper follow-through.
Discuss why stepping forward on the opposite foot is so important.
Review what a completed pass is.
Discuss why a completed pass is important.

Assessment

Observe each player throwing and catching, coaching students throughout the lesson. If students are able to reach each other at five yards, they can move on to the next lesson.

Football Lesson 2   Beginner level

Performance Goals

Students will

be able to throw from 5 yards and 10 yards to a stationary partner;
catch while stationary; and
run, catch, and throw to someone running a hook pattern.

Cognitive Goals

Students will

become more confident in their accuracy and ability to catch a football, and learn a hook pattern.

Warm-Up

Students will

1. Play catch with a friend—allow 10 minutes for this today, making sure to coach and seeking out students having difficulty
2. Practice football throwing mimetics: grip, wrist snap, elbow-level and arm follow-through, shoulder rotation, stepping forward
3. Practice catching a football: lining up behind the path of the ball, the hand position, watching the ball into hands, pulling the ball into body
4. Complete large-body agility movements:
   - Respond to teacher instruction
   - Respond to directional calls
   - Plant the foot before a sharp turn
5. Perform stretches

Motivation

Since no one stands still to catch a football (why is that?), in this lesson, students are going to learn how to throw to someone running away from them and to catch while on the run. They'll learn their first football pattern: the hook.

Lesson Sequence

1. Demonstrate running the hook pattern so that students see how it looks.
2. Emphasize running with the back to the quarterback and then planting the forward foot to turn. Tell students to:
   - Watch the ball into their hands
   - Realize that the quarterback must anticipate the need to throw the ball fewer than five yards
3. Have students alternate throwing and receiving. Proceed from five yards first. After a minimum of three successes at five yards, have the students increase the running distance and throwing distance. See figure 12.3 for how the setup can be arranged: the diagram shows the second in line being the quarterback, the first going out for the pass, and the last waiting his turn to become quarterback.

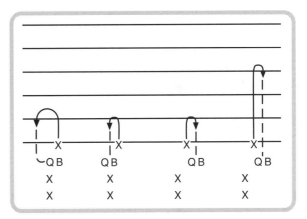

Figure 12.3—Hook pattern path of 5 yards.

4. After some practice, stop the class to emphasize the need for:
   - running straight forward without looking at the ball,
   - turning on a dime,
   - running back to the ball, and
   - completing the catch.
5. Assist students whose needs are more individual.
6. Make a practice contest so students do not get bored or drop from exhaustion. Change goals to maintain interest; for example, group two pairs together (teams of four):
   - One quarterback throws five yards for completions to each of the three players running hook patterns, then becomes the first receiver for the next quarterback, who also throws to everyone on the team. When everyone has been quarterback, and every quarterback has thrown to every receiver, the team is done. Find out who gets done first.
   - See who can move the line of scrimmage the farthest in four plays.
   - Ask students if they can catch the ball if they run a 10-yard hook.

- Find out what quarterback and receiver can complete at 15 yards.
- Ask which group can get to the opposite side of the field first.

Review

Ask the class what makes the hook pattern different from players throwing to someone standing in front of them.

Ask why they should learn how to throw to someone who is moving.

Review what the receiver should concentrate on while running the pattern.

Discuss what the receiver should concentrate on while trying to catch the ball.

Ask what the quarterback needs to do differently.

Assessment

Observe each student, coaching throughout the lesson. Students need to hold on to their catches at 5 and 10 yards and have the stamina to run the plays. More work will be done on this in the next lesson.

Football Lesson 3 — Beginner level

Performance Goal

Students will be able to throw from 5 yards and 10 yards to a partner on the run.

Cognitive Goals

Students will

learn to run a squared pattern,
improve their confidence in throwing and catching, and
improve their confidence in running a hook pattern.

Lesson Safety

Before beginning the square left and right patterns and practice, remind students of their left and right. This will avoid collisions of classmates running into each other and someone else's pass.

Warm-Up

Students will

1. Play catch with a friend
2. Practice football throwing mimetics
3. Practice catching mimetics

4. Jog and turn left on signal, right on signal, and so on
5. Perform stretches

Motivation

Tell the class that if everyone only ran a hook pattern, the defense would not be too confused. In this lesson you will teach another pattern so that students have a few choices once games begin.

Lesson Sequence

1. Demonstrate the square left (figure 12.4):
   • How the pattern should look to the quarterback
   • Where and which foot to cut on
   • When the quarterback should throw
2. Reemphasize
   • planting the forward foot before the cut,
   • watching the ball into the hands, and
   • the quarterback throwing in front of the receiver.
3. Have students alternate throwing and receiving. Start from five yards, and allow repetition and success before increasing the running and throwing distance.
4. After some practice, stop the class to emphasize whatever coaching hints still would help the majority. Go to students whose needs are more individual.
5. Have students practice the square right pattern.
6. Pair two couples together so that practice is now in groups of four, and create some interest by becoming the play caller for the class. Vary the distance that students have to run before they "cut," and the direction—right, left, or hooking back in.

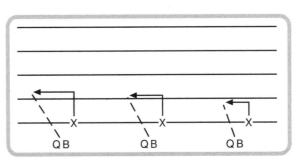

Figure 12.4—Square left path at 5 yards.

Review

Ask the class why it is important to have different patterns.

Ask if anyone knows what an interception is.

Discuss what would happen if the quarterback called a play, expected the receiver to run it, and the receiver went the wrong way.

Review why it is important to throw the ball where the receiver is going, not where she is.

Ask who would rather be a quarterback and who would rather be a receiver.

Football Lesson 4

Beginner level

Lesson Setup

Facility

Game area bounded by lines or cones indicating sidelines, end zone, and first downs

Equipment

Three cones for each game area and each squad of students
Belts and flags for each student

Performance Goals

Students will

learn and practice defensive techniques, and
learn and practice the handoff.

Cognitive Goals

Students will

learn why accuracy is important (they will be throwing through the defense), and
learn defensive priorities in person-to-person defense.

Lesson Safety

Clearly disallow rough play.

Warm-Up

Students will

1. Play catch with a friend
2. Complete agility runs—side to side, quick change of direction
3. Perform stretches

Motivation

Now that the students are becoming good at throwing and catching the ball, tell them it is time for a little confusion. Ask if they knew that a team can advance the ball by running with it and never taking the chance of throwing it. Handoffs or quarterback sneaks occur all the time in the game. Ask students how they can stop opponents who are running with the ball in their hands when, as mentioned at the beginning of the unit, they will not be contacting anyone, much less knocking them down. Find out if anyone knows what the flags are for. First teach them how to give and receive a handoff—then they'll use the flags.

Lesson Sequence

1. Teach the handoff:
   - Demonstrate how to hand it and receive it.
   - Organize class in groups of three, as shown in figure 12.5.
   - Practice handoffs a few times, so the receiver runs several steps after reception.
2. Demonstrate how to legally wear the belt and flags, with the applicable rules:
   - The flags must be loose and unobstructed, as shown in figure 12.6.
   - They cannot be wrapped around the belt.
   - They cannot be covered by clothes, tied on, or blocked by the arms.
   - The ball carrier cannot stiff-arm his opponents.
   - Players should put on the belts first, then the matching flags.
3. With the cones set up in three per group, 10 yards apart, teach and do the defensive drill (figure 12.7):

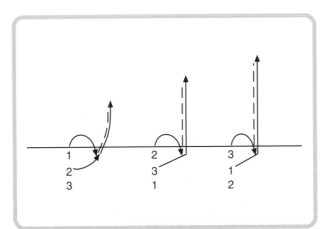

Figure 12.5—Groups of three practicing the handoff.

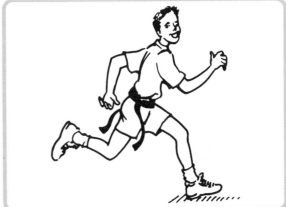

Figure 12.6—Student with flags on waist.

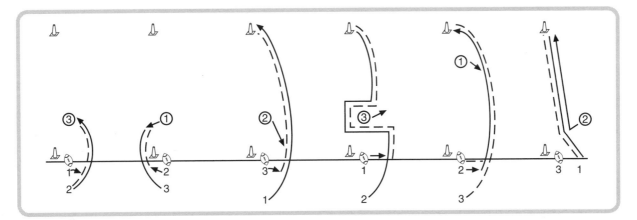

Figure 12.7—Practicing defense against the run. The defensive player is circled.

- Set up the drills so that the quarterback, ball carrier, and defender rotate.
- Explain the goals:
   The ball carrier gets to the cone.
   The defender gets the flag of the ball carrier before the ball carrier arrives at his destination.
- After one round, give defender hints and allow more practice:
   Have players stay between the ball carrier and the cone.
   Tell them to focus on the direction of their hips to know where they are going.
   Instruct them to reach for the flags only.
- Tell players to defend against the pass, and rotate the quarterback, receiver, and defender. See the setup shown in figure 12.8.
- The receiver wants to
   catch the ball, and
   run to the cone after the catch without the flags being pulled.
- Defending players want to
   not let the receiver get behind them;
   reach the ball, bat it down or catch it if they can; and
   if not, grab the flags on the catch.
- The quarterback wants an accurate pass.

Review

Ask the class how one legally stops a player from advancing the ball.
Ask if a player can run after catching the ball, and how one can stop her.
Review whether there is only one right way to wear the belt and flags—and how.
Discuss the penalties if these are not worn properly.

Assessment

Observe each student as he throws and catches, providing coaching to the class throughout the lesson.

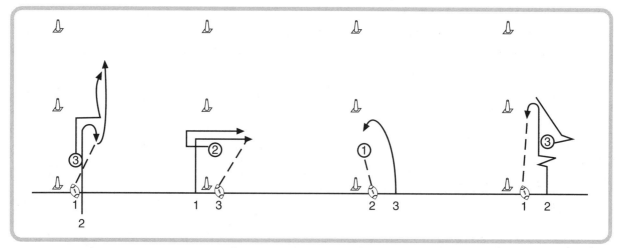

Figure 12.8—Practicing defense against the pass. The defensive person is circled.

Football Lesson 5   Beginner level

Lesson Setup

Facility

Game area bounded by lines or cones indicating sidelines, end zone, and first downs (figure 12.9)

Equipment

Eight cones for each game area, marked off with game boundaries and a method of spotting first downs. Adjacent areas may share the same set of cones marking the sidelines.

Designated teams of five or six players with flags and belts of the same color for each team

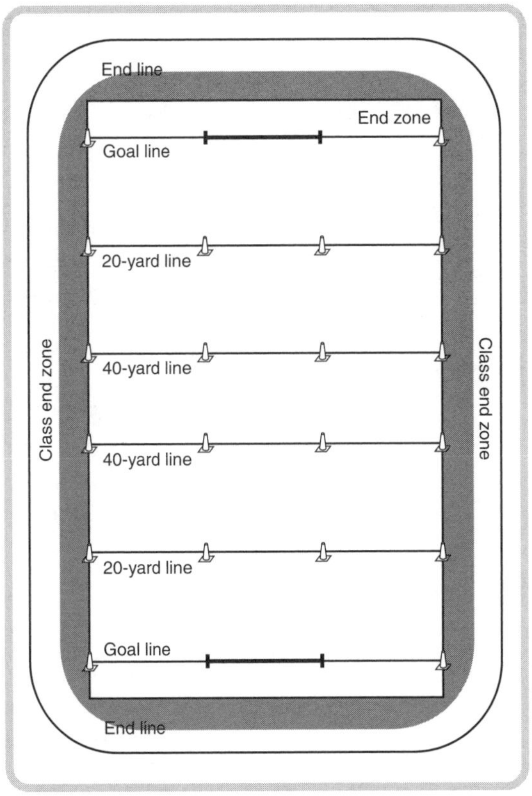

Performance Goals

Students will

use their skills in a game, continue improving their skills and confidence, and

play by the possession rules, giving up the ball to opponents if the ball was intercepted, or the team could not go 10 yards in 4 carries.

Figure 12.9—Football field with several alleys for simultaneous games.

Cognitive Goals

Students will learn

to line up with their own team on their own side of the ball—the line of scrimmage;

the relevant rules and penalty—offsides;

to keep possession of the ball until they get in the end zone and the relevant rules to do so:
  • First down
  • Fourth down
  • End zone
  • Touchdown

the consequences of not moving forward 10 yards in 4 attempts.

Lesson Safety

Clearly disallow rough play.

Teach in a positive way that rules are set up to allow safe and equitable play.

Encourage appropriate penalties when rules are broken so that safety issues are attended to and do not get out of hand.

Be ready to remove students who disregard safety until you are satisfied they will be more careful or until the next lesson.

Warm-Up

Students will

1. Play catch with a friend
2. Perform stretches
3. Complete general calisthenics, including mimetics for the throw and catch

Motivation

Tell students that from now on, they will have to work to get the ball. Let them know that they all have done well, and now it's time to try it in a game. Explain how to play the game.

Lesson Sequence

1. Group the class in temporary teams of five or six, making sure to put one or two experienced football students on each team:
   - Announce the colors that each group should wear.
   - Give students time to put the belts on properly.
2. Teach the following:
   - The possession rules for the day (based on red and yellow flags):
     All reds will have the ball first.
     Games will begin at midfield for red's first down.
     After a touchdown, yellow takes over at midfield for its first down.
   - The possession rules for every day:
     After a play, all players must return to the line of scrimmage.
     Opponents take over when they stop the opposition from reaching the first down marker in four plays.
3. Assign fields and start the games, reminding everyone that there will be no kickoff on this day. Play begins at midfield with red in possession.

Review

Ask the class if any questions or arguments arose during the game.

Ask how many teams scored.

Discuss whether anyone was able to prevent their opponents from getting a first down.

Ask if the teams used the pass only.

Review who was able to run for a score.

Ask if anyone caught the ball and was able to gain even more yardage by running with it afterward.

Assessment

Observe for common problems that can be addressed in the summary or at the beginning of the next class.

Teacher Homework

Divide the class into equally skilled teams, making sure to place the same number of students on each team who have

football experience,

throwing accuracy,

the ability to catch on the run a ball thrown from more than 10 yards away, and

running speed.

Football Lesson 6 — Beginner level

Performance Goals

Students will

get into a game-playing routine, and

play with their tournament teams.

Cognitive Goals

Students will

understand the reason for efficient game preparation and what the routine is:
- Getting on the belts
- Listening to or reading the schedule for the opponent assigned and the field assigned
- Declaring colors and all team members wearing the same color flags
- Choosing for sides or possession

decide who guards whom based on size, speed, and knowledge of game; and learn
- when rushing the quarterback is allowed and why it is important,
- scoring on touchdown and the point after,
- how to start the game—the kickoff and its rules, and
- about identifying their natural team leader.

Lesson Safety

Be available to disallow rough play and arguments.

Warm-Up

Students will

1. Play catch with a friend
2. Perform stretches

Motivation

Inform your students that you have made up their permanent tournament teams. Before announcing them, let the class know that this is the last lesson before the tournament starts, which means that the games will not count. Suggest that the teams take time to organize and learn to work together before official games begin. Not only do they need to learn a few things about starting a game and preparing for the tournament but also they need time to get to know their new teammates and figure out how best to work together.

Lesson Sequence

1. Announce the teams and allow time for students to put on belts:
   - Explain that from now on, they should put them on during free play.
   - Inform them that their captains or games schedules can tell them their color.
2. Review or teach the following:
   - The kickoff rules (a throw-off until the punt is taught)
   - The score value of a touchdown, with no point after
   - The importance of setting up a good defensive matchup, based on speed, size, and knowledge of the game
3. Direct opposing teams to the field for a game.
4. Start games with a throw-off and have students continue playing until the groups are called together.
5. Encourage teams to elect captains before they leave.

Review

Have students elect captains and co-captains. The captains should report names to you.

Summarize how to return equipment properly, how to report scores, and the rules of throw-off and score values.

Answer questions.

Teacher Homework

Make and post the tournament schedule and tournament standings chart. Tournament charts and schedules can be found in appendix A.

Football Lesson 7 — Beginner level

Lesson Setup

Equipment

A round-robin tournament schedule and standings chart posted so students can follow the schedule and see their standings. Examples can be found in appendix A.

Performance Goals

Students will

play games that rush the quarterback legally, and
begin the first round of their tournament.

Cognitive Goals

Students will be taught about the quarterback rush:

Why the quarterback rush is used
How to use the quarterback rush—"seven Mississippi" and then rush:
  • Students must learn that the quarterback's passing time is protected by a seven-second count.
  • Once "seven Mississippi" is counted out loud, the quarterback can run instead of throw, and the player covering can cross over the line of scrimmage to grab the quarterback's flag while she still has the ball and is behind the line of scrimmage.
Who does the rushing
What it allows the quarterback to do
The penalties if players rush too early

In competition, winning counts. The class should be guided toward playing with good sporting behavior and by the rules.

Lesson Safety

Be available to disallow rough play and arguments.

Warm-Up

Students will

1. Play catch with a friend
2. Perform stretches

Motivation

Announce to the class that the first round of their tournament is beginning. But before the players start, you will be teaching about the quarterback rush. (Cover the material in the cognitive goals section of this lesson.)

Once the games start, if the teams are having difficulty agreeing with their opponents, the best and first way to try to sort it out is to have the captains attempt to work out the problems together. If that is not possible, tell them to call you away from the game you're at. You will be available if anyone needs any help.

Wish the class luck, and that the teams that best play together, win.

Lesson Sequence

1. Allow time for students to put on belts properly if they did not do so during the free-play warm-up period.
2. Teach the quarterback rush:
   - The disadvantage of not rushing and why the rush is important
   - How to legally cross the line of scrimmage at "seven Mississippi"
   - The penalties for breaking the rule
3. Guide the class through game preparation (captains choose side or possession).
4. Announce the teams and team numbers and direct students to the field for game 1.
5. Start the games with a throw-off and have students continue playing until the groups are called together.
6. Attend each game, inviting students to work out their problems within the rules.
7. Call out a "last minute of play" warning so that teams can use the time wisely.

Review

Ask students why they should leave someone back to rush the quarterback.

Ask when one is legally allowed to cross the line of scrimmage to rush the quarterback.

Discuss the penalty for going in too soon.

Review problems or rules questions.

Compliment good judgment and sporting behavior.

Collect game scores for the first round of the tournament.

Football Lesson 8   Beginner level

Lesson Setup

Equipment

An updated round-robin tournament standings chart

Performance Goals

Students will

learn to defend against the pass and play by the relevant rules, and play round 2 of their tournament.

Cognitive Goals

Students will

review the strategy for defense against the pass:
  • The number one rule for good defense: Never let your opponent get behind you.
  • Grab the receiver's flag.
  • Try and knock down the ball.
  • Intercept.
learn the rules for a pass interference, and
learn that good sporting behavior and playing by the rules are highly valued.

Warm-Up

Students will

1. Play catch with a friend
2. Perform stretches

Motivation

Tell students that they are in round 2 of their tournament. Announce what the standings are after one round. Remind them that the teams that best play together, win.

Lesson Sequence

1. Allow time for students to put on belts properly if they did not do so during the free-play warm-up period.
2. Teach or review defense against the pass in terms of priorities and relevant rules:

- Tell players to stay behind the receiver and grab her flags.
- If they can reach the ball, they should knock it to the ground.
- If they can catch it, it's an interception—that is great.
3. Announce the team field assignments and direct students to begin round 2.
4. Coach each game, praising good defense and whatever is impressive.
5. Call out a "last minute of play" warning so teams can use the time wisely.

Review

Ask the class the three ways a player can defend against the receiver getting yardage and scoring.
Discuss the difference between knocking down the ball and pass interference and how it is penalized.
Review problems or rules questions.
Compliment good judgment and sporting behavior.
Collect game scores for the second round of the tournament.

Football Lesson 9 — Beginner level

Performance Goals

Students will

review and use quarterback options, and
play round 3 of their tournament.

Cognitive Goals

Students will be reminded of three ways the quarterback can move the ball forward:

Passing
Handing off
Running after "seven Mississippi" (the quarterback sneak)

Students will be encouraged to mix up their strategies to keep the defense guessing.

Warm-Up

Students will

1. Play catch with a friend
2. Perform stretches

Motivation

Tell the class that this is round 3 of the tournament. Announce what the standings are after two rounds. Ask if any team wants special coaching hints.

Lesson Sequence

1. Students should put on belts properly during the free-play warm-up period.
2. Teach or review three quarterback options:
   - Handing off
   - Running themselves
   - Passing
3. Announce the teams and team numbers and direct students to the field for the round 3 game.
4. Coach each game, praising variety in offensive play making and good moments.
5. Call out the "last minute of play" warning so teams can use the time wisely.

Review

Ask the class what three choices are available to every team on every play.
Review problems or rules questions.
Compliment good judgment and sporting behavior.
Collect game scores for the third round of the tournament.

Football Lesson 10   Beginner level

Performance Goals

Students will

play with a defensive "safety," and
play round 4 of their tournament.

Cognitive Goal

Students will learn flexible defensive strategy and the need for considering it.

Warm-Up

Students will

1. Play catch with a friend
2. Perform stretches

Motivation

Remind the students that you have posted a chart for them to follow by themselves. Suggest they take a look at it. Announce that this is round 4 of the tournament and what the standings are after three rounds.

As students begin round 4, wish them all good luck and remind them, once again, that if they are frustrated or need any special coaching hints, to let you know and you'll respond right away. This might be a good time to teach them how to deal with the ball handler who always seems to get away from his opponent, leaving the rest huffing to catch up. Some teams face this every day and cannot stop that person from scoring. Discuss what some teams do—use their "safety."

Lesson Sequence

1. Students should put on belts properly during the free-play warm-up period.
2. Teach the strategy behind creating the position of "safety":
   - Use to protect one's team against the breakdown in person-to-person defense
   - Helpful if someone is too fast to be covered by anyone on the team
   - What a safety is
3. Announce field assignments and direct students to the field for the round 4 game to begin.
4. Coach each game, encouraging the use of a safety and praising good moments.
5. Call out the "last minute of play" warning so teams can use the time wisely.

Review

Ask the class if person-to-person defense always works.

Ask students if they are helpless when the other team has a player who is too good for any one player of theirs.

Discuss some alternatives.

Review problems or rules questions that came up

Compliment good judgment and sporting behavior.

Collect game scores for the fourth round of the tournament.

Football Lessons 11-16 or tournament conclusion — Beginner level

Lesson Setup

Equipment

An updated round-robin tournament chart posted so students can follow the schedule and see their standings

Posted football performance assessment rubric for beginner level (on page 416)

Performance Goals

Students will

learn to plan and play as a team,
complete a round-robin tournament as developed, and
continue improving their football skills.

Cognitive Goals

Students will

understand routine class procedure, evidenced by their self-direction;
exhibit good sporting and ethical behavior;
develop an appreciation for the strengths and weaknesses of teammates and
   learn to adapt to them; and
continue improving their confidence and understanding.

Warm-Up

Students will

1. Play catch with a friend
2. Perform stretches

Motivation

Announce the standings after so many rounds. Ask if any team wants special coaching hints.

Lesson Sequence

1. Students should put on belts properly during the free-play warm-up period.
2. Announce the teams and team numbers and direct students to the field for the continuing rounds.
3. Coach each game, drawing attention to individual achievements and teamwork.
4. Call out the "last minute of play" warning so teams can use the time wisely.

Review

Announce that the class will be having a short football quiz on the next rainy day. Since that can happen at any time, tell students to remember their questions and feel free to ask them at any time. It might be a question on the quiz.

Review problems or rules questions that occurred during the games.
Compliment good judgment and sporting behavior.
Collect the game scores.

Assessment

Assign a skills grading value for the minimum performance standard you might want to grade. Some examples include the following:
- The student can accurately throw a ball to someone five yards away.
- The student can catch a ball thrown within the target area.
- The student will leave the line of scrimmage once the ball is snapped.
- The student can run some type of pattern.
- The student assumes responsibility on defense by staying with the person or zone she is assigned to cover.

Or, follow the football performance assessment rubric (table 12.2). Further general assessment rubrics can be found in appendix B. Whichever you choose, announce the standards well in advance of grading the students.
Observe students as they play to see if they meet the standards.
Conclude the marking period with a quiz (see page 438).

TABLE 12.2 Beginner Football Performance Assessment Rubric

STUDENT NAME _____

	0	1	2	3	4	5
Throw	No effort	• Uses proper body mechanics • Uses correct grip, forward foot, and follow-through	• Ball wobbles in flight • Ball drops before reaching a five-yard target	• Ball reaches a stationary 5-yard target accurately	• Ball reaches a moving target • Is accurate to 10 yards	• Has accurate variable range • Changes speed, maintaining accuracy
Catch	No effort	• Changes position so is lined up behind the ball • Watches the ball in flight • Uses proper hand position	• Brings ball into body • Catches an accurate 10-yard pass while standing • Watches the ball into hands	• Runs and catches a ball thrown to a target	• Adjusts to an inaccurate throw up to three steps from the target area • Does not need to stop running in order to catch	• Catches a ball thrown over head • Catches while running full stride • Catches a ball thrown with speed and/or distance
Pass pattern	No effort	• On command, runs hook or square left/right patterns • Turns at the proper times and in the correct direction	• Makes clean cuts • Doesn't watch the ball until cut	• Loses opponent and still keeps the pattern • Reliably runs a 10-yard pattern and catch a ball thrown accurately	• Instinctively knows when to cut back to the ball • Runs short and long patterns well	• Changes running patterns without confusion • Fakes opponent before making the cut • If open, will catch ball on target

Football Lesson 1   Intermediate level

Lesson Setup

Facility

Large, unobscured playing space

Equipment

One football for every two students

Performance Goals

Students will review and practice

football throwing and catching, and
different football patterns.

Cognitive Goal

Students will understand what to do when told to run a hook, a square left, or a square right pattern.

Lesson Safety

Set up the practice area so that

each squad or working group is a minimum of five yards from one another,
all groups are moving in the same line of direction, and
the line of scrimmage is the same for everyone.

Warm-Up

Students will

1. Play catch with a friend
2. Perform stretches

Motivation

As students get older and stronger, you can expect them to be accurate at longer distances and faster speeds. You also can expect that if someone calls a play and says, "Go out 10 yards and square left," the player knows what is meant and how to do it. Tell students to practice now so that they can.

Lesson Sequence

1. Have students line up behind the designated line of scrimmage.
2. Demonstrate a square left: emphasize the fundamentals of footwork, eyes, and throwing.
3. Have students practice what is demonstrated—each as a passer and a receiver for several trials. Call the snap for the whole class at once.
4. Do the same with square right patterns and then with hook patterns.
5. Mix up the calls (hook, square left, square right) and the distances.
6. Have squads rotate quarterback. Allow each quarterback to call the plays himself, telling the receiver how far to go down and what pattern to run before he cuts.

Review

Review the rules that keep everyone behind the line of scrimmage before the snap.

Review the fundamentals of planting the foot, the eyes on the ball into the hand, and so forth.

Answer any questions the class may have.

Assessment

Continue practicing until most class members have demonstrated mastery before changing the receiving patterns. Determine this by observation.

Football Lesson 2 — Intermediate level

Performance Goals

Students will

increase the number of running patterns they recognize and can perform,
practice throwing at increasing distances, and
assume responsibility for calling their own patterns and following their own quarterbacks.

Cognitive Goal

Students will understand what to do if told to run a slant or post pattern.

Lesson Safety

Make certain there is appropriate space between each working pair or squad.

Warm-Up

Students will

1. Play catch with a friend
2. Perform stretches

Motivation

Ask your students if any of them have seen a football game in person: it looks different in person than on TV. Why? In person, one gets to see all the pass receivers going in different directions. The quarterback has a choice but very few seconds to make it. That is why, before a play, he tells his primary receiver what to run, and he has secondary plays ready if the primary receiver cannot shake his defender. Ask the class, if a quarterback tells one of them to hook at the 15 and another to square out at the 10, will they know what to do? Can they catch the ball if it was thrown to them? They will need to in order to have successful games. Have them spend a little more time practicing before they get into real competition.

Lesson Sequence

1. Have students line up behind the designated line of scrimmage.
2. Demonstrate the slant: emphasize the fundamentals of footwork, eyes, and throwing.
3. Have students practice what is demonstrated, both as a passer and a receiver for several trials. Call the snap for the whole class at once.
4. Do the same with post patterns.
5. Mix up the calls and the distances.
6. Leave the last 10 minutes of class for the quarterback in each practice group to decide how far the receiver should go and what pattern to run.

Review

Review the rules that keep everyone behind the line of scrimmage before the snap.
Review the fundamentals of planting the foot, the eyes on the ball into the hand, and so forth.
Answer any questions the class may have.

Assessment

Continue the practice, looking for mastery from 90 percent of the class before changing the patterns.

Football Lesson 3 — Intermediate level

Lesson Setup

Equipment

Two cones for each group: one for the line of scrimmage and the other to mark the goal to run to after the catch
Belts and flags

Performance Goals

Students will

learn to snap the ball to the quarterback,
wear the flags and belts, and
practice patterns with defenders.

Cognitive Goals

Students will know

the purpose and execution of defensive strategy,
the rules of
• possession,
• the start of the game, and
• the end zone
about belts and flags:
• How to wear them legally
• The penalties for illegal belts or flags

Lesson Safety

Students will need more space between groups to work safely. Be prepared to double the usual space or to make adjustments during the course of this practice.

Warm-Up

Students will

1. Play catch with a friend
2. Perform stretches

Motivation

Tell the class that unless the quarterback can "thread the needle," the nonreceiver can get the ball, interrupt the success of the pass, and get the flag. In this lesson, students will learn how accurate they can be with their throwing when someone else is there who wants the ball.

Lesson Sequence

1. Have students put on belts, reviewing how to put them on legally:
   - Explain that belts should not hang but flags should.
   - Explain the penalty for shielding flags.
2. Teach the snap:
   - Demonstrate.
   - Allow several practices between partners.
   - Teach the relevant rules:
       That the snap begins the "seven Mississippi" count
       The rules for fumbles behind the line of scrimmage
3. Have students get in groups of three and line up behind the line of scrimmage and inside their own set of cones. This will be a three-way practice (figure 12.10)—a quarterback, a receiver, and a defender. You call the snap:
   - The person snapping is the only eligible receiver during this practice.
   - The quarterback calls the pass pattern.
   - The defender tries to prevent the ball carrier from reaching the cone with the ball.
   - Everyone alternates roles each play.
4. Set up contests:
   - Which defender can score the most points:
       Interception—four
       Batted-down ball—three
       Flags pulled on the catch—two
       Flag pulled before the opponent reached the cone—one
   - For variety, you can change it to asking which receiver can score the most points:

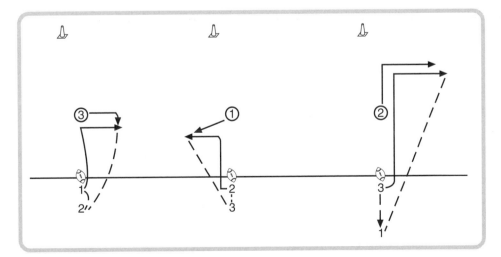

Figure 12.10—Practicing snap, passing, and defense.

> Catches—one
> Catches the pass and makes it to the cone—two
> • Which quarterback can score the most points in the class:
>   Receives the snap without a fumble—one
>   The throw is completed—two

Review

Review with the class what the penalties are for tied-on flags and illegal belts, for obstructed flags, and for pass interference.
Ask students what usually happens when a defender goes for the ball but comes up empty.

Teacher Homework

Make up teams, dividing students on the basis of their skills, so that each team is equal. If you do not feel comfortable doing this yet, because you do not know the skills of the class well enough, wait another day. It is important to make sure you do not make any one team too strong or too weak: knowing your students and how they play is essential before doing this. Place a good passer and receiver on each team, divide up the people with speed, and separate all those knowledgeable about football and place them each on different teams as well.

Football Lesson 4 — Intermediate level

Lesson Setup

Facility

Designated game areas should be marked and separated for every two competing teams:

> Cones to mark side boundaries and first-down markers
> A designated goal line

Performance Goal

Students will play a scrimmage game with teacher-assigned tournament teams.

Cognitive Goal

Students will learn rules for rushing the quarterback, fumbling, unnecessary roughness, and the kickoff.

Lesson Safety

There should be clearly marked lanes for each game so game areas do not overlap.

Warm-Up

Students will

1. Play catch with a friend
2. Perform stretches

Motivation

In this lesson you will announce the tournament teams. Tell them it is time to get organized because the tournament will begin soon.

Lesson Sequence

1. Have students gather to learn teams and get belts and flags. Instruct them to choose their own captains.
2. Review the rules not yet taught:
   - The throw-off process to start a game
   - No rushing or quarterback sneaks until "seven Mississippi"
   - The penalties for unnecessary roughness:
     Offense—loss of a down and sent back 10 yards
     Defense—opponents advance 15 yards
     Person involved—one warning, and if it happens again, "out"
3. Assign fields and ask that students begin their games right away.
4. Get to each group, officiating where necessary and providing positive feedback when possible.

Review

Ask the class if there were any disagreements over the rules. (Share something that came up that might be useful for the rest of the class to know.)
Ask who used a handoff.
Discuss who caught a pass.
Go over who got a flag.
Ask who won.

Assessment

Try to make sure that all teams were relatively equal in skill. If not, make a decision to switch some players now before the tournament starts.
Look for common problems in skill, strategy, or rule observation that can be addressed during the summary or at the beginning of the next class.

Football Lesson 5 — Intermediate level

Performance Goals

Students will

learn the punt, and
play another practice game.

Cognitive Goals

Students will

learn about the punt,
learn how to get points after they score a touchdown,
learn where to set up the line of scrimmage,
learn how they can choose between a one-point and two-point play, and
be part of a group effort in a football tournament.

Warm-Up

Students will

1. Play catch with a friend
2. Perform stretches

Motivation

This lesson will be a practice game. That way, your students have a bit more time to get to know their teammates and how best to organize for the tournament team. It also will give them time to learn and put into practice two things they did not do the previous year—using the punt and going for points afterward.

Announce that the tournament begins in the next class. In this class, you would like them to get used to beginning the game and play after a touchdown by starting with a kickoff, using a punt instead of a throw, and doing it from the second cone. But before they go any further, they should give the punt a try, and you should explain their teams' options after scoring a touchdown.

Lesson Sequence

1. Instruct students to put on belts when they arrive and worry about flags once their captains arrive to tell them which color flags to wear.
2. Demonstrate the punt:
   • Allow students to practice with partners from sideline to sideline.
   • Review the kickoff rules.
3. Review the points for touchdown and safety.

4. Introduce point after play from the next to last cone.
5. Assign fields and have students begin games.
6. Cover all games, one at a time. Remind the players about punting and the point after, encourage good defensive matches, and praise anything noteworthy—such as good blocks, pass coverage, and containing the quarterback.

Review

Ask the class if anyone's team got points after the touchdown.
Review the fact that players are allowed an additional play after the touchdown is scored.
Ask who won.

Teacher Homework

Prepare and post the tournament charts that show game schedules and updated team standings. Tournament charts and schedules can be found in appendix A.

Football Lesson 6   Intermediate level

Lesson Setup

Equipment

A posted roster of captains, game assignments, and tournament standings (see appendix A)

Performance Goal

Students will play round 1 of the tournament using all legal options for their game strategy.

Cognitive Goals

Students will

learn how the quarterback can become a receiver;
review three other options a team can use for moving the ball:
  • The handoff
  • The quarterback sneak
  • The pass
learn that catching short passes and then running can be more successful than long passes.

Lesson Safety

Now that the tournament has started, be vigilant about excessive aggression that will endanger the physical or mental health of the students. Be prompt to respond with

a simple general verbal correction,

a pointed verbal correction, mentioning a specific behavior or incident you do not want repeated, or

a special action to stop the behavior of a specific student.

Warm-Up

Students will

1. Play catch with a friend
2. Perform stretches

Motivation

Announce that this is round 1 of the tournament. As always, you will be getting to each game during the period. Tell students that if you have not yet arrived at their game and there is a problem to get your attention. Mention that if any team has questions, needs advice, or needs some more ideas, you will get there to help. Wish them luck.

Lesson Sequence

1. Have students put their belts on during the free-play warm-up period and wait to get their team color flags.
2. Review strategies:
   • Quarterback options—ask how the quarterback can become a receiver, and review other options
   • The short pass strategy—catch and run
3. Have students meet their opponents on the assigned fields and begin games.
4. Act as class coach and rules adviser, encouraging controlling the ball and using a variety of options.

Review

Ask the class which quarterback rushed for yardage.
Review what got farther—the long run, the long pass, or the short pass.
Discuss whether it's better to go for the touchdown or the first down.
Ask which teams won.

Football Lesson 7   Intermediate level

Lesson Setup

Equipment

Updated tournament standings charts

Performance Goals

Students will

implement defensive strategies, and
play round 2 of the tournament.

Cognitive Goals

Students will

be clear about defensive priorities:
- Pulling flags
- Knocking down the ball
- Intercepting

recognize that they are improving their endurance and fitness.

Warm-Up

Students will

1. Play catch with a friend
2. Perform stretches

Motivation

Tell the class that you cannot help but notice that each student looks a little stronger and less winded at the end of a play. Ask how many feel that they are in better shape now than when they began the school year. It is great when they can improve their health and fitness while they are enjoying themselves.

Announce what the standings are after the first round of the tournament. Remind students that if any team needs advice to call you over. Wish them luck.

Lesson Sequence

1. Have students put their belts on during the free-play warm-up period and wait to get their team color flags.

2. Review defensive strategies and priorities.
3. Have students meet their opponents on the assigned fields and begin their games.
4. Act as the class coach and rules adviser.

Review

Ask the class what students gained yardage after the catch.
Review who caught a ball and had her flags ripped off.
Ask who grabbed a flag.
Discuss whether anyone was able to knock a ball to the ground that was intended for her opponent.
Ask if anyone intercepted and discuss the advantage of an interception.
Ask which teams won.

Assessment

In evaluating student performance achievement, you can begin by observing for minimal standards as defined by the intermediate football assessment rubric that appears on page 430. This will be a several-day process. Have students take a quiz (see page 439) on the first rainy day of the tournament.

Football Lessons 8-10 or tournament conclusion   Intermediate level

Lesson Setup

Equipment

Cones for game area
Daily updated tournament standings charts
A posted intermediate performance rubric

Performance Goals

Students will

use a variety of offensive and defensive strategies, and
play the remaining rounds—3, 4, and 5—of the tournament.

Cognitive Goal

Students will learn to plan their team's response to different teams when the differences make their execution more difficult, and when the differences make defending against them in the same way too frustrating.

Lesson Safety

Be vigilant about competitive behavior, making sure it is safe and emotionally appropriate.

Warm-Up

Students will

1. Play catch with a friend
2. Perform stretches

Motivation

Announce the standings after so many rounds of the tournament. Wish your students luck, and tell them that, as always, you will be there if they need some friendly advice.

Lesson Sequence

1. Have students put their belts on during the free-play warm-up period and wait to get their team color flags.
2. Announce the standings and what goals to aim for.
3. Have students meet their opponents on the assigned fields and begin their games.
4. Act as coach and rules adviser, and praise everything worthy of recognition:
   - Team strategy (even if it doesn't work out)
   - Team cohesiveness
   - Skills during play
   - Sporting behavior
   - Reliability

Review

Ask students what they can do when an opponent is the fastest person on the field, and how they can stop someone who can outrun everyone on their team.

Review why players want someone equally fast to stay back with the quarterback.

Ask if anyone on their team blocked for them when they carried the ball.

Discuss whether there's an advantage to punting rather than throwing off.

Inform the students that if they are interested in how they are being evaluated, you have posted the intermediate performance standards on the board. They also should know that the minute it rains, you will be giving them a short quiz before playing any games. So, if they have any questions, they should ask.

Assessment

Continue observing students to assess their achievement based on the definition and standards in the performance assessment rubric for their grade level (table 12.3). For further general assessment rubrics, see appendix B.

TABLE 12.3   Intermediate Football Performance Assessment Rubric

STUDENT NAME _____

	0	1	2	3	4	5
Skill of possession	No effort	• Generally directs or controls the football • Knows the team's general objective and uses skills to help meet it • Gets back to the line of scrimmage at the end of each play	• If given the ball, maintains possession • Assists the team in maintaining possession by faking, blocking, or getting open	• Plays the game within the context of the rules • Has good sense of the boundaries, the end zone, and the first down markers • Able to implement team strategies	• Adapts to short or long plays • Blocks for the ball carrier • Uses speed and agility to avoid a "tackle" • Plays a flowing game	• Understands responsibility and how it relates to the rest of the team • Is able to call plays and adjust if the play does not work the way planned • Finds a way to get the next first-down score
Skill for defense	No effort	• Knows to stop the ball carrier by pulling flags or tagging • Leaves the line of scrimmage • Uses hands to reach for ball carrier or ball	• Is capable of covering a player of equal speed and size • Covers the assigned zone • Able to occasionally interrupt opponent's play	• Reacts to a handoff at the line of scrimmage • Does not let the opponent get behind him • Drops person or zone once the ball is up and go after the carrier • Plays within the rules	• Knows how to use positioning to cut off opponent's lanes • If unable to prevent the completed pass, prevents additional yardage • Runs down the ball carrier who gets away from teammate	• Is able to inter-cept passes and change the direction of the game • Is effective in regaining posses-sion of the ball • Anticipates opposition • Helps teammates focus on the things to stop
Running, catching, and throwing	No effort	• Is very reliable up to five yards on offense • Is very reliable up to 10 yards on defense • Prepares for the game (with flags or pinnies) and arrives on the correct field in a timely fashion	• Offensively effective to 10 yards • Defensively effective to 15 yards if the opponent they cover carries the ball or if the ball reaches the zone they cover	• Leaves own defensive assignment only if the ball is up • Has stamina to play aggressively • Is reliable to go to with the ball when open • Gets open and turns evasively	• Plays aggressively within the rules • Runs a variety of plays in front and behind the line of scrimmage • Focuses and catches the ball in a crowd • Though not the designated quarterback can pass accurately down the field	• Throws accurately long or short • Catches a ball thrown fast, high, low, or off target a few steps • Handles power, speed, and long distances with ease • Changes direction immediately

Football Lesson 1 — Advanced level

Lesson Setup

Facility

Clear, unobstructed field

Equipment

One ball for every two students

Performance Goals

Students will

warm up their football skills,
improve the depth and accuracy of their throw, and
review football patterns and play calls.

Cognitive Goals

Students will

learn how and why to fake, and
learn the advantage of and how to execute a zone defense.

Lesson Safety

Practicing pairs should be spaced out so there are no collisions between students. The line of direction should remain the same for all couples, with everyone starting along the same line.

Warm-Up

Students will

1. Jog around the field
2. Play catch with a friend
3. Perform stretches

Motivation

The students now are older and have a few years of playing flag football under their belts. However, they do need a little warm-up to reacquaint themselves with the football before they get into competition. Tell them you also want to introduce some ideas that they might not have had before. First have them practice the things they have already learned. If they feel they need more practice, there is no rush to get into games right away. They just need to let you know, and you will let them be your guide.

Lesson Sequence

1. Have students work in groups of two, practicing patterns.
2. Have passers switch, calling plays for their receiver.
3. Bring the class together for instruction and remind everyone of the quarterback's options.
4. Lead them through the additional practice of
   - a few snaps with the quarterback dropping back,
   - a few handoffs,
   - some long and short passes, and
   - some laterals.
5. After each change above, bring students together to discuss
   - the skills they use,
   - relevant rules, and
   - problems to anticipate.
6. Have students practice some punts.

Review

Invite questions.
Review problems.
Compliment good performance, effort, and improvement.

Assessment

Observe for familiarity, checking the level of comfort with each skill and rule.

Teacher Homework

If you are familiar with your class, the students, and their skills, make up the teams, being sure to distribute talents so that teams are as competitively equal as possible. If you are not yet familiar enough with the class, delay this process or elicit help from the students who seem most aware and have been in the school the longest time.

Football Lesson 2   Advanced level

Lesson Setup

Equipment

Cones to divide the field into game stations for every two teams
Belts and flags for each student

Performance Goals

Students will

play with their teams for the remainder of the tournament, and
work on using their skills as teams to compete successfully against their opponents.

Cognitive Goals

Students will

learn or review the rules for
- the use of flags,
- the kickoff,
- rushing the quarterback,
- offsides, and
- unnecessary roughness
review defensive strategies and the particular advantage of each:
- Zone
- One-on-one
- One-on-one with safety

Lesson Safety

Monitor play for unnecessary roughness.

Warm-Up

Students will

1. Play catch with a friend
2. Perform stretches

Motivation

Announce the teams and tell students you made sure to make them as equal as possible. Now it is their job to decide who will lead them, to determine what responsibilities each has on offense and defense, and to play with all the skills and intelligence they have. Tell them you will be there to help coach and officiate. If you are not on their field when a problem arises, ask them to try to resolve it themselves; if they cannot, they should call for you.

Lesson Sequence

1. Have students practice in pairs to warm up.
2. Announce the teams after reviewing the rules and procedures.
3. Once the students are in teams, assign the fields and begin the scrimmage games.

Review

Review problems or rules questions that occurred during practice. Compliment good performance, effort, and improvement.

Teacher Homework

Prepare and post a tournament schedule and team standings chart. Tournament schedules and charts can be found in appendix A.

Football Lessons 3-8 or tournament conclusion — Advanced level

Lesson Setup

Facility

Game stations for each two teams in the group

Equipment

Cones for dividing up the field
A team standings chart and posted tournament schedule (appendix A)

Performance Goals

Students will

use their personal skills to an advantage on their teams,
play by the rules and regulations for flag football games, and
play up to six rounds of a football tournament.

Cognitive Goals

Development throughout the tournament will focus on one of the following groups each day:

The quarterback:
  • Practicing throwing to the open player
  • Using short passes to retain possession
  • Exercising all options so not too predictable
  • Learning it is better to run than to throw and be intercepted
The defense:
  • Practicing pressuring the quarterback
  • Not letting people get behind them
  • Calling to the team when the ball is thrown so it can refocus defense
  • Using zones or a "safety" when playing person to person

The receiver:
  • Practicing keeping an eye on the ball
  • Breaking to the outside
  • Making cuts and faking to lose opponents
  • Running behind teammates so they block or screen
The offense:
  • Making a plan that includes everyone, even if not a ball carrier

Lesson Safety

Monitor for unnecessary roughness and emotionally stressful behavior, and correct it.

Warm-Up

Students will

1. Play catch with a friend
2. Perform stretches
3. Complete agility drills

Motivation

The teams that do well are the ones that utilize everyone on the team. Tell the students that those who depend on the biggest and fastest player on their team will learn quickly that their star player can easily be shut down by alert opposition. Smart teams make sure everyone contributes to the team.

Mention that this is for fun. Tell the class to go out there and see if their wits and skills can keep them in the game. Offer your help if they need it.

Lesson Sequence

1. Have students practice in pairs during the warm-up.
2. Post the tournament game schedule near the locker room. It should include the following:
   • The round of the tournament
   • The team identity numbers and whom they will play (1 plays 4, etc.)
   • The color of the flags to pick up
   • Which field the game will be played on
3. Post the team standings near the locker room. They should include the following:
   • The team identifying numbers
   • The captain and co-captains' names
   • The game record
4. After the players stretch, make announcements that introduce ideas for strategy, focusing on a new strategy every day (attendance should be taken during the game):

- Students go to the field of play.
- They choose to receive or choose which side of the field they will play on for the period.
- They begin their tournament games.

5. During the course of the class, while officiating and coaching games, focus on the strategy brought to everyone's attention during the announcements.

Review

How did the class think the day's strategy got played out?
Which team successfully incorporated the day's strategy?
How could they make the strategy work better?
How did the strategy break down? Have them give examples.
Answer questions and collect scores.

Assessment

The unit should conclude with a quiz that questions knowledge of rules, fundamental strategies, and fundamentals of movement. Since the unit is short, it is probably best to select questions from all the activities done in the fall before testing. A short quiz appears on page 440.

Skills grading can be done in a number of ways:

Announce minimal standards and award points for
- proper positioning on defense,
- moving to the open field,
- cutting to lose opponent,
- blocking for teammates or making a catch of a ball thrown accurately, and
- responding to the team game plan

Follow the system of points in the advanced football performance assessment rubric in table 12.4. For further general assessment rubrics, see appendix B.

Assign self-assessment. At this age level, you might consider letting the students evaluate themselves, based on the performance assessment rubric, or even have their teammates pair off and do it for each other.

TABLE 12.4 Advanced Football Performance Assessment Rubric

STUDENT NAME _____

	0	1	2	3	4	5
Sporting behavior	No effort	• Blames others • Needs supervision to stay on task • Interferes with others	• Is self-directed: knows the rules, knows how games begin, and is prepared to start without hampering the routine or arguing about possession, position, or own function on the team	• Participates respectfully with others • Relies on skill and strategy to win, not intimidation	• Shows concern for others despite a desire for the team to win • Accepts own strengths and limitations and works with others to strengthen the team	• Assists others to achieve • Increases team spirit and members' self-confidence • Displays leadership and self-confidence
Maturity and leadership	No effort	• Arrives on the field prepared and in team colors • Plays within the rules • Is ready for each play	• Accepts offensive or defensive assignments and plays them • Implements team strategies	• Adjusts to a new team strategy when necessary • Accommodates the needs of the team despite personal desires	• Develops or suggests new team strategies • Helps the team maintain group focus and cohesiveness	• Makes sure equipment is where it needs to be at the beginning and end of period • Maintains a positive attitude • Bolsters the feelings and self-concept of team members
Skill	No effort	• Generally is successful in an uncrowded field • Is competent up to 10 yards	• Occasionally is successful in a competitive, crowded field • Is competent up to 15 yards	• Is undeterred from the primary objective • Does not compromise the team • Is relatively consistent to 20 yards	• Performs despite distractions • Is consistent at most distances • Is more competent on either offense or defense	• Plays both offense and defense equally well • Is strongest and fastest on the team • Is big play maker

Football Quiz–Beginner level

NAME _____ TEACHER _____

DATE _____ CLASS PERIOD _____

True or False: Read each statement below carefully. If the statement is true, put a check under the True box in the column to the left of the statement. If the statement is false, put a check under the False box in the column to the left of the statement. If using a grid sheet, blacken in the appropriate column for each question, making sure to use the correctly numbered line for each question and its answer.

True	False	
☐	☐	1. To keep possession of the ball, a team must be able to move the line of scrimmage forward at least 10 yards in 4 downs.
☐	☐	2. Opposing players can wait for the next play on either side of the line of scrimmage.
☐	☐	3. Passes, handoffs, running the ball, and blocking for the ball carrier are plays of the defensive team.
☐	☐	4. A team scores a touchdown when it carries or catches the ball in its opponent's end zone.
☐	☐	5. Once the ball is moved in front of the line of scrimmage, the ball carrier can pass it forward to a different teammate.
☐	☐	6. If the ball changes hands while it is still behind the line of scrimmage, the defensive team may rush the carrier of the ball even though "seven Mississippi" has not been called.
☐	☐	7. In order to legally stop the ball carrier from gaining more yardage, one must pull a flag off the ball carrier's belt.
☐	☐	8. To be a good defensive player, you should never let the person you cover get behind you.
☐	☐	9. If a ball that is passed is not caught, the line of scrimmage does not move forward and all players must return to the same spot they were in before for the next play.
☐	☐	10. If a player runs out of bounds with the ball, the new line of scrimmage is no closer to the end zone than where the ball was taken out of bounds.

Extra Credit: Match the columns:

_____1. Catching the ball   **a.** Illegal in class

_____2. Interception   **b.** Push off left foot

_____3. Tackling   **c.** Watch the ball into your hands

_____4. Square right   **d.** Starting the game

_____5. Kickoff/throw-off   **e.** The defense catches the ball

From *Complete Physical Education Plans for Grades 7–12* by Isobel Kleinman, 2001, Champaign, IL: Human Kinetics.

Football Quiz—Intermediate level

NAME _____ TEACHER _____

DATE _____ CLASS PERIOD _____

True or False: Read each statement below carefully. If the statement is true, put a check under the True box in the column to the left of the statement. If the statement is false, put a check under the False box in the column to the left of the statement. If using a grid sheet, blacken in the appropriate column for each question, making sure to use the correctly numbered line for each question and its answer.

True   False

☐   ☐   1. Teams should choose to punt on the fourth down when on their own 20-yard line.

☐   ☐   2. An offsides penalty results when a team player is ahead of the ball before the play begins.

☐   ☐   3. A receiver who is told to "square in" must line up closer to the sideline than the center of the field.

☐   ☐   4. The defense can score, even without the ball, if its opponent's flag is pulled while still holding the ball and still inside her own end zone.

☐   ☐   5. Once the ball is in front of the line of scrimmage, the ball carrier can throw it to someone behind him or next to him.

☐   ☐   6. The player who stays back to count "seven Mississippi" gives the quarterback endless time to throw the ball and the receivers unlimited time to get open.

☐   ☐   7. A player unable to intercept a pass but able to touch the ball should try to bat the ball down to the ground.

☐   ☐   8. Defensive players should keep their own end zone to their back and the player they are responsible for in front of them.

☐   ☐   9. It is better to punt so that the ball lands in bounds at the 10-yard line before bouncing out-of-bounds than it is to have it land in the end zone.

☐   ☐   10. No one on the offensive team can pass the ball if the quarterback gives the ball to a teammate and runs in front of the line of scrimmage.

Extra Credit: Match the columns.

_____1. Pass interference   a. Moving the ball from the ground to the quarterback

_____2. The snap   b. Protecting the quarterback without a defensive line

_____3. The punt   c. Illegal, loss of yardage, play repeated

_____4. "Seven Mississippi"   d. Pushing the receiver away from the ball

_____5. Hidden flags   e. A kick that takes place behind the line of scrimmage

From *Complete Physical Education Plans for Grades 7–12* by Isobel Kleinman, 2001, Champaign, IL: Human Kinetics.

Football Quiz—Advanced level

NAME _____   TEACHER _____

DATE _____   CLASS PERIOD _____

True or False: Read each statement below carefully. If the statement is true, put a check under the True box in the column to the left of the statement. If the statement is false, put a check under the False box in the column to the left of the statement. If using a grid sheet, blacken in the appropriate column for each question, making sure to use the correctly numbered line for each question and its answer.

True **False**

☐ ☐ 1. Teams should punt on the fourth down when on their opponent's 10-yard line.

☐ ☐ 2. Grabbing opponents' clothes or tackling is considered unnecessarily rough play in flag football.

☐ ☐ 3. A receiver told to "square in" should line up closer to the sideline than the center of the field.

☐ ☐ 4. A player who has the ball and is stopped in her own end zone has permitted her opponents to score even though they never had possession of the ball.

☐ ☐ 5. A ball in front of the line of scrimmage can be passed as long as the pass is lateral or moves backward.

☐ ☐ 6. The player who counts "seven Mississippi" should count with his hands at his sides.

☐ ☐ 7. A player able to touch the ball but unable to intercept should bat the ball to the ground.

☐ ☐ 8. Defensive players should keep their own end zone to their back and the player they are responsible for in front of them.

☐ ☐ 9. It is better to punt so that the ball lands in bounds at the 10-yard line before bouncing out-of-bounds than it is to have it land in the end zone.

☐ ☐ 10. If the quarterback gives the ball to a teammate behind the line of scrimmage and then runs in front of the line of scrimmage, the defense should go after the new ball carrier because no one on the offensive team can pass the ball.

Match the columns:

_____ **11.** Safety

_____ **12.** Offsides

_____ **13.** Blocking

_____ **14.** Defensive center

_____ **15.** Right foot

a. Ahead of the ball before it is snapped

b. Anticipates the ball on the scrimmage line after counting to seven Mississippi

c. Runner should plant it before cutting to the left

d. Player covering an area that is behind the rest of his team's defense

e. Creating a moving wall between your own teammate and an opponent

Diagram: From the diagram, identify the running pattern that best describes the question and then put the correct number in the margin to the left.

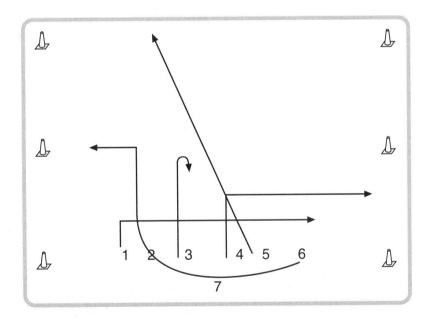

_____ **16.** Which is a slant pattern?

_____ **17.** Which player's pattern allows the quarterback to hand off to him early or, if not, throw later?

_____ **18.** Which pattern has the receiver running in front of the quarterback?

_____ **19.** If the cones to the left represent first down markers, which receiver is running to receive the ball at the next first down?

_____ **20.** Which receiver is expecting to come back to the ball?

From *Complete Physical Education Plans for Grades 7–12* by Isobel Kleinman, 2001, Champaign, IL: Human Kinetics.

Football Answer Key—Beginner level

True or False

1. T

2. F. This is offsides. There is a penalty for whoever is at fault.

3. F. Each is a strategy that requires possession of the ball. If a team has possession, it is the offensive team.

4. T

5. F. Forward passes are only allowed if the thrower is behind the line of scrimmage.

6. T. Counting to "seven Mississippi" is for protecting the quarterback and giving him time to find a receiver downfield. After "seven Mississippi," if the ball is still in the quarterback's hands, then players can cross the line and get the flags. If the quarterback gives up the ball, the non-rush rule no longer applies.

7. T

8. T

9. T

10. T

Extra Credit

1. c

2. e

3. a

4. b

5. d

Football Answer Key—Intermediate level

1. T. If opponents take over, they are only 20 yards from the end zone in which they score.

2. T. Penalties result when a team breaks a rule—in this case, the offsides rule.

3. T. "Squaring in" requires running across the middle.

4. T. This would be a safety.

5. T. No forward pass is allowed; these are not going forward.

6. F. "Seven Mississippi" is the limited time the quarterback has without fearing being rushed.

7. T. If the ball hits the ground, there is no chance of the opponent getting a completion.

8. T. Never let your person get behind you.

9. T. There is no chance of a runback.

10. F. The quarterback or anyone else can receive as long as the ball is behind the line of scrimmage.

Extra Credit:

1. d

2. a

3. e

4. b

5. c

Football Answer Key—Advanced level

1. F. They cannot hope to get their opponents any further back than they already are, and they can use the fourth down to possibly score.

2. T

3. T

4. T

5. T

6. F. The player should always try to block the throwing lanes of the quarterback.

7. T

8. T. Good defense means never letting your opponent get behind you.

9. T. This avoids a touchback and bringing the ball out to the 20-yard line.

10. F. Because the ball is still behind the line of scrimmage, it can be passed. The defense should continue to keep its responsibilities until the ball is up or over the line of scrimmage.

11. D

12. A

13. E

14. B

15. C

16. 5

17. 6

18. 1. The "square in"

19. 6

20. 3

Soccer

Unit Overview

1. Allow students the chance to learn a skill by providing a lot of repetition with the ball as well as encouraging them to understand the advantage of using their skills within game rules and strategies.

2. Teach the instep kicking pass (footwork, point of contact, firm leg) and the foot trap (heel-down position, lining up behind the ball) and the applicable rules (such as it being illegal to use one's hands).

3. Teach the soccer positions and their special responsibilities (forward line, midfielders, fullbacks, goalies) and applicable rules (offsides, penalty area, lineup on kick-off).

4. Teach the place kick, body trap, knee trap, and heading.

5. Teach the goalie's punt and the drop kick.

6. Incorporate soccer terminology while the skills are being learned.

7. Introduce whatever rules have not been introduced during skills lessons (throw-in, penalty kick, direct kick, indirect kick, corner kick, goal kick).

8. Teach the common penalties for rules violations so that students can assist in the games of others or monitor their own games, knowing when something is illegal and what penalty is awarded the violated team.

9. Teach the fundamental game strategies for defense:
   - Zone or person-to-person defense—marking one's person
   - The outlet pass

10. Teach the fundamental offensive strategies:
    - Centering the ball
    - Moving forward with the ball or moving ahead of the ball with two opponents between the player and the goal

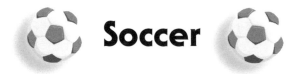

Soccer

HISTORY

Soccer, or football as it is known in most of the world, is thought to have begun around 200 BC. The Chinese played the game early on as a form of military training. Eskimos played aqsaqtuk, in which they played football with goals 10 miles apart. During the 1300s, football became popular in England. And in 1863, the London Football Association was formed. Then, in 1904, the Fédération Internationale de Football Association was founded in Paris.

FUN FACTS

➜ Mia Hamm is the all-time leading international goal scorer for females.

➜ Just Fontaine, who scored 13 goals in the 1958 World Cup, still holds the record for the most goals.

➜ The United States Youth Soccer Association has more than 3 million members.

➜ The United Soccer League was founded in 1986 to help players develop a higher level of play.

➜ Men's Major League Soccer began in 1996.

BENEFITS OF PLAYING

1. Soccer provides you with a great cardiovascular workout.
2. Playing soccer is a great way to condition your legs.
3. Soccer is a good team activity that teaches you how to work together.
4. You can play soccer in a gym or outdoors.
5. Soccer is fun!

TIME TO SURF!

Web Site	Web Site Address
United States Soccer Federation	http://www.us-soccer.com/
United States Youth Soccer Association	http://www.usysa.org/
Fédération Internationale de Football Association	http://www.fifa.com/

From *Complete Physical Education Plans for Grades 7–12* by Isobel Kleinman, 2001, Champaign, IL: Human Kinetics.

Soccer Unit Extension Project

NAME _____ CLASS _____

Equipment needed to play soccer

Item	Where you would purchase it (be specific)	Cost

Where you would play soccer

Please explain where in the community you would play soccer. Be specific. Are there any organized leagues for adults. Are there soccer fields available for the public. Are there open spaces where you might set up your own field?

Health benefits of playing soccer

Please explain the health benefits of playing soccer. Include how much soccer you would need to play each week to gain these benefits.

Reflection question

Do you think soccer is an activity you would like to play as an adult? Why or why not? And if you believe you'd like to play soccer, would you rather play in an organized recreation league, in pick-up games at a park, or in your own backyard with friends and family?

From *Complete Physical Education Plans for Grades 7–12* by Isobel Kleinman, 2001, Champaign, IL: Human Kinetics.

Soccer Teaching Tips

1. Plan to teach the rules appropriate to the skill when the skill is introduced.
2. Allow sufficient noncompetitive practice time with equipment for students to learn and improve their skills without additional performance pressure.
3. Use movements specific to soccer during the warm-up phase of the lesson.
4. After several lessons, and when you have a feel for the depth of skill of the class, divide up the class into equal teams on the basis of skill, gender, and number, and begin to encourage working together as a unit, establishing leadership within the group, and promoting feelings of belonging and being needed.
5. Develop a short tournament, having all students involved by assigning each of them to a team or, if they're unable to participate, giving them the jobs of officiating, marking the ball, or keeping score:
   - Students clearly will have different prior experiences with soccer. Advanced soccer athletes should be encouraged to help others and to improve their own goals while following class instructions. They should be looking to improve consistency, accuracy, distance, time, and speed.
   - Every effort should be made to assure students that improvement is what is valued, not a predisposition to be a great athlete.
6. If students are unable to participate fully in class activities, remember that they can be involved by coaching, officiating, keeping score, or conducting a research project.

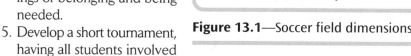

Figure 13.1—Soccer field dimensions.

Unit Setup

Facility

When indoors, use a large space unencumbered by obstruction, allowing movement of a minimum of 30 yards forward and 10 yards right and left, without running into a wall, person, or temporary obstructions

Clear boundaries for each concurrent game

An outdoor field marked for soccer, with soccer goals, 100 yards by 50 yards, for every 22 players

Equipment

One soccer ball for every two students

Pinnies to identify opposing teams

A visual aid (blackboard, chart, or magnetic board) and writing implements

Paper for each student

Unit Timeline

One unit of 12 to 16 lessons for the younger age groups has been developed here:

6 lessons to develop skill competency in the fundamentals and the basic game concept

6 to 10 lessons to complete an event using the fundamentals in a challenging way

Unit Assessment

A student portfolio checklist is provided here for student use (table 13.1). Encourage students to track their progress as they master new skills. Students will conclude the unit with a quiz. Their performance will be based on the soccer performance rubric.

TABLE 13.1 Soccer Student Portfolio Checklist

STUDENT NAME _____

☐ Is able to stop a soccer ball

☐ Is able to pass a soccer ball 10 yards

☐ Can dribble, using a tight soccer dribble

☐ Understands the goal of the team in possession of the ball

☐ Understands the goal of the team without the ball

☐ Understands basic soccer terminology

☐ Understands where offensive players without the ball should go

☐ Knows how to and can attempt to disrupt the successful play of opponents

☐ Is able to follow basic soccer rules

☐ Is able to exhibit good sporting behavior

☐ Can play without endangering the safety of others

From *Complete Physical Education Plans for Grades 7–12* by Isobel Kleinman, 2001, Champaign, IL: Human Kinetics

Additional Resources

Herbst, Dan. 1999. *Soccer: How to Play the Game: The Official Playing and Coaching Manual of the United States Soccer Federation*. New York: Universe Press.

McGettigan, James. 1989. *Soccer Drills for Individual and Team Play*. West Nyack, NY: Prentice Hall Direct.

Rees, Roy, and Cor Van Der Meer. 1997. *Coaching Soccer Successfully*. Champaign, IL: Human Kinetics.

Soccer Lesson 1 — Beginner level

Lesson Setup

Facility

Clear, unobstructed field

Equipment

One ball for every two players

Performance Goals

Students will

use their feet to pass and trap a soccer ball, and
practice the loose and tight soccer dribble.

Cognitive Goals

Students will learn

that passing with the left or right instep gives them a choice,
why they should not lift their foot to trap a ball, and
several ways to advance the ball.

Lesson Safety

Practice areas should be separated by a minimum of five yards per group with a ball.
The line of direction of practice should be the same.

Warm-Up

Students will

1. Jog around the playing area
2. Practice soccer-kick mimetics: body position, leg position, follow-through

3. Practice trapping a soccer ball
4. Perform stretches

Motivation

Most of your students probably have kicked a ball before. Ask them to see if they can kick the ball to someone and have that person stop it without losing it.

Lesson Sequence

1. Demonstrate a proper instep pass and foot trap.
2. Have students get a partner and practice kicking back and forth; start close so that passes are accurate. Increase the distance a few feet at a time until students are 20 feet apart.
3. Demonstrate the dribble and have students practice the tight dribble and the loose dribble. This will be a review for most.
4. Make a contest of this practice so students do not get bored while improving these skills. Change the goals to maintain interest. Some examples:
   - Whoever can stop five passes first is the winner.
   - See who can dribble to the other side first.
   - See who can dribble the ball halfway and pass to his partner accurately.

Review

Review where a player's foot should contact the ball.
Ask who can show the class a proper follow-through.
Ask students to explain why keeping the heel down is so important when trapping the ball.
Discuss the advantages of a tight dribble and a loose dribble.

Assessment

Observe each student, providing individualized coaching hints to improve a tight dribble or loose dribble.
Check the kick, making sure students have a low swinging motion and meet the ball with a firm foot.

Soccer Lesson 2 — Beginner level

Performance Goals

Students will

use their foot to trap the ball when an opponent is dribbling with it—a straight-on tackle;
perform a body trap; and
practice passing the ball using the instep and top of foot.

Cognitive Goals

Students will learn the rules

relevant to a body trap—no hands may touch the ball; and
relevant to a straight-on tackle—it is illegal to
- kick one's opponent,
- slide-tackle, and
- use unnecessary roughness.

Lesson Safety

Make certain that practice groups are five yards apart for simple drills. Once the mini-competitions start, separate groups by 10 yards.

Warm-Up

Students will

1. Practice soccer-kick mimetics: body position, leg position, follow-through
2. Practice trapping a soccer ball
3. Dribble a soccer ball
4. Perform stretches

Motivation

There are a few skills that the students absolutely need to play a soccer game: They have to be able to move the ball forward—they did this one way when they practiced the dribble. They also have to get it in order to move it forward. Ask students how they can get the ball from an opponent legally. That is what they are going to find out in this lesson.

Lesson Sequence

1. Demonstrate a straight-on tackle and have students try it.
2. Have students get a partner and a ball and dribble slowly to each other. The one without the ball should stop the ball while the partner is dribbling:
   - Have each player try it slowly first, and repeat several times.
   - Ask them to increase the speed so it is more like a game, and repeat several times.
3. Demonstrate a place kick (the top of the foot contacts the ball) and have students practice.
4. If students seem to be getting bored, make a contest, changing the goals to maintain interest. For example, combine groups of partners so they are working in fours:
   - Ask who can kick a place kick (top of the foot) farthest.
   - See if they can dribble the ball halfway and pass to their partner accurately.
   - In groups of four, have students count off one through four. Teams are based on the odd and even numbers. Then begin an odd/even drill.

Give the ball to the odd team first. Their job is to dribble from their cone to the cone on the other side. If they do, they get a point for their team. At the same time the even-team players are trying to get the ball from the odd team. Instruct students to use the straight-on tackle to come up with the ball (figure 13.2). If they do, they are to dribble to the opposite cone and try to get a point. The group has 20 seconds. If neither of the two groups gets the ball to the opposite side, then no one gets a point.

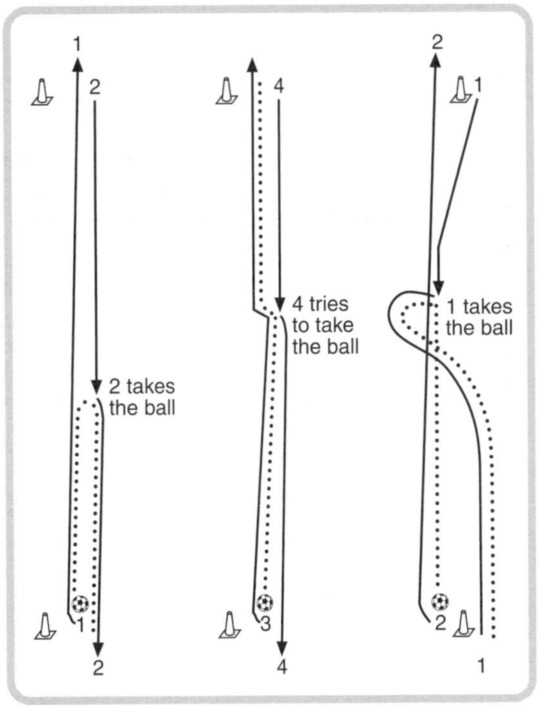

Review

Ask students where their foot should contact the ball on a place kick and on a straight-on tackle.

Instruct them that at the beginning of the next class they should help themselves to the equipment, get a partner, and do a lap around the field, dribbling and passing back and forth with their partner. When they are done, they should practice passing.

Figure 13.2—Practicing the straight on tackle.

Soccer Lesson 3   Beginner level

Lesson Setup

Facility

Goalposts and a game area for every two teams

Equipment

Scrimmage vests for half the class

Performance Goals

Students will

move the ball by heading and knee-volleying, and play a game.

Cognitive Goals

Students will

learn why, when, and where they use their head to contact the ball;
learn a legal way to redirect a ball coming at their body; and
begin to understand why jobs on the soccer field are differentiated.

Lesson Safety

The fields should be clean of debris and set up with visible goalposts.

Warm-Up

Students will

1. Dribble and pass a soccer ball with a partner once around the outside of the soccer field
2. Practice passing with partners
3. Perform stretches

Motivation

Tell students that one of the interesting things about learning to play soccer is that the player can use every single part of the body to move the ball except for the part he is probably most used to using: the hands. In this lesson they will learn to use a few more parts of the body. Then they will try to run around and do what everyone else tries to do when playing a soccer game: score.

Lesson Sequence

1. Demonstrate heading:
   - Have students rehearse looking up at an imaginary ball, lining up under it, and heading it.
   - Then have them try with an actual ball, allowing students to first head from a self-toss.
   - Have partners toss the ball to them and try to head it back.
2. Demonstrate the knee volley. Use the same procedure to practice it as above.
3. Divide the class into teams for the day.
4. Prepare them for a game:
   - Indicate the boundaries.
   - Have one team put on pinnies.
   - Assign the pinny team to kick the ball on your whistle, and let them play—with no other instructions.

Review

Tell the class that their game looked difficult. Ask students if they can dribble in a crowd. Tell them no, they really cannot get very far.

Ask them how they knew when to go after the ball.

Review whether it works to have all of them go after the ball at once—22 people trying to get the ball. Ask what their chances are: How can they get the ball out of that crowded mess? If a player kicks it and everyone is with her trying to get the ball, ask who will get the pass.

Admit that it is confusing and that in the next class you will try to clear up the confusion and teach them how to divide up the responsibilities on the field so they are not so frustrated.

Assessment

Observe the class during its practice, providing individualized coaching. Watch the game, stopping it to call penalties, scores, or throw-ins and observing what team strategies players are lacking. Plan on focusing on those strategies in the next lesson.

Soccer Lesson 4 — Beginner level

Lesson Setup

Equipment

Blackboard, chart, or magnetic board

Performance Goals

Students will

begin games with a proper kickoff, and
be in soccer positions at kickoff and play their positions during a game.

Cognitive Goals

Students will

learn why and how jobs on the field are different for the forward line, midfielders, and backs;
take one of the jobs on the field and learn it; and
learn how, why, and the applicable rules for a throw-in.

Lesson Safety

There should be clean and clear game areas with visible goals.
Be prepared to stop any dangerous play, particularly once competition starts.

Warm-Up

Students will

1. Dribble and pass ball with partners one lap around the field then engage in free play
2. Perform stretches as a class

Motivation

Tell the class that if everyone tried to do it all, there would be 22 people around the ball and no one away from it to pass to. In this lesson, you will teach students that in soccer—a game that can travel 5,000 square yards in any given moment—no one player tries to do it all. Team members divide up the responsibilities and then back each other up in case the game plan doesn't work.

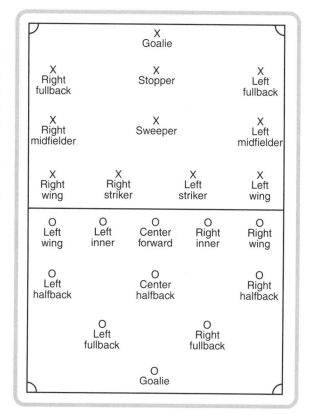

Figure 13.3—Starting line-up on the soccer field.

Lesson Sequence

1. Diagram the team positions at kickoff (figure 13.3):
   • Show where players start off at kickoff and after every score.
   • Give the positions their name and a general idea of their responsibility:
      The forwards work together to score.
      The halfbacks sometimes join them, but mostly try to get the ball back once it is lost to opponents.
      The backs are there to stop the ones who get away and are becoming a scoring threat.
      The goalies are the last line of defense.
2. Change the diagram so that it shows each position once the ball moves down the field.
3. Divide the class into game teams, indicate boundaries, and have one team put on pinnies.

4. Start the games with a kickoff.
5. During games, coach students to remember the side of the field they should be on.
6. After 10 minutes of play, stop the game:
   - Demonstrate a proper throw-in.
   - Explain when it is used and what happens if it is not done correctly.
7. Continue the game until it's time for review.

Review

Ask students what they should do when the ball goes out of bounds on the sidelines.

Ask the class who played on the forward line, who played as wings, and who were strikers. Ask who shot at the goal.

Review who the midfielders were, and if they remembered to defend their own goal before worrying about scoring.

Ask if the goalie made any saves.

Ask if the backs moved up or if they were glued to the penalty area.

Assessment

If this is too much material to cover in one day, spend a second day on it before going on to the next lesson.

Soccer Lesson 5 — Beginner level

Performance Goals

Students will play a game, returning the ball to play

after a score with a kickoff,
after a failed shot for the goal with a goal kick, and
after it goes on the sideline with a throw-in.

Cognitive Goals

Students will

learn what skills work best for the players
- on the left side of the field, and
- on the right side of the field
begin to learn what special skills are more useful in different soccer positions:
- Fast runners with good ball-handling skills—the wings
- Good basketball skills with no fear of being hit—the goalies
learn the how, why, and applicable rules for
- the goal kick,
- the kickoff after the score, and
- the throw-in.

Warm-Up

Students will

1. Practice passing and dribbling with partners
2. Practice mimetics for heading, body trap (figure 13.4), knee volley, and shoulder volley

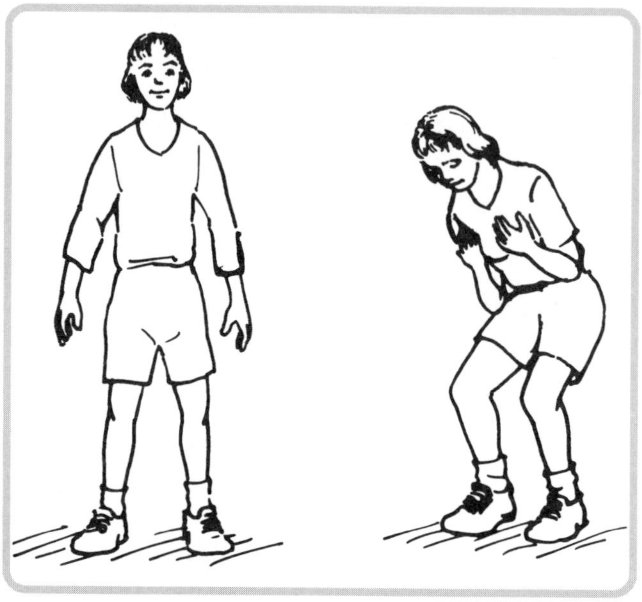

Motivation

Tell the class that everyone is different and can make special contributions to his team that perhaps he never thought of. People who are strong-footed on one side and not the other, people with great anticipation of their opponents, people with good reach and quick reflexes with their hands, people who have long driving kicks, and people with good foot speed and a love of keeping the ball to themselves as they razzle-dazzle everyone with great footwork—they all would fit well in different positions on the soccer field.

In this lesson, students will learn where each would fit best, so their strengths can be taken the most advantage of.

Figure 13.4—Mimetic for a body trap.

Lesson Sequence

1. Explain how personal assets can be used more easily in certain positions:
   - Assign those able to kick to the right to positions on the left side of the field.
   - Since the breakaway position is the wing, the fastest dribbler with the best footwork should be a wing.
   - Since the most complex job on the field is the center halfback, assign the most knowledgeable player on the team to that position.
   - Since the goalies need to use their hands, stretch to get everything near the goal, and bend down to stop a ball that someone is intent on kicking, they need guts and good basketball skills such as jumping and catching.
   - Since the least amount of running is done by the backs, students who don't love to run and who have a strong kick should enjoy that position best.
   - Since the people in the middle must be able to pass well to the left and the right, those sent for the job should not be one-footed.

2. Explain how to put the ball in play after a team shoots and scores or misses the goal.
3. Either use the teams from the previous class or divide the class again, having one team put on pinnies.
4. Point out the boundaries before the games begin.
5. Start the games with a kickoff.
6. Coach from the sidelines:
   - Make sure that all balls that go out of bounds are returned properly.
   - Remind the class about positions and where the players should be on the field.
   - Call obvious rules violations.

Review

If someone shoots and misses, ask the class how the ball gets put back into play.

If someone shoots and scores, ask how the ball gets put back into play.

Have students discuss who is the fastest on their team that day, and ask if that person played wing or sweeper. Ask if that player got to use her speed.

Advise students to bring in a sweatshirt or sweater that they can leave in their locker for any chilly days outside.

Teacher Homework

Divide up the class into equally skilled tournament teams.

Soccer Lesson 6 — Beginner level

Performance Goals

Students will

be able to put the ball back into play after personal violations, and

play a game using a penalty shot for the goal if the offense is fouled in the penalty area.

Cognitive Goals

Students will learn

what is meant by high kicking, dangerous play, sliding tackles, pushing, holding, kicking, and offsides;

when and why penalties are harsh—for example, a penalty shot for the goal; and

their tournament teams.

Warm-Up

Students will

1. Practice with equipment—complete a dribbling lap with partners passing back and forth
2. Practice mimetics for a body trap, heading, knee volley, shoulder volley, foot trap, and knee trap

Motivation

Explain to the class that rules make it possible for everyone to play a fair and safe game. Review the rules, especially now that the students are getting ready to start their tournament. Then, announce the teams.

Lesson Sequence

1. Explain the following:
   - High kicking and why it is dangerous
   - Dangerous play, especially around the goalie
   - Sliding tackles
   - Pushing, holding, and kicking
   - Offsides
2. Explain penalties: the direct kick, indirect kick, penalty shot for goal
3. Announce the teams and allow them to pick their captains.
4. Start the games with a kickoff.
5. Coach the positions and call obvious rules violations.

Review

Ask the class what would cause a penalty shot for the goal.
Ask if offsides would be dangerous.
Ask someone to explain offsides.
Review whether a player can be offsides when he is no closer to the goal than the ball.
Review whether he can be offsides if his dribble passed everyone on the field.

Soccer Lessons 7-12 or tournament conclusion   Beginner level

Lesson Setup

Equipment

A posted tournament schedule. Tournament schedules and charts can be found in appendix A.

Posted team standings, updated daily
Game ball for each game

Performance Goals

Students will

play one match each day,
play their positions and assume team responsibilities,
play by the rules, and
exhibit good sporting behavior.

Cognitive Goals

Students will

improve their knowledge of team interaction,
understand what an outlet pass and an inlet pass are and when to use each,
    and
understand the rules.

Lesson Safety

Correct and redirect competitive behavior that takes a bad turn and starts to endanger the physical and psychological health of the students.

Warm-Up

Students will

1. Pass, trap, and dribble with partners during free-play practice
2. Perform class stretches

Motivation

Announce the standings of the tournament. Tell students that you will be at every field, but if you are not there when they need you, they should call. Wish them luck, and may the team that best plays together, win.

Lesson Sequence

1. Explain and show the following (diagrammed in figure 13.5, which shows two suitable defensive passes and one not-so-suitable pass for defense):
   • The value of passing the ball out to the closest side of the field while on defense
   • The value of centering or passing it in on offense
2. Announce the standings and the new team matchups and what field they play on.

3. Have captains choose a side or pinnies (the pinny team wins the kickoff).
4. Start the games with a kickoff, coach the positions, and call obvious rules violations.

Review

Ask if the class has any questions.
Review who won.

Assessment

Observe and compliment the following: good passes, good anticipation, good field positioning, a great stop, a great assist, a good try, good sporting behavior, good team leadership, and so forth.

Give a quiz, saving it for the first rainy day. If there is none, give it on the last day of the unit.

Post the defined performance goals and observe for standards as per the performance assessment rubric for soccer (table 13.2). For further general assessment rubrics, see appendix B.

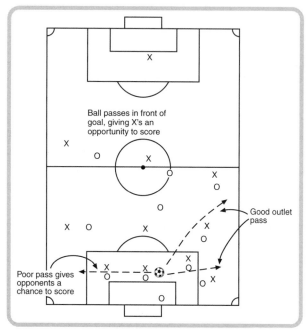

Figure 13.5—Team O uses an outlet pass to position the ball near the side of the field. Passing the ball to the left centers it for Team X, giving them the opportunity to score.

TABLE 13.2 Beginner Soccer Performance Assessment Rubric

STUDENT NAME _____

	0	1	2	3
Trapping	No effort	• Uses proper body mechanics • Lines up with the ball	• Foot-traps an accurate pass • Blocks an inaccurate ball up to three feet away	• Sucessfully uses body traps • Controls the ball and direction
Dribble	No effort	• Uses proper body mechanics • Moves the ball forward	• Uses a tight dribble • Moves the ball at top speed	• Chooses to use a loose or tight dribble at the proper times
Pass	No effort	• Uses proper body mechanics • Is accurate up to 10 yards away	• Moves the ball forward— left or right • Passes from a dribble • Moves the ball to 30 yards away	• Uses many body parts to pass • Follows a trap with an accurate pass • Varies speed and distance
Position or direction	No effort	• Knows where to go to score • Tries to move the ball in the correct direction	• Uses an outlet pass on defense and an inlet pass on offense • Shifts in the direction of play • Maintains distance between teammates	• Interchanges position • Senses when help is needed • Anticipates opponents
Teamwork and sporting behavior	No effort	• Gets to the field on time • Gets along with teammates • Hogs the ball or blames others	• Tries to play within the rules • Does not hog the ball • Makes an effort to improve weaknesses	• Leads the team constructively • Plays within the rules • Is the go-to person

Soccer Quiz–Beginner level

NAME _____   TEACHER _____

DATE _____   CLASS PERIOD _____

Multiple Choice: Read each question and each answer carefully. Be sure to choose the best answer that fits the statement preceding it. When you have made your choice, put the appropriate letter on the line to the left of the numbered question.

_____1. The soccer dribble is a skill that allows
    a. the player to bounce the ball from his hands to the ground
    b. the player to move with the ball by tapping the ball with his instep
    c. the player to kick the ball to the goal for a possible score
    d. the ball to get clean while the tops of the player's sneakers get dirty

_____2. An outlet pass
    a. is out of bounds
    b. is best used by the forward line as they get nearer the goal
    c. is an attempt to get the ball out of an opponent's scoring position
    d. all of the above

_____3. The reason every position on the field should be covered regardless of where the ball is, is that
    a. the teacher will get mad if everyone does not get a chance
    b. it gives players more places and players to pass to when in danger of being stripped of the ball
    c. defensive players are not allowed to shoot for the goal
    d. all of the above

_____4. The body trap should result in the ball
    a. dropping near your feet so that you can dribble or pass it if you want to
    b. bouncing away from your body, with the hope that a teammate will get it
    c. hitting your shoulder before bouncing on the ground
    d. being covered by the goalie until everyone clears the penalty area

_____5. When a ball goes out of bounds at a sideline, the game stops and an opponent must
    a. run out of bounds, put it down on the line, and kick it in
    b. run out of bounds to get it and dribble it into play
    c. run to get it and throw it in using both hands, with both feet on the ground
    d. wait for the official to roll it into play

_____6. The penalty area is
    a. the area in which the goalie may pick up the ball in her hands
    b. where penalty shots are awarded the offense because the defense fouled them
    c. the area in which the goal box is marked
    d. all of the above

_____7. The kickoff is
    a. used at the beginning of the game
    b. used to start play at the beginning of each playing period and after a goal is scored
    c. awarded to the team that did not just score
    d. all of the above

_____8. To properly head the ball, you should
    a. drop your head just before the ball touches it
    b. keep your eyes up, get under the ball, and allow the ball to meet your hairline
    c. be prepared to scream a lot but feel good about helping the team
    d. understand that anyone who uses his head other than to think is nuts

_____9. The left wing position should be taken by the fastest person on the team because
   a. most people kick to the left more easily than to their right, so more passes go to the left wing
   b. the field is usually more empty on the sides than in the middle and there is room for the wing to use her speed
   c. if she really gets a "breakaway," she always can run to the goal
   d. all of the above

_____10. The player most likely to both play defense and score is the
   a. goalie
   b. sweeper/center halfback/center midfielder
   c. stopper/fullback
   d. all of the above

Extra Credit: Eleven players on the X team are diagrammed as if spread out during play. Find the correct number on the diagram to correspond with the questions and put your answer on the line to the left.

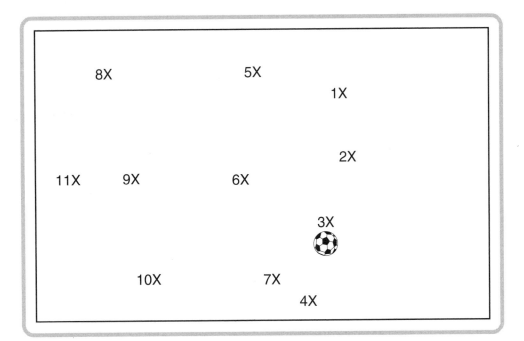

_____1. X team goalie
_____2. X team left wing
_____3. X stopper

_____4. The name of 3x
_____5. X right midfielder

From *Complete Physical Education Plans for Grades 7–12* by Isobel Kleinman, 2001, Champaign, IL: Human Kinetics.

Soccer Answer Key—Beginner level

1. B. A dribble is intended to move forward while keeping control of the ball.
2. C. Outlet passes move the ball away from the goal to the side of the field, getting the ball out of the scoring position.
3. B
4. A. The purpose of trapping a ball is to get control of it.
5. C. A throw-in is the required method of returning a ball that goes out of bounds on the sideline.
6. D
7. D
8. B
9. D
10. B

Extra Credit:

1. 11x
2. 1x
3. 9x
4. Right striker
5. 7x

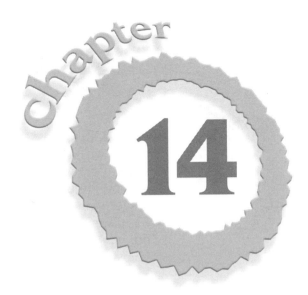

Softball

Unit Overview

1. One new concept should be introduced and developed each lesson. The early lessons tend to practice more than one skill, which avoids muscle overuse and flattening of the learning curve because of boredom.

2. Teach skills by providing a lot of repetition with the ball. Teach the advantages of using skills within a game and rule strategies:

   - Throwing (grip, stance, arm motion, follow-through) for accuracy, speed, and distance
   - Catching (glove position, eye contact, footwork) for grounders, fly balls, and drives
   - Pitching terminology, rules, and strategies; the strike zone
   - Batting—a full swing, a bunt
   - Base running—tagging inside of the bag, overrunning first, sliding, and leading off
   - Fielding strategies and rules:
     Going for the automatic out at first
     Force plays
     Squeeze plays
     Throwing ahead of the runner to get the out
     What to do after catching a fly ball
     Anticipating coverages
     Limiting the bases run by throwing to second
     The cutoff person
     When a tag is necessary
   - Offensive strategies—batting-order strategies and base running
   - Game rules—three outs, full innings, scoring, when a game is over
   - Coeducational rule modifications:
     Infield covered by an equal number of males and females
     Batting order so it alternates male and female
     Alternate male and female pitchers after every two innings
     Have girls pitch to girls, boys pitch to boys
   - Common penalties for rules violations:
     Balking
     Interfering with a base runner
     Batter out of batter's box
     Overrunning second or third

467

Softball

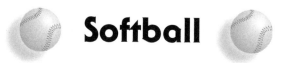

HISTORY

In Chicago in 1887, Yale had just beat Harvard in a football game. This sparked a Yale alumnus to throw a boxing glove at a Harvard alumnus, igniting the beginnings of softball. Reporter George Hancock saw the Ivy League interaction and invented an indoor game of baseball. His game later was taken outdoors, where eventually the name became kitten ball. Finally, the name softball was given to the game in 1926 by Walter Hakanson, a Denver YMCA official.

FUN FACTS

➜ More than 40 million people play softball each summer in the United States.

➜ Softball is the number one team sport participated in in the United States.

➜ More than 1.2 million boys and girls play American Softball Association Junior Olympic Softball each year.

➜ The USA won the first-ever Olympic Gold Medal in softball in 1996.

➜ Women can play professional fast-pitch softball.

BENEFITS OF PLAYING

1. Softball is great for hand-eye coordination.
2. Softball helps you develop teamwork skills.
3. There are many recreational softball leagues that people can participate in.
4. You can play softball at almost any age.
5. It is fun!

TIME TO SURF!

Web Site	Web Site Address
Amateur Softball Association	http://www.softball.org/
Women's Pro Softball League	http://www.prosoftball.com/
USA Softball	http://www.usasoftball.com/

From *Complete Physical Education Plans for Grades 7–12* by Isobel Kleinman, 2001, Champaign, IL: Human Kinetics.

Softball Unit Extension Project

NAME _____ CLASS _____

Equipment needed to play softball

Item	Where you would purchase it (be specific)	Cost

Where you would play softball

Please explain where in the community you would play softball. Be specific.

Health benefits of playing softball

Please explain the health benefits of playing softball. Include how much softball you would need to play each week to gain these benefits.

Reflection question

Do you think softball is an activity you would like to play as an adult? Why or why not? And if you believe you'd like to play softball, would you rather play in an organized recreation league or in pick-up games at a park with friends and family?

From *Complete Physical Education Plans for Grades 7–12* by Isobel Kleinman, 2001, Champaign, IL: Human Kinetics.

Softball Teaching Tips

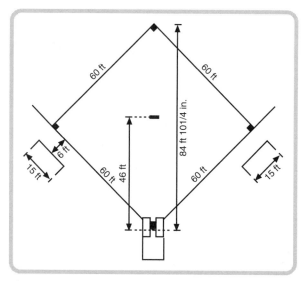

Figure 14.1—Softball field dimensions.

1. Plan to teach the rules appropriate to the skill when the skill is introduced and practiced. For example, when emphasizing the importance of catching a softball when it is in the air, teach the advantages of the automatic out, and that the base runners who advanced before the ball was caught must return to the previous base.

2. Allow noncompetitive practice time with equipment so that students can improve their skills without performance pressure.

3. Have the class use the proper footwork and muscle sequence during the warm-up phase of the lesson.

4. After several lessons, when you have a feel for the depth of skill of the class, divide up the class into equal teams, on the basis of skill, gender, and number, and begin to encourage working together as a unit, promoting leadership within the group and feelings of belonging.

5. Develop a short tournament that includes all students. If students are unable to play in the game, assign a job of calling balls and strikes, umpiring in the field, or keeping the score book:
   - Students clearly will have different experiences with softball and baseball. Advanced players should be encouraged to help others and to improve the quality of the same skills the class is being taught. They should be looking to improve consistency, accuracy, distance, time, and speed.
   - Every effort should be made to assure students that improvement is what is valued, not a predisposition to be a great athlete.

6. If students are unable to participate fully in class activities, remember that they can be involved by coaching, officiating, keeping score, or conducting a research project.

Unit Safety

The following safety rules will make all softball games safer:

The catcher must wear protective equipment.

Fielders should each have a softball glove.

Sliding will not be allowed during class.

Fielding practice throws and catches will be restricted to the beginning of the inning.

No one can practice batting; the swinging of bats is restricted to whoever is on deck.

Unit Timeline

There are three units of softball in this chapter:

15 lessons for seventh- and eighth-graders:
- Four to develop skill competency
- Four to learn to use them in a game
- Seven days set aside for three official games of softball, a class tournament, and a quiz

12 lessons for 9th- and 10th-graders:
- Six for skills and game practice
- Six for a small class tournament of three official games

10 lessons for 11th- and 12th-graders:
- Four for skills and game practice
- Six for three official games

Unit Setup

Facility

A large space, unencumbered by obstruction and free of rocks and garbage

A backstop, first baseline, and third baseline—at a minimum—if a real softball field not available

A visual aid—blackboard, softball magnetic board, or chart of fielders' positions

Equipment

One softball for every two students

One glove for every student

Catcher's equipment—a mask, chest protector, shin guards, and glove

A set of bases and a pitcher's mound

Bats of varying lengths and weights. Make sure there are bats short and light enough for even the smallest student in your class. They should be able to hold the bat up and swing it horizontally without the head of the bat tipping down. Also, make sure there are bats adequate for the tallest and strongest students. Each team should have a complete set of bats.

Round-robin tournament schedules and charts (see appendix A)

Unit Assessment

A student portfolio checklist is provided here for student use (table 14.1). Encourage students to track their progress as they master new skills. The unit concludes with a quiz and a softball performance assessment rubric for each grade level. Additional general assessment rubrics can be found is appendix B.

Additional Resources

American Sport Education Program. 1996. *Coaching Youth Softball*. Champaign, IL: Human Kinetics.

Craig, Susan, and Ken Johnson. 1985. *The Softball Handbook*. Champaign, IL: Leisure Press.

Meyer, Gladys C. 1984. *Softball for Girls and Women*. New York: IDG Books Worldwide.

Potter, Diane L., and Gretchen A. Brockmeyer. 1999. *Softball: Steps to Success* (2nd ed.). Champaign, IL: Human Kinetics.

TABLE 14.1   Softball Student Portfolio Checklist

STUDENT NAME _____

- ☐ Is able to throw a softball accurately a minimum of 60 feet
- ☐ Is able to catch a softball thrown to a target
- ☐ Can run the bases
- ☐ Can stop ground balls
- ☐ Can catch pop-ups within a four-step radius
- ☐ Has learned and can assume responsibility for one defensive position
- ☐ Has learned softball rules
- ☐ Has learned the batter's stance and how to swing and meet the ball
- ☐ Can identify the strike zone
- ☐ Is able to exhibit good sporting behavior
- ☐ Can play without endangering the safety of others

From *Complete Physical Education Plans for Grades 7–12* by Isobel Kleinman, 2001, Champaign, IL: Human Kinetics

Softball Lesson 1   Beginner level

Lesson Setup

Facility

Practice lanes separated by a minimum of five yards per couple
Four bases set up in a diamond, 60 feet from each other, preferably on a softball baseline

Equipment

Blooper softballs, if there are not enough gloves to go around
One softball glove per student
One ball for every two students

Performance Goals

Students will

hold and throw a softball;
catch, using their weak hand while wearing a softball glove; and
run around and tag the bases.

Cognitive Goals

Students will learn

a little history of softball,
what gives the ball direction and speed,
why the catch is so important in the field, and
why they should tag the inside corner of the base when rounding it.

Lesson Safety

Practice should be in the same line of direction.
All students should have softball gloves. Those who do not should not have to
catch anything but a blooper ball.

Warm-Up

Students will

1. Jog the bases, tagging the inside corner of the bag
2. Practice softball throwing mimetics: first the grip, adding, one at a time, the
   wrist snap, elbow and arm follow-through, shoulder rotation, and step forward, practicing in proper sequence as each new item is added
3. Practice mimetics for catching with the weak hand: lining up behind the
   path of the ball, the weak hand's position, watching the ball into the glove,
   and pulling the ball out with the throwing hand
4. Perform stretches, paying particular attention to the shoulder joint (figure
   14.2, a-b)

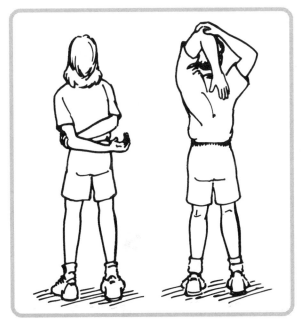

Figure 14.2—Stretching the shoulder.

473

Motivation

Americans invented baseball in the early 1800s, but the Canadians contributed softball to our game chest. Tell the class that the two games are very similar, but there are differences: the size of the field, the size of the ball, when runners may steal base, and how the pitch is thrown. In modern days, another form of softball has gained popularity: slow pitch. But the students will be learning the fastpitch game—the game used during interscholastic competition.

The class will be starting with the skills that, if well developed, will allow one's team to get to bat pretty fast. Tell them that if they cannot catch and throw the ball to the base person to put the batter out, they will be in the field all day. Have you played in a game where the offense took control and the defense didn't get to bat for a long time? Share the story with your students, or feel free to use my story.

I was one of a few teachers to participate in a teacher's group that decided to challenge our girl's junior high school interscholastic team to a game. Only three of us teachers could catch and throw a ball. We had taught and coached these girls so well, a winning team by the way, that they kept hitting our pitches like they were having batting practice. We, their teachers, were out in the field for over an hour before we ever got to bat!

Lesson Sequence

1. Having taught the proper softball throwing motion during warm-ups, emphasize catching first:
   - Have students get a partner and practice throwing back and forth:
      Emphasize reaching the target at chest height.
      Emphasize using the weak hand wearing the glove to reach for the catch.
   - Start at short distances that everyone can master easily, moving back a few steps at a time.
2. Teach students to remove the ball from the glove quickly. Use a contest to emphasize the importance of accuracy and speed and to make practice more fun:
   - From the sound of a whistle, see who can throw the ball to his partner fastest; from the same distance, see which partners get the most throws in 10 seconds
   - Do the same contest, but at a larger distance.
   - Be careful that the class does not overdo this muscle group—change the skills.
3. Teach catching grounders, having the thrower use an underhand motion to give arm relief:
   - The position
   - Moving in to get the ball
   - The mechanics of getting it out of the glove and throwing quickly

Review

Ask the students how their fingers should be on the ball.
Ask if someone can show a proper follow-through.
Discuss why stepping forward on the opposite foot is so important.
Review what is making the catch important.
Ask what is the most important thing to make sure to do when going after a ground ball.

Softball Lesson 2   Beginner level

Performance Goals

Students will

improve their throw and catch, and
simulate a softball game using only throwing and catching skills.

Cognitive Goals

Students will

realize the value of accurate throwing and being able to catch;
learn how the fly ball affects base-running rules, forces, and tags; and
learn that three outs is half an inning and what a full inning is.

Lesson Safety

Use the same line of direction for well-spaced-out practice.
Begin developing proper safety habits during softball by having the batting team at least 10 yards from the first or third baselines and no one but the catcher and the batter inside the backstop.

Warm-Up

Students will

1. Play catch with all equipment available during free-play time
2. Jog the bases once, then run them, tagging the inside corner of the bags
3. Practice softball throwing and catching mimetics with footwork

Motivation

Tell your students that they worked so hard at their throwing and catching in the last class that it's time for a little treat. First, you will give them a few minutes to warm up and practice a little more, so they'll never drop the ball. Then they are going to play an interesting game.

Lesson Sequence

1. Have the class practice throwing and catching (10 to 15 minutes).
2. Teach a "throw" softball game, in which the batter catches the pitch and throws the ball to become the base runner (figure 14.3):
   - The fielders must follow all the rules of softball:

     The ball must beat the runner to the bases to get the runner out.

     Runners who round first, with no one behind them, must be tagged out.

     Fly balls are an automatic out, and advancing runners must return to the base.

     Baserunners may not leave to advance to the next base until the ball is thrown by the next person "at bat."
   - The players up at home plate have one chance to catch a throw to the plate. If they drop the ball, they are out:

     Everyone gets a number in the batter order and must go in sequence.

     The batter can throw anywhere, but the ball cannot go higher than her head.

     The batter has to be put out at base unless she is put out at the plate, or her throw into the field is caught as a fly ball.
3. Divide the class in half; send half out to the field and half to the bench, and have them play the game.
4. When both teams have gotten their three outs, announce the end of the inning.
5. If there is time for more than one inning, make sure all students bat before anyone gets up a second time.

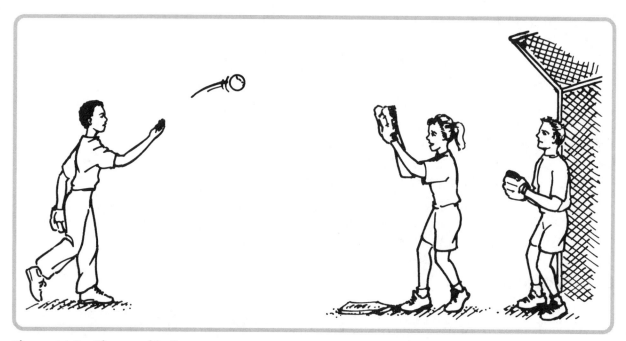

Figure 14.3—Throw softball game.

Review

Ask students which base they can overrun without being tagged.
Ask if anyone can explain a force play.
For the inning to be over discuss whether both teams have to get up.

Softball Lesson 3   Beginner level

Performance Goals

Students will

throw for distance,
catch pop-ups, and
simulate a softball game using only throwing and catching skills.

Cognitive Goals

Students will

realize the value of accurate throwing and the ability to catch a ball without
letting it drop;
review rules that apply to a fly ball—runners go back, an automatic out; and
learn what a batting order is and how to follow it.

Warm-Up

Students will

1. Play catch with all equipment available during free-play time
2. Jog the base once, then run them, tagging the inside corner of the bags
3. Practice softball throwing and running forward and back to catch fly
   balls

Motivation

Tell students that in this lesson they will try catching fly balls. For some, it may
be a little intimidating—but fly balls are great. If a player catches one, he gets an
automatic out. If he throws the ball to the base that a runner left before he
caught the fly, he might actually get that person out, too. And the nicest part is
that for every second the ball stays in the air, the player has more time to get
to it.

Actually, most of the class should be pretty good at getting under fly balls,
because the positioning for catching one is the same as getting ready for a setup
pass in volleyball. Suggest that the students get comfortable with these kinds of
catches and try them in a game.

Lesson Sequence

1. Have the class practice throwing pop-ups and catching them:
   - Explain that players can get greater throwing distance if the release of the ball is at a 45-degree angle from the horizontal plane their arm makes to the ground. (To figure this angle, have students stand with their throwing arms straight out horizontally. Then, have them raise their arms straight up. The mid-way distance between the two arm positions is 45 degrees.)
   - Tell them they should get under the ball so it looks like it's falling in their eyes, then block the ball with their glove.
2. Review the "throw" softball game:
   - The fielders must follow all the rules of softball:
     The ball must beat the runner to the bases to get the runner out.
     Runners who round first, with no one behind, must be tagged out.
     Fly balls are an automatic out, and advancing runners must return to the base.
     When the ball is "batted" into the outfield, runners can tag up. Discuss the strategy and why it is considered when the ball is in the outfield.
   - Players up at home plate have one chance to catch a throw to the plate. If they drop the ball, they are out:
     The batter throws anywhere on the field, but in today's game the ball must be a high throw.
     The batter must be thrown out at the base if the ball is not caught.
     A foul ball is an automatic out.
3. With the same teams, have the students who did not get up take their turn at the plate. The lineup continues:
   - Coach the player in the batter's box.
   - Before the batter hits, ask the team in the field where the lead runner is going.
   - Compliment everything that is right—the way the players ran, caught, got ready, and so forth.
4. Announce the scores at the top and bottom of the inning, reinforcing the concept of an inning.

Review

Ask the class why it is better to catch a ball while out in the field.
Ask what a fielder should do with a caught fly ball if the runner who was on second base ran to third and is still there.
Review what should be done with the ball if it is dropped in the outfield and the runner has already reached first base.
Review what should be done if there is no runner on first base, the player on second is coming to third, and an outfielder caught the ball.

Lesson Setup

Facility

A backstop for each group practicing batting, if possible
Batters on the same line with each other

Equipment

Two different-size bats for each group of four
A plate for each group of four
A pitcher's mound for each group of four

Performance Goals

Students will

bat, and
improve their throwing and catching skills.

Cognitive Goals

Students will learn

what the strike zone is,
how to address the plate,
how to choose a bat that is right for them,
how to swing a bat, and
batting rules.

Lesson Safety

Batters all must be on the same horizontal plane, with catchers behind them,
since there is no catcher's equipment for each catcher of a practice group.
Students should not fling the bat or let go while swinging. They must learn to
keep two hands on the bat at all times.
Groups should be at least 20 yards from each other.

Warm-Up

Students will

1. Play catch with all equipment available during free-play time
2. Practice pitching and batting swing mimetics

Motivation

Tell students that they have worked so much on throwing that it is now time to bat. You'll be teaching how to take full swings and and hit balls within their reach so they are confident to swing at pitches and not just hope the pitcher will walk them.

Lesson Sequence

1. After the warm-ups and pitching mimetics, gather the group around home plate. Teach the following:
   - Choosing a bat
   - Addressing the plate
   - The grip and stance
   - The swing
   - What happens in a game if a player gets hit inside the batter's box
2. Explain the procedures for practicing batting with the following reminders. Whoever is pitching should stay as far out as necessary to get the ball in the striker's zone:
   - Explain the strike zone and how the hitter can get out without swinging.
   - For this lesson, encourage swinging at everything students think they can reach.
   - Each batter must get three hits before leaving the plate. If one student is taking too long, students should notify you so you can help the batter get his timing and focus and complete successful hits.
3. Have students work in groups of four that rotate from one position to another after the batter gets three hits. Encourage, as pictured in figure 14.4, all outfielders to respond to another group's batted ball when it enters their area by getting it and throwing it back to the pitcher of the group that hit it. Each group of four consists of:
   - One catcher behind the plate setting a target for the pitcher
   - A batter
   - A pitcher
   - An outfielder
4. Before sending the students to practice, explain that getting the ball back to the pitcher fast will enable them to get more turns at bat. In order to do that, all the outfielders for all the groups should help relay stray balls back to the pitcher calling for them. Class cooperation will make the practice more meaningful.

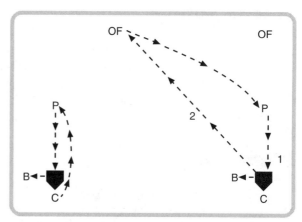

Figure 14.4—Class batting practice with the catcher (c) behind plate, the batter (b), pitcher (p), and outfilder (of).

Review

Ask the class what addressing the plate means.

Ask which is the power hand on the bat.

Review which hip of a right-handed player faces the pitcher.

Discuss whether the feet are supposed to help give the swing more power: Both of them, or just one? If one, which one?

Review where the strike zone is.

Ask the class whether a ball has to come down the middle of the plate if the pitcher wants it to be a strike.

Tell students to imagine the ball coming across their knees.

Softball Lesson 5 — Beginner level

Lesson Setup

Facility

Strike-zone targets painted, chalked, taped, or otherwise put on a wall

Equipment

A plate for each group of four
A pitching mound for each group

Performance Goals

Students will

pitch to a wall target, and
continue batting.

Cognitive Goal

Students will learn what fastpitch is and how it differs from slow-pitch softball.

Lesson Safety

Make sure students use the same line of direction in practice.
All fielders should wear a softball glove.

Warm-Up

Students will

1. Play catch with all equipment available during free-play time
2. Practice pitching and batting swing mimetics

Motivation

In this lesson, students need to develop potential pitchers. To do that, everyone can't keep lobbing the ball to the plate. If they did that in a game, the outfielders wouldn't like it too much—the players at bat would be hitting the ball all day and the fielding team would have a hard time getting them out and coming up to bat.

So, the class should practice pitching for a bit. Then, reconstruct batting practice the way it was done in the last class. But this time, instead of everyone pitching, the best pitcher should pitch, but from further back.

Lesson Sequence

1. After warm-ups and pitching mimetics, have the class go to the wall where the targets are visible:
   - Have each student in the group pitch three pitches, fast, aiming for the target.
   - They should rotate after every three successive pitches.
   - Continue this practice until the line goes through three times.
   - The next time, keep score. Give five pitches and see who hits the target most.
2. Distribute the equipment for batting (including a pitching mound):
   - Set up as the day before.
   - Encourage the group to let the best pitcher pitch during batting practice.
   - Use the pitching mound to keep the pitcher further away from the batter.
   - Ask someone behind the batter to give the pitcher a hand target to focus on.
   - Repeat batting practice.

Review

Ask the students what they should change if their pitches are too high.
Ask whether a batter should change anything about her swing if the pitch is coming in faster.
Review whether it is easier to hit a pop-up when the pitch is high or low.
Ask how big the strike zone is.

Teacher Homework

Divide up the class into teams.

Softball Lesson 6 — Beginner level

Lesson Setup

Facility

A designated softball field for each game

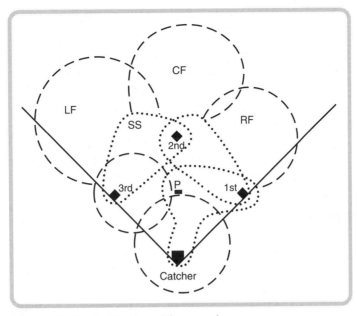

Figure 14.5—Softball positions and coverage.

Equipment

Blackboard or chart of fielding positions and coverages (figure 14.5)
A set of bases and a pitcher's mound for each game
A catcher's mask and equipment for each game
A list of each team's players

Performance Goal

Students will play a softball game with the teams they will be on for the tournament.

Cognitive Goals

Students will learn

the different fielding positions and the basic coverages, and
how to work with the eight other members of their team.

Lesson Safety

Catchers must wear safety equipment.
All fielders must wear a softball glove.
There is to be no sliding.

Warm-Up

Students will play catch with all equipment available during free-play time

Motivation

Tell students that they have been doing well. Now it is time to put it all together and get out on the field for a game. Before announcing the teams, go over one rule change—the foul ball in softball. The class played it out in "throw" softball, but in softball and baseball, it is only out on the third strike if a player is bunting or if it is a fly ball and is caught. All other fouls just count as a strike and one can never foul out. Now discuss the positions in the field: show the class how such a large field is essentially covered by just eight players (not counting the catcher, the ninth player).

Lesson Sequence

1. After the warm-ups, explain the following:
   - Why the catcher should wear the proper equipment during a game and how to put it on
   - The pre-hit positioning of base people and fielder and why
   - Who and how to back up
2. Announce the teams:
   - Send the first team out to the field so they can set up the bases. These students play defense first.
   - Announce the other team. The should set up their batting order and send their first batter to home plate.
3. Begin games right away. You might want to modify pitching rules for the first day.

Review

If a player is a base person and a grounder comes near her, review whether she should get the ball or cover the base. Have the class explain.

Softball Lesson 7 — Beginner level

Lesson Setup

Equipment

Blackboard or chart with enlarged lineup, score sheet, and field positions
Clipboards, pencils, clean score sheets, and lineup sheets for each team (table 14.2)

Performance Goal

Students will play a softball game.

TABLE 14.2 Softball Score Sheet

	1	2	3	4	5	6	7		1	2	3	4	5	6	7
1								1							
2								2							
3								3							
4								4							
5								5							
6								6							
7								7							
8								8							
9								9							
Runs in inning								**Runs in inning**							
Cumulative score								**Cumulative score**							

Codes

O	Got to first safely
/	Out
>	Got to second safely
■	Scored a run
◇	Got to third safely

Cognitive Goals

Students will
  review fielding positions and the basic coverages,
  review how to make a lineup and follow it, and
  work on teamwork with their teammates.

Warm-Up

Students will play catch with all equipment available during free-play time

Motivation

Now that students have spent a little time with their team, it is time to learn to organize it in the most profitable way possible. Tell them you will teach about making a lineup so that they have the best chance of scoring all the players who get to base, without leaving them stranded. They will have a little time to decide their lineup before starting the real games. As students play in this class, they should think about things like who they want to have as captain, who should "lead off," and who should be the "cleanup" batter. Have them take a look at the blackboard and see what is suggested. Tell them you will leave both the fielding positions and the lineup suggestions on the board so they can check it when they like.

Lesson Sequence

1. After warm-ups, explain about setting up a lineup:
   • Leading off with player strengths
   • Position three and four in the batting order and the rationale for placing players
2. Begin games right away, assigning someone to call balls and strikes.

Review

If students haven't yet decided on a captain and co-captain, ask them to do it now.

Review whether anyone got to first base without hitting the ball.

Ask if anyone heard, "A walk is as good as a hit." Discuss whether that means if they see a bad pitch, they should hit it anyway.

Softball Lesson 8 — Beginner level

Performance Goal

Students will work on their softball skills.

Cognitive Goals

Students will learn

how to read a score sheet,
to resume a game where it left off, and
how games that are "called" because of being out of time are recorded.

Lesson Safety

Batting team members must remain outside the backstop until their turn to bat.

Catchers should wear all the safety equipment.
All fielders should wear a softball glove.
No sliding or bat flinging is allowed.

Warm-Up

Students will play catch with all equipment available during free-play time

Motivation

When students play softball in class, by the time they get warmed up, they have just about 20 minutes for a game. Ask how many complete innings their teams played in the last class: not many. Ask if anyone knows how many innings represent a completed softball game: seven. If a game gets called because of dark or bad weather and it already had started, discuss how many innings have to be played for it to count: five. Ask students what they propose to do to make the games complete: they should take more than one day to play them.

In this class, you will teach them how to read the score sheet so that they begin where they left off. You should set aside two class periods for every game so that there are at least five complete innings before the game winner is called victorious.

Lesson Sequence

1. After the warm-ups, teach how things are represented on a score sheet:
   • Outs and runs
   • Players on base
2. Begin games right away, with someone—a student leader, a medically excused student, or someone on the batting team—keeping the score sheet.

Review

Review how many innings students completed that day.
Collect team score sheets with their line-ups.

Teacher Homework

Make up and post the tournament schedules and standings. Tournament schedules and charts are available in appendix A.

Softball Lesson 9 — Beginner level

Lesson Setup

Equipment

Posted tournament schedules and standings (see appendix A)

Performance Goal

Students will play softball, beginning their first official game.

Cognitive Goals

Students will

improve their understanding of fielding positions and basic coverages,
learn to coach their own base running, and
learn to play competitively within the rules and with good conduct.

Warm-Up

Students will play catch with all equipment available during free-play time

Motivation

Announce that the students are about to begin their first games. Whatever lineup they write on the score sheet is the one they must use throughout the game, even if they're not happy with it. Instruct them to think about all the members of their teams and where they can best take advantage of their skills so they make the best lineup possible.

The class is about ready to have the games count. Tell students you have posted their schedules so they can follow them on their own. Suggest that from now on, they practice their fielding and pitching once they are on the softball field. It will help them avoid overthrows. They should get used to doing that while the pitcher is warming up before the batter comes up to bat.

Tell them they have been doing great and it's time to see how they do as teams.

Lesson Sequence

1. Allow throwing practice as a warm-up.
2. Begin the games right after the motivation.

Review

Ask if the class has any questions.
Ask which team is in the lead at the end of class.

Ask which team was winning at the end of the last complete inning.

Make sure all the score sheets are complete for the day—they show who starts out as batter, who is on base, and the latest score.

Softball Lessons 10-15   Beginner level

Lesson Setup

Equipment

The posted performance assessment rubric for seventh and eighth grades

Performance Goal

Students will play the second half of their first official softball game. In the remaining four lessons, they will play two other official softball games.

Cognitive Goals

Students will

learn more about their fielding responsibilities in relation to their team and backing teammates up;

learn a batting strategy;

coach themselves on defense, learning to remind each other of the following:
- Where the next fielding play is
- Whom the lead runner is
- Where the force is
- If they can go for a double play
- If they need pitching changes

coach themselves on offense:
- Covering base running
- Designing their own lineups

learn how to come back from a first day's deficit to try and turn the table.

Lesson Safety

Behavior that endangers the class either physically or psychologically should be stopped immediately.

Warm-Up

Students will play catch with all equipment available during free-play time

Motivation

Announce after so many innings which team is leading and with how many runs. Say who leads off and who are on base. Challenge the team that is behind to make a comeback. Tell students to enjoy themselves.

Lesson Sequence

1. Allow throwing practice as a warm-up.
2. Begin the games right after the motivation.

Review

Ask if the class has any questions.

Ask students to be prepared for a quiz on the first rainy day.

Ask which teams are winning at the end of the last complete inning.

Make sure all the score sheets are complete for the day—they show who starts out as batter, who is on base, and the latest score.

Assessment

There is a softball quiz to assess knowledge on page 512. You can also use the softball performance assessment rubric (table 14.3) to assess student performance. For further general assessment rubrics, see appendix B.

TABLE 14.3 Beginner Softball Performance Assessment Rubric

STUDENT NAME _____

	0	1	2	3
Throwing	No effort	• Uses proper body mechanics • Keeps eye on target • Reaches a 30-foot target	• Is accurate up to 60 feet • Throws with speed • Is smooth from catch to throw	• Has a fast throw • Is accurate at 80 feet and higher • Has a quick release after a catch
Catching	No effort	• Uses proper body mechanics • Catches soft throws • Aligns body with the ball	• Moves forward for pop-ups • Catches on the move • Blocks grounders with body	• Runs four or more steps to catch • Uses glove proficiently • Is usually successful
Batting	No effort	• Uses proper grip, stance, and swing • Keeps eyes on the ball • Swings at balls in zone	• Connects with the ball • Takes a walk • Does not fling bat	• Gets a hit often • Hits grounders on demand • Is not deterred by varied pitches
Fielding	No effort	• Gets to position quickly • Attempts to block the ball	• Backs up plays in sector • Moves quickly to cover the ball • Is frequently successful	• Is respsonsible for outs • Has solid coverage of position
Base running	No effort	• Runs to first base after hitting • Runs in the correct order • Touches each base	• Holds up on fly balls • Leads after each pitch • Is aware of base runner in front	• Tags inside of corner • Rounds base aggressively • Takes advantage of rules

Softball Lesson 1 — Intermediate level

Lesson Setup

Facility

A designated softball field

Equipment

A blackboard, magnetic board, or chart of fielders' positions
One ball for every two students
One softball glove for every student
Bases and pitcher mound

Performance Goals

Students will

practice and improve their softball throws;
practice catching pop-ups, grounders, and fast-thrown balls;
run the bases; and
if time remains, play a "throw" softball game.

Cognitive Goals

Students will

review fielding skills, knowledge, and rules; and
understand the importance of catching.

Lesson Safety

Have students use the same line of direction when practicing.
Space out the practice group so there is a minimum of 10-foot separation.

Warm-Up

Students will

1. Play catch—equipment should be available as soon as students arrive
2. Jog the bases:
   • Tag the inside corner of the bags
   • Overrun first
3. Practice softball throwing mimetics for all kinds of throws necessary in a game

4. Practice catching a pop-up, grounder, and low throw, adding footwork for the pickup and release to throw
5. Perform stretches, with particular attention to the shoulder joint

Motivation

Since most of the students haven't touched a softball or glove in a year, use this class to have them warm up their throwing arm, get familiar with the glove again, and dig into their memory banks for what they already have learned. Tell them that after a good review, they can set up for a game without batting if time remains.

Lesson Sequence

1. Have students practice throwing fast to a partner, increasing the distance 10 feet at a time until everyone is doing well at 60 feet.
2. Take a time-out from throwing, to
   • run the bases, and
   • stretch the shoulder, as shown in figure 14.2.
3. Explain the need to throw farther than players are sometimes comfortable with, and teach how to get greater distance.
4. Take a time-out from throwing, to
   • run the bases, and
   • stretch the shoulder again.
5. Have students practice getting down for grounders and releasing the ball quickly and accurately. Be careful that they don't overdo this muscle group by changing the skills.
6. Review the positions, using the blackboard, chart, or magnetic board brought out to the field.
7. Review the object of the fielding team—to get three outs quickly.
8. Start a short "throw" game.

Review

Review whether the pitcher was able to get the batter out, even when pitching straight to the strike zone.
Ask which worked more effectively for getting on base—fly balls or grounders.
Discuss if it's best to attack the left field or the right field if a player is going to first.

Assessment

The progress of this lesson depends on the skills level of the class. Unless the skills are good and the practice seems routine, it might be best to make this two lessons. If your class needs two lessons, you might want to work on fly balls first, and have a "throw" softball game, allowing the batter to throw only fly balls. The next day, work on grounders and have the batter only throw grounders.

Softball Lesson 2   Intermediate level

Lesson Setup

Equipment

Bats—one long, one short—for every four people
Two plates for each practice group

Performance Goals

Students will

practice and improve their softball throwing and catching,
learn how to bunt, and
practice batting.

Cognitive Goals

Students will learn

rules relating to bunting:
- Striking out if the bunt goes foul on the third strike
- The footwork in relationship to the plate
batting strategy.

Lesson Safety

The batting groups should be separated by 10 yards.
Have each home plate set up on the same horizontal plane.
Do not allow anyone to swing away if the class is learning to bunt. Any hint of
a student swinging and attempting to hit a home run should be stopped.

Warm-Up

Students will

1. Play catch—equipment available as soon as students arrive
2. Jog the bases:
   - Students tag the inside corner of the bags.
   - They overrun first.
3. Practice mimetics for the bunt

Motivation

Most people get up to bat and hope to hit a home run. But few actually do, and
those that try frequently hit a fly ball and get out. Batting has its own strategies.

493

Among them is the option to hit a soft, slow-moving infield ball—the bunt. In this class, students will learn how to bunt.

Lesson Sequence

1. Demonstrate and teach the bunt—the grip on the bat, the stance, direction, and purpose.
2. Set up a drill group of four—one first-base person, one pitcher, one batter, and one catcher—and rotate positions (see figure 14.4):
   • Allow the bunter three successes before the rotation.
   • Encourage the catcher to play the bunt and throw down to first.
   • Remind the pitcher of his fielding responsibility if the bunt gets more than halfway to him.
   • Talk about the suicide position at third base (figure 14.6), how the third base person usually plays into the infield, anticipating a bunt, and how it can be when the batter fakes a bunt and chooses to hit.
   • Allow several group rotations, so that students have a minimum of six successes.
3. Call the groups in. Review full-swing mimetics. Return to practice:
   • Have students prac-
   tice hitting away.
   • Switch the first-base person to the out-field.
   • Ask all the outfield-ers to retrieve and return balls from other groups if the ball is hit in their al-ley.

Review

Ask if anyone in the class can list the mechanical differences between a bunt and a full-swing footwork strategy.

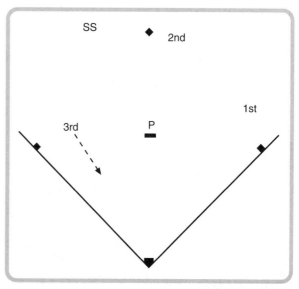

Figure 14.6—The suicide position with the third base person anticipating a bunt.

Softball Lesson 3   Intermediate level

Performance Goals

Students will

practice and improve their softball skills,
learn how to steal, and
play a game.

Cognitive Goals

Students will learn

what a leadoff is in softball,
about stealing:
- How to do it
- How to defend against it

what a balk is.

Lesson Safety

Students who are not batters or catchers are not allowed inside the backstop.

Warm-Up

Students will

1. Play catch—equipment available as soon as students arrive
2. Practice mimetics for the pitch
3. Complete footwork drills with emphasis on a change of direction

Motivation

Ask students how many watch baseball. Find out if they know who the leading stealer in baseball is. Tell them that you're drawing their attention to baseball so that all those wonderful stealing plays don't go to their heads. If they tried to steal base in softball the way they do in baseball, they would be *out*. But, yes, they can steal bases in softball. Explain how they can do it legally, and then they will have a game.

Lesson Sequence

1. Demonstrate the leadoff in relationship to the pitch and explain the related rules:
   - The pitcher who begins the motion must complete it or it is a balk. A balk entitles the base runner to advance one base.
   - The runner cannot leave the base until the pitcher releases the ball. After the pitch she can go to the next base or stay on the base she's at.
   - The only player who can throw the runner out is the catcher, not the pitcher as in baseball.
   - The batter cannot interfere with the catcher.
2. Divide the class into teams and begin a game.

Review

Ask the class what the difference is between stealing in baseball and in softball.
Ask why only the catcher can throw out the base runner.
Find out if anyone can tell the class the advantage of being able to steal.

Softball Lesson 4   Intermediate level

Lesson Setup

Equipment

A large diagram of the field on blackboard, magnetic board, or chart (see figure 14.5)
Catcher's equipment

Performance Goals

Students will

practice and improve their softball skills, and
back up each other in the field while playing a game.

Cognitive Goals

Students will

learn their secondary responsibilities in the field, and
start learning to anticipate hits and shift for them.

Lesson Safety

Make sure the catcher is wearing the proper equipment. For further safety, the batter should be the only offensive player allowed in the backstop. The batting team must be on a bench or seated 10 feet beyond the first and third base lines. No one can practice swinging unless they are on deck.

Warm-Up

Students will

1. Play catch
2. Practice mimetics for everything
3. Perform stretches

Motivation

Tell the class that the great thing about playing on a team is if one makes a little mistake out on the field, someone should be there a few seconds later to get the ball. The fact is, players should not allow themselves to feel bad when they miss the ball if they tried to cut it off early. They were doing the right thing. But, if they turn and run after the ball they missed and do not see someone coming in for it—well, then, there is someone who is doing the wrong thing. Review everyone's secondary field responsibilities. Some positions are confusing when it comes to secondary responsibilities, but have the class try learning them; then by the end of the unit, it all will be clear and automatic.

Lesson Sequence

1. Review the coverages of
   - outfielders;
   - third, shortstop, and second; and
   - pitcher, catcher, and first.
2. Review the rule of safety equipment for the catcher and why it exists.
3. Explain shifting with the ball—how, depending on where the fielded ball is going, the coverages might change.
4. Ask students to see if they can remember what direction the batter hit the ball in the last class and shift there.
5. Have the students play games with the same group as the last class. Before the games begin, remind students about the safety regulations.

Review

Ask students if there were any confusing plays in their games—review each play and what should have been done.

Ask if they were able to spot a consistency in the batter that helped them cover the field better.

Teacher Homework

Make equal teams, being certain to split good pitchers, hitters, outfielders, and base people.

Softball Lesson 5   Intermediate level

Lesson Setup

Facility

One designated field with a backstop for each game

Equipment

Team lists
Clipboards with pens and pencils and the team score sheet

Performance Goals

Students will

improve their softball skills,
improve their agility and reflexes, and
play games with their new team members.

Cognitive Goals

Students will

learn to play with new tournament teams;
recognize, choose, and follow a team leader; and
review the concepts involved in making and following a lineup.

Warm-Up

Students will

1. Play catch
2. Complete footwork drills (for fielding properly) and base running
3. Perform stretches

Motivation

Tell students that you have made their teams as usual: Every team has the same ability so winning is not a sure bet like in the days of the Yankees, when they bought the best players in baseball and hardly ever lost a game. The students will have to use all their skills, plan well, and work as a team to come out ahead. Then talk about setting up a lineup that works for them before getting started with the last practice days before the round-robin tournament.

Lesson Sequence

1. Announce the teams and have them pick a captain and co-captain.
2. Review:
   • The use of the score sheet
       Making a lineup, the need to follow it, and how it's recorded
       Entering positions on base and the number of runs and outs
   • The aim to play five or more innings in two class lessons before declaring a winner
3. Distribute clipboards with score sheets (see table 14.2).
4. Have the class play games with the new teams.

Review

Ask students for their completed score sheets.
Discuss any questions.
Ask if there were any stolen bases, any advances by tagging up, or any bunts.

Softball Lesson 6   Intermediate level

Lesson Setup

Equipment

A clean team score sheet for every new game
Posted team schedules and standings

Performance Goals

Students will

lead off and steal bases, and
play games with their tournament teams

Cognitive Goals

Students will learn

to coach their base runners:
  • A proper leadoff
  • When to hold
  • Overrunning first
  • Stopping on the bag
  • When to go
the penalty for a pitcher's balk,
the penalty for leading off too soon, and
how to stop the steal:
  • Who throws the ball
  • Who covers the base
  • Who backs up the base
  • If a tag is necessary

Warm-Up

Students will

1. Play catch
2. Complete footwork drills or base running
3. Perform stretches

Motivation

Ask students whether they get to first faster if they run to it without being
afraid of overrunning it, or if they turn, preparing to head for second base.
Ask whether they run faster if they look straight ahead or if they have their

heads going back and forth between facing forward and to the side. The reason you're asking is that you want to know if it is better for a base runner to just go or to have to decide while he is going whether to go or stop.

Teach students about coaching the base runner and leaving the decision to someone on their team who is looking at the whole field while the base runner is running.

Lesson Sequence

1. Teach the strategy of base running.
2. Teach rules that apply to coaches.
3. Distribute clipboards with score sheets.
4. Have students play games with their new teams.

Review

Ask students for their completed score sheets.
Discuss any questions.
Ask if any runner was told to go on and scored.
Ask if any runner advanced who would not have.
Find out if any runner got out.

Softball Lesson 7 — Intermediate level

Lesson Setup

Equipment

Round-robin tournament schedules and charts (see appendix A)

Performance Goals

Students will

improve their softball skills,
play the first half of the first official game of their tournament,
play by the rules,
coach each other, and
exhibit good sporting behavior.

Cognitive Goals

Students will

learn what constitutes a game in this tournament,

improve their knowledge and appreciation of softball, and learn to be team players.

Warm-Up

Students will

1. Play catch
2. Perform stretches

Motivation

Announce to the students that they are about to start their tournament. You will be around to call balls and strikes and to answer any questions or give them hints. Suggest that in the interest of fairness, if there is no neutral third party to umpire, they should allow someone with a good eye on the batting team to do it. Tell them to enjoy themselves.

Lesson Sequence

1. Have students practice throwing down to a base when they take their positions in the field.
2. Games should commence as soon as possible.
3. Call a time-out and explain what a game is:
   • It has five or more complete innings.
   • Games will continue over a two-day period.
   • The score sheet must show how many outs there are in an inning, and who is on base. (Review these entries if the class does not know how to make them.)
4. Let the games continue.

Review

Ask if the class has any questions.
Ask for the completed score sheets. Explain that they are needed because the next time the class meets students will play the same team, but they'll start where they left off.

Softball Lessons 8-12　　　　　Intermediate level

Lesson Setup

Equipment

Updated team standings

Performance Goals

Students will

complete the first official game during lesson 8, and play two additional games.

Cognitive Goal

Students will learn to be team players.

Warm-Up

Students will

1. Play catch
2. Perform stretches

Motivation

Announce that after so many innings or games of softball, which team is in the lead so far. Tell students what that day's games are and how many outs and how many runs they have. Announce the game standings and tell players to enjoy themselves.

Lesson Sequence

1. Have students practice throwing down to a base when they take their position in the field.
2. Games should commence as soon as possible.
3. Use the teachable moment, reacting to an event during the game to teach or reinforce something taught before.

Review

Tell students that if any questions come up, they should ask.
There will be a quiz on the next rainy day.
Ask for their completed score sheets.

Assessment

Observe the students to determine what needs to be reemphasized. Post the softball performance assessment rubric, which is the standard for skills grading (table 14.4). General assessment rubrics can be found in appendix B. Give a quiz on a rainy day. Since it will only take a few minutes, continue the games afterward. If it is raining, you might continue the tournament inside by using Wiffle balls and bats.

TABLE 14.4 Intermediate Softball Performance Assessment Rubric

STUDENT NAME _____

	0	1	2	3
Offensive skills	No effort	• Has good batting form • Moves forward on the hit	• Gets to base—with a hit or a walk • Runs the bases aggressively	• Is consistent • Is able to direct hits or bunts
Defensive skills	No effort	• Blocks the ball • Has inconsistent catching	• Has good catching and throwing skills • Is aware of base runners • Throws ahead of the lead runner	• Moves to cover a hit properly • Makes big catches or plays
Fielding	No effort	• Gets to position • Is focused on the game	• Throws ahead of the lead runner • Anticipates hits	• Tries for a double play • Backs up teammates
Team strategy	No effort	• Understands the basic game • Is improving specific skills	• Keeps the chances for scoring alive • Uses base-running rules	• Sets goals that individual teammates can meet
Sporting behavior	No effort	• Is frequently in disagreements • Blames others • Breaks rules to win	• Tries to develop and improve • Works well with the team • Violations are unintentional	• Plays within the rules • Is a team leader • Helps others

Softball Lesson 1 — Advanced level

Lesson Setup

Facility

A designated field large enough to set up several different squad areas

Equipment

A complete set of bases for each group of 11 students working on a field
A blackboard, magnetic board, or chart of fielders' positions
Several different sized bats
Catcher's equipment
One glove for every student
One softball for every two students

Performance Goals

Students will

practice catching pop-ups, grounders, and fast balls; and practice batting.

Cognitive Goal

Students will review fielding and batting skills.

Lesson Safety

Make sure the line of direction of the ball's throws or hits will not compromise the safety of or interfere with any squad working on something else in a neighboring area.

Warm-Up

Students will

1. Play catch—equipment available as soon as students arrive
2. Perform stretches, with particular attention to the shoulder joint

Motivation

Since most of the students haven't touched a softball or glove in a year, have them warm up their throwing arm, get familiar with the glove again, and review what they already have learned.

Lesson Sequence

1. Divide the group up so that students work at different practice stations. They should rotate every eight minutes:
   • Pitching–bunting–catching backup person (figure 14.7a)
   • Catching–pitching–batting (figure 14.7b)
   • Accurate throwing to bases (figure 14.7c)
   • Catching pop-ups and throwing to bases (figure 14.7d)
2. Call the class together to summarize and review the rules:
   • Base running, when to advance, when to return, tagging up
   • Force plays and the reason for tags
   • The strike zone
   • Fouls and fouling out if bunting
   • Stealing

Review

Promise that in the next class students will get to play a game.

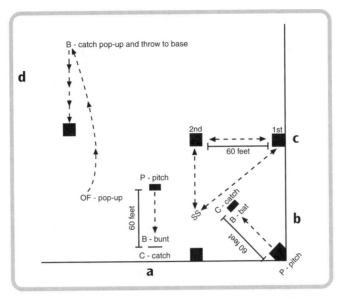

Figure 14.7—Practice stations for *(a)* bunting, *(b)* batting, *(c)* throwing, and *(d)* catching.

Assessment

Observe students' throwing and catching to determine how much practice is necessary and if the class would do well to repeat this lesson the next time.

Softball Lesson 2   Advanced level

Performance Goals

Students will

practice softball skills, and
play a game.

Cognitive Goals

Students will

learn to understand the third-strike rule and see if they can take advantage of it, and
review rules as they come up during the game.

Lesson Safety

Students should observe game rules that are meant for their safety:

Catchers must wear protective equipment.
All fielders must wear softball gloves.

Only the batter, catcher, and umpire belong in the backstop while the ball is being pitched.

Spectators and the at-bat team should sit 10 feet outside of the baseline.

There is no batting warm-up once the game begins.

The fielding warm-up can only take place when the team goes onto the field before the first batter comes up.

Warm-Up

Students will

1. Play catch—equipment available as soon as students arrive
2. Perform stretches, with particular attention to the shoulder joint

Motivation

The students may feel they know just about everything there is to know about softball, but before the games, see if you can teach them something they might not already know. Ask if they knew that a player can get to base without a hit, without having four balls pitched to him, even, in fact, if he swings and misses. It's called the third-strike rule.

Lesson Sequence

1. Explain the third-strike rule.
2. Divide the class into teams and send them out to play.
3. Make an appearance at each game and use the teachable moment to reinforce and review rules and/or coaching hints for fielding.

Review

Although the third-strike situation does not come up too often, ask students if it did in this class.

Review when the third-strike rule is in effect.

Ask, if players are on base whether they also can advance.

Discuss whether the batter can leave the batter's box and then decide to run to first.

Softball Lesson 3   Advanced level

Performance Goals

Students will

learn and practice a rundown, and
play a game.

Cognitive Goals

Students will

understand how to make it easier to strand runners for the tag, and review and practice stealing.

Lesson Safety

Have the rundown drill groups working in the same line of direction.

Warm-Up

Students will

1. Play catch—equipment available as soon as students arrive
2. Perform stretches, with particular attention to the shoulder joint

Motivation

Ask students how many have turned the corner, driving to the next base, only to find the base person waiting there with the ball. Discuss what they do: they turn back if they are not forced out, because the base person has to tag them. Ask how many of them have been the base person.

Some students know from watching baseball just what to do; others may not have the foggiest idea. Have the students play a little "monkey in the middle," just so they can get the feel of squeezing that runner in between them until they easily can reach out and tag her. This is called a rundown.

Lesson Sequence

1. Demonstrate a rundown and set groups of three out to practice, rotating the "monkey in the middle." (This makes a wonderful rainy-day lesson; you might want to save it until it rains.)
2. Review the stealing rules and strategies.
3. Send the same teams out to play, changing the field and opponent if there are more than two teams.

Review

Ask the class if anyone got caught in a rundown.
Ask students to put into words what the defenders should do during a rundown.
Review whether the dropped third strike rule came up.
Discuss whether the batter remembered to go to first.
Ask if the catcher was able to get the batter out at first.

Softball Lesson 4 — Advanced level

Performance Goals

Students will

slide to base (optional and dependent on what students generally wear to class), and
play a game.

Cognitive Goals

Students will

understand why sliding is done and the difficulty of the tag, and
learn to use a "relay" person to feed balls to second base, third base, and home from the outfield.

Lesson Safety

Because of the potential for abrasions, this lesson will not be practiced outdoors unless students are wearing the appropriate clothing to protect their legs.

Warm-Up

Students will

1. Play catch
2. Perform stretches, with particular attention to the shoulder joint

Motivation

In this lesson, before the games, students are going to understand and see a proper slide. But unless they are in sweatpants, they shouldn't practice this in the dirt. Tell them that on the next rainy day, they can practice this on mats indoors. If students ask why, tell that that injuries are possible. Tell them a story of your being injured while sliding, or feel free to use my story.

Years ago, a colleague of mine came in one morning to tell me that one of our girls had broken her leg on the field. I asked how. She told me she was so excited during the game, she slid into first.

Lesson Sequence

1. Demonstrate and explain the "slide":
   • It attempts to evade a tag.
   • It helps the runner stop on the bag.
   • It should not be practiced unless indoors using mats or students are in long pants.

2. Review all the new rules learned this year and answer questions about old ones.
3. Reinforce the use of a relay person when the ball is hit into the out-field.
4. Send the same teams out to play, changing the field and opponent.

Review

Ask the class if there were any rundown plays or any plays in which a slide would have been helpful.

Ask the class if they think the catcher's job is still as easy as they once thought, now that stealing is allowed. Ask if the third-strike rule makes the catcher's job even harder.

Tell students that they will receive their team assignments in the next class.

Teacher Homework

Divide the class into teams that are equally skilled. Write the team lists separately for each team on top of a score sheet for distribution to the team in the next class. Examples of round-robin teams and schedules can be found in appendix A.

Softball Lessons 5-10   Advanced level

Lesson Setup

Equipment

Blackboard or enlarged chart of the score sheet
A clipboard with the score sheet for each team (see table 14.2)
A pen or pencil for each clipboard
Round-robin tournament charts and schedules (appendix A)

Performance Goal

Students will compete in a tournament of three games over six days.

Cognitive Goals

Students will

read and make entries on the score sheet, and
understand and exhibit the following:
  • Leadership
  • Responsibility
  • Good sporting behavior
  • Teamwork

Warm-Up

Students will

1. Play catch—equipment available as soon as students arrive
2. Perform stretches, with particular attention to the shoulder joint

Motivation

Announce to the class that the tournament is going to start. Students have been with each other long enough to know who the cleanup batters are, who will get on base, and who should pitch, play first, cover shortstop, take center field, and take the massive job of catcher. Remind them of the procedure they'll use to get the most out of their class time. You will be announcing the teams and letting them go play. Tell them games will take place over a two-day period. You will give the selected captains the clipboards so they can insert their lineups and keep score, but first show them a score sheet and how to use it.

Lesson Sequence

1. Announce the teams and give each team their score sheet with their team roster on it.
2. Using a visual aid, go over the score sheet and the types of entries that are necessary (lineup, outs, runs).
3. Announce the general procedure of the tournament:
   - Students should read the game schedule and get out to their assigned field for warm-ups on time every day.
   - Games are to start after the pitcher gets warmed up.
   - Fielding teams are responsible for setting up and breaking down the field. They must bring out three or four balls.
   - Batting teams should bring out several sizes of bats for their field and the clipboards, pens, and score sheets.
   - Balls and strikes should be called by a neutral umpire if available or a person from the batting team.
   - Students are responsible for coaching their base runners.
   - Games will continue for a second day in exactly the position they left off on the first.
4. Have the teams choose captains and co-captains and start the tournament.
5. Use teachable moments during the game to give input on strategies, coverages, rules, and mechanics.

Review

Ask if there are any questions. Remind students that they will have to be prepared for a rainy-day quiz, so they shouldn't sit with unanswered questions. Ask if the score sheets are up to the minute.

Assessment

Give the quiz on the first rainy day (page 514). Also, have the students use the softball performance assessment rubric (table 14.5) and either grade themselves or someone on their team. Allow this self-assessment on the last day of the unit. There are also general assessment rubrics in appendix B that can be used for further assessment.

TABLE 14.5 Advanced Softball Performance Assessment Rubric

STUDENT NAME _____

	0	1	2	3	4	5
Skills	No effort	• Has proper swing • Has inconsistent skills • Does erratic throws • Walks instead of runs	• Swings meet ball • Blocks the batted ball in the field • Has slow, accurate throw to 60 feet • Catches slow balls thrown accurately	• Gets to base • Moves to the ball quickly • Swings at pitches in the strike zone only • Does legal base running	• Has fast, accurate throw • Makes solid hits • Has smooth, quick catch and throw • Uses proper movement in the field on a hit	• Is a big hitter • Bats in runs • Secures the out • Uses knowledge to make the most of base running
Teamwork	No effort	• Concentrates • Arrives promptly • Is temperamental	• Plays the assigned position • Forgets to back up the team and where the lead runner goes	• Responds to coaching hints • Backs up the team • Remembers the play	• Anticipates hits and fielding coverage • Uses skills to advance team, not self	• Helps the team focus • Takes a leadership role
Attitude	No effort	• Blames others • Needs supervision to stay on task • Interferes with the other team • Tries to take over	• Gets to the court on time • Warms up with the team • Plays within the rules	• Works well with teamates • Plays within the rules • Takes responsibility for position	• Consistently tries to play at personal best • Recognizes good teammate effort and success • Has good sporting behavior	• Inspires the team • Backs up, not takes over, for teammates • Provides reliable, consistent leadership • Assists individual team members to improve

Softball Quiz—Beginner level

NAME _____ TEACHER _____

DATE _____ CLASS PERIOD _____

True or False: Read each statement below carefully. If the statement is true, put a check under the True box in the column to the left of the statement. If the statement is false, put a check under the False box in the column to the left of the statement. If using a grid sheet, blacken in the appropriate column for each question, making sure to use the correctly numbered line for each question and its answer.

True   False

☐ ☐ 1. A hit ball traveling in foul territory is a strike.

☐ ☐ 2. After a hit, the force play is usually at first base.

☐ ☐ 3. Runners leaving a base before a ball is caught on a fly must return.

☐ ☐ 4. You may overrun third base without fear of being tagged out.

☐ ☐ 5. Base people should forget their base and stop the batted ball from going into the outfield.

☐ ☐ 6. Most people at bat miss the ball because they do not watch it drop over the plate.

☐ ☐ 7. A ball that passes above the outside corner of home plate at the batter's waist level is a "ball."

☐ ☐ 8. The shortstop covers second base almost as often as the second-base person does.

☐ ☐ 9. The cleanup batter is usually the ninth person in the lineup.

☐ ☐ 10. Batters cannot leave home plate and get on first base legally unless they have a fair hit.

☐ ☐ 11. Official softball games are seven complete innings.

☐ ☐ 12. When getting grounders, you should get down in a squat so your body blocks the ball if it takes a bad bounce.

☐ ☐ 13. Right-handers wear their softball gloves on their right hand.

☐ ☐ 14. When reaching to catch a ball below the waist, your fingers should point to the ground.

☐ ☐ 15. The team that is leading 10-5 when the game is called wins, even though they scored 6 of their 10 runs at the top of the sixth inning and the game was called without their opponents getting to bat.

From *Complete Physical Education Plans for Grades 7–12* by Isobel Kleinman, 2001, Champaign, IL: Human Kinetics.

Softball Quiz—Intermediate level

NAME _____ TEACHER _____

DATE _____ CLASS PERIOD _____

Multiple Choice: Read each question and each answer carefully. Be sure to choose the best answer that fits the words or statement preceding it. When you have made your choice, put the appropriate letter on the line to the left of the numbered question.

_____ 1. When the batter hits the ball down the first-base line,
   a. the first-base person should get the ball and run back to cover first
   b. the first-base person should stay on first and let the pitcher and catcher worry about the ball
   c. the shortstop goes to second, second goes to first, first and pitcher react to the ball
   d. everyone should move in to the ball, letting whoever gets it run to first

_____ 2. The second-base runner takes off after the pitch:
   a. The catcher should throw to second base.
   b. Third covers third, shortstop backs up the throw to third, catcher throws to third.
   c. The shortstop should run into the baseline to slow down the runner.
   d. All of the above.

_____ 3. If there is a player on second,
   a. the batter should bunt to third
   b. the batter should bunt to first

   c. the batter should hope to get walked
   d. all of the above

_____ 4. A ball is hit long and high into right field:
   a. The runner on third should go home no matter what.
   b. The runner on third should stay on third and wait for the next batter to come up.
   c. The runner should run home after the ball is caught.
   d. The runner should go back to second.

_____ 5. The batter has two strikes and three balls. Choose the strategy he should *not* use:
   a. The batter should swing at every ball if he thinks he can hit it.
   b. The batter should leave a ball that looks as if it is out of the strike zone.
   c. The batter should bunt.
   d. The batter should fake a bunt and swing away.

Matching Questions: Read one numbered item at a time. Then look at each of the possible choices in the column on the right. Decide which item in the right-hand column best matches up with that of the left-hand column. Put the corresponding letter on the blank space to the left of the number it best matches.

_____ 6. Tagging up   **a.** Over the plate, above the knees, and below the armpits

_____ 7. Bunting   **b.** The suicide position

_____ 8. The catcher   **c.** Advancing to the next base after a ball is caught on a fly

_____ 9. Strike   **d.** Makes the throw to put the stealer out

_____ 10. The third-base person   **e.** Sliding the hands up the grip

From *Complete Physical Education Plans for Grades 7–12* by Isobel Kleinman, 2001, Champaign, IL: Human Kinetics.

Softball Quiz—Advanced level

NAME _____ TEACHER _____

DATE _____ CLASS PERIOD _____

True or False: Read each statement below carefully. If the statement is true, put a check under the True box in the column to the left of the statement. If the statement is false, put a check under the False box in the column to the left of the statement. If using a grid sheet, blacken in the appropriate column for each question, making sure to use the correctly numbered line for each question and its answer.

True   False

☐ ☐ 1. Batters who bunt-foul on the third strike are out.

☐ ☐ 2. Taking a lead *before* the pitch is advised on every pitch.

☐ ☐ 3. The third-base runner should stay on third after a fly has been caught in deep center field.

☐ ☐ 4. With runners on second and third and two outs, the fielder should throw to first.

☐ ☐ 5. The only position on the field where catching is everything and throwing is second-rate is first base.

☐ ☐ 6. There are runners on first and second. The shortstop should catch a line drive and wisely throw to first.

☐ ☐ 7. With an unforced runner between two bases, the leading base person should stay on base, waiting for the runner and throw.

☐ ☐ 8. Bunting toward first when a player is on third is a great sacrifice strategy to score the third-base runner.

☐ ☐ 9. The third-base person is usually the relay person.

☐ ☐ 10. Sliding when you are forced to run to the base is taking a health risk for no reason.

Matching Questions: Read one numbered item at a time. Then look at each of the possible choices in the column on the right. Decide which item in the right-hand column best matches that of the left-hand column and put the corresponding letter on the blank space to the left of the number it best matches.

_____ **11.** Comes from the left hand of a right-handed player

_____ **12.** Covers first base on grounders toward the right side of the field

_____ **13.** Advancing to the next base after a ball is caught on a fly

_____ **14.** Conditions allowing a batter to run after striking out

_____ **15.** The runner closest to scoring

a. The second-base person

b. The lead runner

c. Tagging up

d. Batter's power

e. The third-strike rule

Diagram Questions: This diagram represents a score sheet turned in after one day of play. Each question is based on the information in the diagram above. Read each question. Be sure to choose the best answer based on all the rules you know and the information in the diagram. When you have made your choice, put the appropriate letter on the line to the left of the numbered question.

STARS	1	2	3	4	5	6	7	HEROES	1	2	3	4	5	6	7
1. Sue	①	♦	/					1. Carol	♦	②					
2. Mike	/	③						2. Lisa	>	/					
3. Hugh	②		♦					3. Mark	/	③					
4. Roger	③		②					4. Steve	①						
5. Cathy		①	♦					5. Alan	②						
6. Iris		♦	♦					6. Daryl	③						
7. Marcus	−	②	♦					7. Kisha		①					
8. Nancy		>	>					8. Ari		♦					
9. Ann		/	①					9. Meg		♦					
Runs/inning	0	2						Runs/inning	1	2					
Total score	0	2						Total score	1	3					

_____ **16.** Nancy has
   a. advanced to second each time she gets up to bat
   b. been left stranded on base
   c. has never been put out
   d. done all of the above

_____ **17.** The Stars believe they are *officially* winning the game.
   a. True
   b. False

_____ **18.** Who leads off for the Heroes?
   a. Carol
   b. Ari
   c. Steve

_____ **19.** The cleanup hitter for the Stars is
   a. Iris
   b. Marcus
   c. Roger

_____ **20.** When this game resumes,
   a. the Stars go into the field
   b. the Stars are up—Sue is on first, Nancy is on second, and Mike is up
   c. Alan from the Heroes leads off
   d. none of the above

From *Complete Physical Education Plans for Grades 7–12* by Isobel Kleinman, 2001, Champaign, IL: Human Kinetics.

Softball Answer Key—Beginner level

1. T
2. T
3. T
4. F
5. T
6. T
7. F
8. T
9. F
10. F
11. T
12. T
13. F
14. T
15. F

Softball Answer Key—Intermediate level

1. C
2. B
3. B
4. C
5. C
6. C
7. E
8. D
9. A
10. B

Softball Answer Key—Advanced level

1. T. A foul ball that is bunted is considered a strike, even if it is the third strike.
2. F. It is illegal to be off the base before the ball is pitched.
3. F. The runner should tag up to try to score.
4. T. Go for the force play.
5. T. First-base people rarely throw, but their ability to catch with a foot on the base is worth its weight!
6. F. The shortstop should throw to first or second only if the runner left the base before the catch was made and had not returned.
7. F. This is a classic rundown situation in which both base people want to get closer until the tag is easy.
8. T. The out at first allows the runner at third to score.
9. F. The relay person is usually the shortstop when the ball is thrown in from center or left field.
10. T. As soon as the ball gets to base, you are out. There is no need for a tag or a slide.
11. D
12. A
13. C
14. E
15. B
16. D
17. B. The official score is that of the last complete inning. In that case it was Stars 2, Heros 3.
18. C
19. C
20. B

Team Handball

Unit Overview

1. Teach the basic skills of soccer, basketball, and handball that apply to this game: throwing, catching, hand dribbling, hits and volleys using knees, shoulders, and head.

2. Teach familiar rules that apply and how:
   - Holding should be for no more than three seconds.
   - If the player is still moving with the ball after three steps, the following choices must be made for it to be legal:

     The basketball dribble
     The basketball dribble followed by three steps
     Passing the ball
     Shooting the ball
   - The following are legal passes (note, no kicking):

     Jump pass
     Bounce bass

   Overhand pass
   Wrist pass

3. Teach the boundaries and field marking and how the rules apply to them:
   - Players cannot use the "when in doubt, it's out" strategy.
   - They cannot enter the goal area unless playing goalie.
   - They may shoot from anywhere, including off the field when throwing in.

4. Teach the goalie's limitations:
   - While inside the goalie area, he cannot grab a stationary ball or rolling ball outside of the goalie area.
   - He cannot intentionally deflect the ball out of bounds once gaining control of it.

5. Teach violations, fouls, and penalties—for example, a player cannot intentionally send the ball out of bounds.

Team Handball

HISTORY

Team handball began in Europe around the late 1920s. The Olympic debut of team handball was in the Berlin Olympics of 1936. The next appearance of team handball was not until the Munich games of 1972, where only men played the game. Finally, in 1976, women's team handball was added to the Olympic Games. In 1984, the United States took its first women's handball team to the Olympics. Today, there are 15 million handball players.

FUN FACTS

→ Team handball has been played in Canada for about 50 years.

→ Team handball is the second most popular sport in the world.

→ The International Handball Federation has 136 member institutions.

→ Finland has 140 youth handball teams.

→ Both females and males play team handball.

BENEFITS OF PLAYING

1. Team handball provides you with a great workout.
2. Playing team handball teaches you about teamwork.
3. Team handball is good for your leg muscles.
4. Team handball is good for your hand-eye coordination.
5. Team handball is a fun, fast-paced sport that is full of running, jumping, throwing, and catching.

TIME TO SURF!

Web Site	Web Site Address
USA Team Handball	http://www.teamhandball.org/
Canadian Team Handball Federation	http://www.handball.ca/
Japan Handball League	http://www.jhl.handball.or.jp/eng/

From *Complete Physical Education Plans for Grades 7–12* by Isobel Kleinman, 2001, Champaign, IL: Human Kinetics.

Team Handball Unit Extension Project

NAME _____ CLASS _____

Equipment needed to play team handball

Item	Where would you purchase it (be specific)	Cost

Where you would play team handball

Please explain where in the community you would play team handball. Be specific.

Health benefits of playing team handball

Please explain the health benefits of playing team handball. Include how much you would need to play each week to gain these benefits. What skills do you learn in team handball that you can apply to other activities?

Reflection question

Is team handball a sport you think you'd enjoy playing in college? If yes, name some colleges that have team handball clubs (hint—use the Internet to search).

From *Complete Physical Education Plans for Grades 7–12* by Isobel Kleinman, 2001, Champaign, IL: Human Kinetics.

Team Handball Teaching Tips

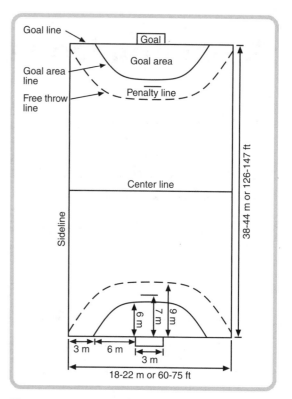

1. This unit has been written for students who already have had soccer and basketball and have developed most of the skills necessary to immediately enjoy getting into team handball. Lessons change insignificantly from one grade to another. They simply review with a mind to getting students into the game as quickly as possible. The unit is quite short, just seven lessons. As a result, you might want to have students assess themselves. A quiz concludes each unit for each grade level.

2. Follow the lessons that combine skills and knowledge acquisition with the game.

3. Review skills with attention to what makes them different from the sport they originally were learned in.

Figure 15.1—Team handball court dimensions.

4. Get students into the game immediately

5. Develop a short tournament, using a different approach to team selection that means changing teams each day and having a different person assume the captainship. This allows each student to be a captain for a day.

6. If students are unable to participate fully in class, remember that they can be involved by coaching, officiating, keeping score, or conducting a research project.

Unit Setup

Facility

A court with goals and a goalie restraining area for every two teams

An area with no obstructions

Equipment

One team handball ball for every two students (figure 15.2)

Scrimmage vests of different colors for every team of six players

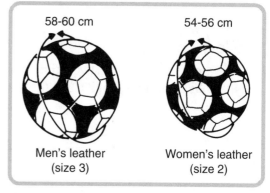

Figure 15.2—Team handballs for males and females.

TABLE 15.1   Team Handball Student Portfolio Checklist

STUDENT NAME _____

- ☐ Has reviewed all methods to legally advance the ball while in possession of it
- ☐ Has reviewed the legal methods to pass or shoot the ball
- ☐ Has learned the rules of scoring
- ☐ Has learned the boundaries for the players and the goalie
- ☐ Understands the specific restrictions for the goalie and the goal area
- ☐ Knows common violations and the procedure for returning the ball to play
- ☐ Knows violations/fouls and their penalties and procedures
- ☐ Has developed offensive and defensive strategies
- ☐ Exhibits responsibility and good sporting behavior during competition

From *Complete Physical Education Plans for Grades 7–12* by Isobel Kleinman, 2001, Champaign, IL: Human Kinetics

Unit Timeline

There is a team handball unit for each of the three levels:
Two lessons to explore the adaptation of basic skills while learning rules and a new game
Four lessons for a class tournament
One lesson for a quiz or culminating activity

Unit Assessment

A student portfolio checklist is provided here for student use (table 15.1). Encourage students to track their progress as they master new skills. Quizzes at the end of this chapter can also be used to assess students' knowledge of the sport.

Additional Resources

Clanton, Reita E., and Mary Phyl Dwight. 1997. *Team Handball: Steps to Success.* Champaign, IL: Human Kinetics.

Hamil, Baha M., and James D. LaPoint. 1994. *Team Handball.* Eddie Bowers Publishing Co.

Team Handball Lesson 1 — Beginner level

Lesson Setup

Facility

An area with no obstructions
One court or playing area for every 12 students

Equipment

Scrimmage vests of a different color for every group of six
One ball for every two students

Performance Goal

Students will legally learn to advance a ball in team handball.

Cognitive Goals

Students will examine the difference between the rules for soccer and for team handball, including

the size of the team,
moving the ball:
  • One cannot use anything below the knees to direct the ball.
  • One cannot touch the ball twice unless it touches something else, such as the floor, the wall, or so on, or is touched by someone else.
when and where one can shoot from, and
the boundaries and using them:
  • One cannot send a ball out of bounds to delay the game.
  • The goalie cannot go out to save a ball outside the restraining line.
  • Players cannot go inside the goalie area.

Lesson Safety

Each participant with a ball should be separated by a minimum of six feet from the next.
A team needs a set of goals and its own court on which to play.

Warm-Up

Students will

1. Complete push-ups and sit-ups
2. Perform stretches
3. Jog while hand dribbling and hand or body passing balls to partners

Motivation

Introduce team handball to your students and tell them it has a big following outside of this country. Here, it is just a trick of adjustment. Let them know they already have learned the skills necessary to play this game, so instead of focusing on skills development, you will just point the way, tell them how things differ a little, and let them adapt on their own with the help of their teammates.

Team handball uses a lot of soccer skills, as long as a player can move the ball without using her feet or shins. For the soccer players in the class, that little difference may drive them crazy. Talk about the allowed skills, inform them that they know the soccer skills they can use, and then it's time to get into a game.

Lesson Sequence

1. Review the allowed skills by calling them out and having partners practice them:
   - The hand dribble
   - The overhand pass (figure 15.3)
   - The wrist pass (figure 15.4)
   - Throw and catch
   - Volley and catch

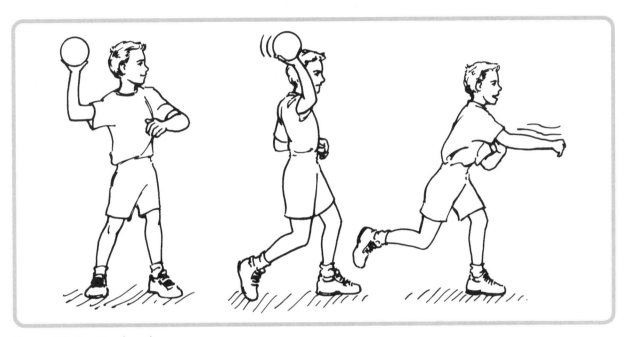

Figure 15.3—Overhand pass.

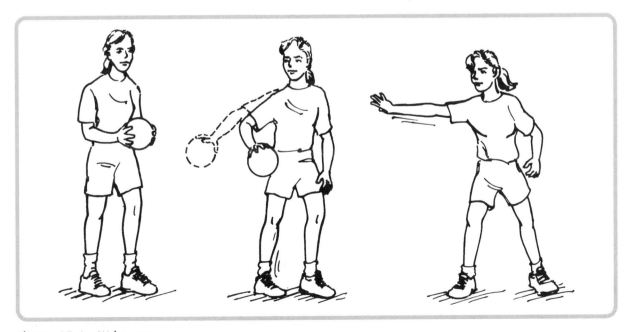

Figure 15.4—Wrist pass.

- Three steps and get rid of the ball
- Head, knee, and shoulder volleys

2. Stop the class to go over boundaries, pointing out the goalie area and applicable rules.
3. Divide the class into teams of six and have them play a game.

Review

Ask students if they like the game.
Discuss how many of them got mixed up.
Ask what was the most difficult skills transition for them to make.

Team Handball Lesson 2 — Beginner level

Performance Goal

Students will play team handball.

Cognitive Goals

Students will

understand that the rules are to keep the game fair and safe, and
learn the rules and penalties in team handball:
- The size of the team
- What constitutes a violation of skills and boundaries
- What constitutes personal fouls
- What the penalties are

Lesson Safety

Each participant with a ball should be separated by a minimum of six feet from others.
A team needs a set of goals and its own court on which to play.

Warm-Up

Students will

1. Participate in free play to get adjusted to the ball's weight and size
2. Complete push-ups and sit-ups
3. Perform stretches

Motivation

Review the rules and how to adjust the game when they are broken. Get the class into the spirit of the game.

Lesson Sequence

1. Review violations and fouls:
   - Skills
   - Boundaries
2. Have the students play.

Review

Ask the class whether players can roll the ball with their feet.
Ask if they can pass by kicking.
Review what the penalty is for doing either.
Ask if they can score from off the field or in the goalie area.
Review what the penalty is.

Teacher Homework

Prepare and post a list of each student in the class. It can be updated to include students' game records and if they have been captain.

Team Handball Lessons 3-6 — Beginner level

Lesson Setup

Equipment

A posted student roster

Performance Goal

Students will play team handball.

Cognitive Goals

Students will

learn to work with a variety of teammates and learn to adapt quickly to each new change,
rotate the responsibility of choosing teams and being captains, and
have an opportunity to have a leadership role.

Lesson Safety

A team needs a set of goals and its own field on which to play.

Warm-Up

Students will

1. Participate in free play to get adjusted to the ball
2. Complete push-ups and sit-ups,
3. Perform stretches

Motivation

Tell the students it might be interesting for them to see what it's like to be a captain. In this unit, everyone is going to be a captain—you'll let them know when. Each captain will get the opportunity to pick one co-captain and another player—they will be picking half their team. You will pick the other half. Then the captain will take charge of assigning field positions and helping to coordinate team strategy.

For a change, since teams are being picked so differently, announce that you will give scores to the individual. Everyone will get a point every day that they play. If they win, they get two points. If they win when they are captain, they get four points; otherwise, the losing captain gets three points. At the end of the unit, the person with the most points is the class champion.

Lesson Sequence

1. During the class's free play period, pick two team captains. The captains should be different each day and should be students with similar abilities. Assign a color to each team. Let each captain choose a co-captain and one other player. Assign three more players at one time to each team by handing out colored scrimmage vests according to which team the students will play on. This guarantees that no student will feel left out by being picked last. Also, by giving out three vests at a time you can even out the playing field by separating the more talented students.
2. Play team handball games.

Review

Ask the class if there are any questions.
Ask students not to leave until you know whether they won and if they were a captain. Tell them you want to make sure they are credited with the right number of points.

Assessment

Observe for physical effort, teamwork, and cooperation. You can use the general performance assessment rubrics in appendix B to further assess your students. This is a short unit, dependent on what students learned in other sports. With a unit this short, teachers may choose to skip the quiz. However, a quiz for this level can be found on page 536.

Teacher Homework

Post all the participants and update their scores after each gym class.

Team Handball Lesson 1 — Intermediate level

Lesson Setup

Facility

One field for every 12 players

Equipment

One ball for every two players
Set of different colored scrimmage vests for each team of six

Performance Goal

Students will legally advance the ball in team handball.

Cognitive Goals

Students will review the differences between basketball or soccer rules and those for team handball, including

the size of the team,
the parts of the body that can be used for moving the ball,
when one can shoot and from where,
the boundaries and using them,
how many steps can be taken, and
how long the ball can be held.

Lesson Safety

A team needs a set of goals and its own field on which to play.

Warm-Up

Students will

1. Jog while hand dribbling and hand or body passing balls to partners
2. Complete push-ups and sit-ups
3. Perform stretches

Motivation

Tell students that team handball uses a lot of skills they already have learned. Using a skill a player learned under another set of rules can be confusing even if it is fun. For instance, explore with the class the differences between how a step taken when pivoting is treated in this game and how it is treated in basketball.

Lesson Sequence

1. Review the rules.
2. Stop the class to go over boundaries, pointing out the goalie area and applicable rules.
3. Divide the class into teams of six and have them play a game.

Review

Ask students how many of them got mixed up.
Ask what was the most difficult skills transition to make.

Team Handball Lesson 2 — Intermediate level

Performance Goal

Students will play team handball.

Cognitive Goals

Students will

understand that the rules are to keep the game fair and safe,
learn the rules and penalties in team handball,
learn what constitutes personal fouls, and
understand the penalties.

Warm-Up

Students will

1. Participate in free play to get adjusted to the new ball's weight and size
2. Complete push-ups and sit-ups
3. Perform stretches

Motivation

Review the rules and how to adjust the game when they are broken. Get the class into the spirit of the game.

Lesson Sequence

1. Have students perform instant activity and warm-ups.
2. Review the fouls.
3. Have them play games.

Review

Ask the class whether players can roll the ball with their feet.
Ask if they can pass by kicking.

Review what the penalty is for doing either.

Ask if they can score from off the field or in the goalie area—and what the penalty is.

Review what happens if a player kicks a ball so it hits someone in the head.

Ask what would happen if the defense bumped into someone trying to score.

Teacher Homework

Prepare and post a list of each student in the class. It can be updated to include students' game records and if they have been captain.

Team Handball Lessons 3-6   Intermediate level

Lesson Setup

Equipment

A posted student roster

Performance Goal

Students will play team handball.

Cognitive Goals

Students will

rotate the responsibility of being captain, assuming a leadership role;
play with different teammates each game; and
use prior knowledge of strategies of basketball, soccer, and team handball to develop a daily strategy.

Warm-Up

Students will

1. Participate in free play to get adjusted to the ball's weight and size
2. Complete push-ups and sit-ups
3. Perform stretches

Motivation

As in the previous year, everyone will get to be a captain and pick half his team with the teacher assigning the other half. Students will again get credited one point individually for playing, two points for winning as a player, three points for being captain for the day, and four points for winning as a captain. Those with the most points at the end will be the class champs.

Lesson Sequence

1. Pick new captains who will choose their teams during free play. As described in the beginner level, this gives students the chance to experience setting up a team, like they might do as adults for a city recreation league.
2. Have the class play team handball games.

Review

Ask the class if there are any questions.

Ask students not to leave until you know whether they won and if they were a captain. Tell them you want to make sure they are credited with the right number of points.

Assessment

Observe for physical effort, teamwork, and cooperation. General performance assessment rubrics are available in appendix B to further assess your students. Also, a short quiz is available (page 537) if you'd like to grade more than students' effort and participation.

Team Handball Lesson 1   Advanced level

Lesson Setup

Facility

An area with no obstructions

Equipment

Scrimmage vests, with a different color for every group of six
A posted student roster
One ball for every two students

Performance Goal

Students will advance the ball.

Cognitive Goals

Students will review the special rules for advancing a ball in team handball:

How many steps can be taken
The parts of the body that can be used in moving the ball
How long the ball can be held

Students will review the rules related to boundaries.

Lesson Safety

A team needs a set of goals and its own field on which to play.

Warm-Up

Students will

1. Jog while hand dribbling and hand or body passing balls to partners
2. Complete push-ups and sit-ups
3. Perform stretches

Motivation

Mention to the class that it's kind of fun to take all the skills already learned and change the rules a little. Team handball levels the playing field a little. It's a relatively new sport for everyone, so you don't have kids breezing through the lessons while others are just learning. Almost everyone should be coming together as novices. Basketball stars have great skills in basketball, but they cannot use them quite the same way here. The same is true of great soccer players. Review the rules with the class and get into the game.

Lesson Sequence

1. Have the class perform instant activity (free play) and then warm-ups.
2. Review the rules:
   - Ball-handling rules
   - The boundaries
   - The goalie area and applicable rules
   - Fouls and penalties
3. Divide the class into teams of six and have them play games.

Review

Find out how many students got mixed up.

Ask the class whether players can roll the ball with their feet.

Ask if they can pass by kicking.

Review what the penalty is for doing either.

Ask if they can score from off the field or in the goalie area. Review what the penalty is.

Review what happens if a player kicks a ball so it hits someone in the head.

Ask what would happen if the defense bumped into someone trying to score.

Discuss what was the most difficult skills transition for students to make from basketball and why.

Ask the same question about soccer players, and ask them to explain why it was so difficult.

Team Handball Lessons 2-6   Advanced level

Performance Goal

Students will play team handball games in an individualized tournament.

Cognitive Goals

Students will

change teammates,
play with the change in teammates, and
rotate the responsibility of choosing teams and being captain.

Warm-Up

Students will

1. Participate in free play to get adjusted to the ball's weight and size
2. Complete push-ups and sit-ups
3. Perform stretches

Motivation

Ask if students remember how the games in team handball were run in the previous year. Tell them that it makes for a nice change each year, so you'll try it again. Everyone will get to be a captain and choose half a team. They all will get a score for each day they participate. Ask if they remember how it was credited: one point for participating, two for winning, three for participating as a captain, and four for being a winning captain. Ask if there are any questions and announce the day's captains.

Lesson Sequence

1. Pick the captains:
   - Have the captains choose two people for their team while everyone is at free play. All students having a turn at putting together a team gives them experience being a leader. Note that you do not let them pick an entire team so nobody has to be selected last, which can be very hurtful to those students.
   - Have captains get a team-color scrimmage vest.
   - Assign the other players to the teams, sending students in equally skilled groups for their team colors and to join teams.
2. Have students play team handball games.

Review

Ask the class if there are any questions.

Ask students not to leave until you know whether they won and if they were a captain. Tell them you want to make sure they are credited with the right number of points.

Assessment

Observe for physical effort, teamwork, and cooperation. General assessment rubrics in appendix B and a quiz (page 538) are available for use in arriving at an objective grade for this short unit.

Teacher Homework

Post all participants and update their scores after each gym class.

Team Handball Quiz—Beginner level

NAME _____ TEACHER _____

DATE _____ CLASS PERIOD _____

True or False: Read each statement below carefully. If the statement is true, put a check under the True box in the column to the left of the statement. If the statement is false, put a check under the False box in the column to the left of the statement. If using a grid sheet, blacken in the appropriate column for each question, making sure to use the correctly numbered line for each question and its answer.

True   False

☐   ☐   1. There are 11 players on an official team.

☐   ☐   2. A player kicking the ball into the goal does not score for her team.

☐   ☐   3. Throwing the ball up in the air and running forward to catch it is a violation.

☐   ☐   4. On a throw-in from out of bounds, the thrown ball goes through the goal post and over the goal line. This is a scored goal.

☐   ☐   5. All the rules of soccer apply in team handball.

☐   ☐   6. The person in possession of the ball is allowed to keep it for five seconds before passing it.

☐   ☐   7. Once you get the ball, you may take three running steps before releasing it to dribble or before passing it off.

☐   ☐   8. If the ball has rolled to a stop outside of the goal area, the goalie cannot go out to get it and bring it back into the restraining area.

☐   ☐   9. If you make a save, your deflecting pass would be best if it stays in the middle, in front of the goal.

☐   ☐   10. In team handball, as in basketball, the player has an unlimited ability to use the pivot step.

From *Complete Physical Education Plans for Grades 7–12* by Isobel Kleinman, 2001, Champaign, IL: Human Kinetics.

Team Handball Quiz—Intermediate level

NAME _____   TEACHER _____

DATE _____   CLASS PERIOD _____

True or False: Read each statement below carefully. If the statement is true, put a check under the True box in the column to the left of the statement. If the statement is false, put a check under the False box in the column to the left of the statement. If using a grid sheet, blacken in the appropriate column for each question, making sure to use the correctly numbered line for each question and its answer.

True	False	
☐	☐	1. All attacking players can enter the goal area while in the process of shooting.
☐	☐	2. A player throwing the ball into the opponent's goal scores if it passes over the line.
☐	☐	3. A knee volley is illegal in team handball.
☐	☐	4. A person off the field may shoot for a goal.
☐	☐	5. The dribbling rules of basketball apply in team handball.
☐	☐	6. The person in possession of the ball is allowed to keep it for five seconds before passing it.
☐	☐	7. Once you get the ball, you may take three running steps before releasing it to dribble or before passing it off.
☐	☐	8. The goalie cannot go out of his restraining area to bring the ball back into it.
☐	☐	9. If you make a save, your deflecting pass would be best if it stays in the middle, in front of the goal.
☐	☐	10. In team handball, as in basketball, the player has an unlimited ability to use the pivot step.

From *Complete Physical Education Plans for Grades 7–12* by Isobel Kleinman, 2001, Champaign, IL: Human Kinetics.

Team Handball Quiz—Advanced level

NAME _____ TEACHER _____

DATE _____ CLASS PERIOD _____

True or False: Read each statement below carefully. If the statement is true, put a check under the True box in the column to the left of the statement. If the statement is false, put a check under the False box in the column to the left of the statement. If using a grid sheet, blacken in the appropriate column for each question, making sure to use the correctly numbered line for each question and its answer.

True   **False**

☐   ☐   1. Only the goalie can play inside his own restraining area.

☐   ☐   2. A player throwing the ball into her own goal scores for the other team.

☐   ☐   3. The foot dribble is illegal in team handball.

☐   ☐   4. On a throw-in from out of bounds, the thrown ball goes through the goal post and over the goal line. This is a scored goal.

☐   ☐   5. The dribbling rules of basketball apply in team handball.

☐   ☐   6. The person in possession of the ball is allowed to keep it for five seconds before passing it.

☐   ☐   7. Once you get the ball, you may take three running steps before releasing it to dribble or before passing it off.

☐   ☐   8. The goalie cannot go out of his restraining area to bring the ball back into it.

☐   ☐   9. If you make a save, your deflecting pass would be best if it stays in the middle, in front of the goal.

☐   ☐   10. In team handball, as in basketball, the player has an unlimited ability to use the pivot step.

From *Complete Physical Education Plans for Grades 7–12* by Isobel Kleinman, 2001, Champaign, IL: Human Kinetics.

Team Handball Answer Key—Beginner level

1. F
2. T. Kicking is illegal in team handball.
3. T. Air dribbles are illegal. The ball must touch someone or something before a player can touch it again.
4. T
5. F. Team handball incorporates some strategies and skills of soccer and basketball, but it has its own rules.
6. F. The ball holder is allowed only three seconds to hold the ball.
7. T
8. T
9. F. Whatever the sport, defensive clearing of the ball is best done using an outlet pass, getting the ball away from the middle and its goal.
10. F

Team Handball Answer Key—Intermediate level

1. T
2. T. To score for her team, the ball must go in the opponent's goal.
3. F. Using anything below the knee is illegal.
4. T
5. F. Players are allowed three steps, not two, before they dribble.
6. F. The ball holder is allowed only three seconds to hold the ball.
7. T
8. T
9. F. Whatever the sport, defensive clearing of the ball is best done using an outlet pass, getting the ball away from the middle and its goal.
10. F

Team Handball Answer Key—Advanced level

1. T
2. T. To score for her team, the ball must go in the opponent's goal.
3. T. Using the foot is illegal.
4. T
5. F. Players are allowed three steps, not two, before they dribble.
6. F. The ball holder is allowed only three seconds to hold the ball.
7. T
8. T
9. F. Whatever the sport, defensive clearing of the ball is best done using an outlet pass, getting the ball away from the middle and its goal.
10. F

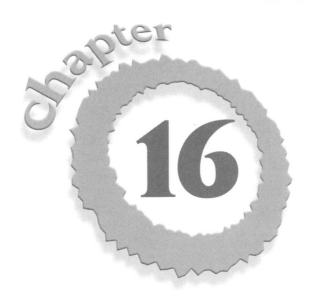

Chapter

Volleyball

Unit Overview

While teaching skills and strategies, conclude each lesson with a game of some kind.

1. Teach skills:

- Serves: underhand, overhead, sidearm
- Passes: bump and set, being able to direct both
- Defensive skills: tip-over, net recovery, block
- Offensive skills: offensive volley, spike, backward set

2. Teach a short history and evolution of volleyball.

3. Teach the importance of teamwork and an acceptance of individual differences.

4. Teach the rules of the game as skills are being taught:

- The difference between legal and illegal taps
- The service rules while learning to serve
- Legal rotation and scoring when ready for the first game
- The rules around the net while learning net recovery, spiking, and blocking

5. Teach the ground rules for your school: boundaries, obstructions

6. Teach strategies:

- Be prepared:
  Keep eyes on the ball
  Good position is dependent on where the ball is
  When receiving, get behind and under the incoming ball
  Pay attention even when it seems the point is over. It is not over until the ball hits the ground
- When in doubt, hit it up
- Offensive strategies include hitting the ball
  to the open court,
  deep,
  to the weakest player,
  with a change of direction, and
  with power and speed,

Volleyball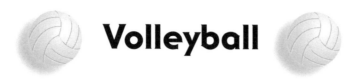

HISTORY

Volleyball was created in 1895 when William G. Morgan, a YMCA instructor in Massachusetts, combined components of basketball, baseball, handball, and tennis to create what he called "mintonette." As observers watched the game, they noted that players were "volleying" the ball back and forth. Thus, mintonette was changed to volleyball. The first game of volleyball was played at Springfield College in 1896. Then, in 1947, the Federation Internationale De Volley-Ball (FIVB) was founded.

FUN FACTS

→ The FIVB added the Beach Volleyball World Championship Series in 1987.

→ A 1992 Antigua and Barbuda stamp features Mickey Mouse and Donald Duck playing beach volleyball.

→ In 1994, an indoor volleyball event at Madison Square Garden had $4 million in total prize money.

→ Both women and men can play professional volleyball.

→ Today, more than 46 million Americans play volleyball.

BENEFITS OF PLAYING

1. Volleyball helps build your leg muscles.
2. It is great for your hand-eye coordination.
3. Volleyball helps you communicate with others and work as a team.
4. You can play indoors or outdoors.
5. It's a lot of fun!

TIME TO SURF!

Web Site	Web Site Address
USA Volleyball	http://www.usavolleyball.org/
Federation Internationale de Volleyball (FIVB)	http://www.fivb.ch/
United States Professional Volleyball (USPV)	http://www.uspv.com/

From *Complete Physical Education Plans for Grades 7–12* by Isobel Kleinman, 2001, Champaign, IL: Human Kinetics.

Volleyball Unit Extension Project

NAME _____ CLASS _____

Equipment needed to play volleyball

Item	Where you would purchase it (be specific)	Cost

Where you would play volleyball

Please explain where in the community you would play volleyball. Be specific.

Health benefits of playing volleyball

Please explain the health benefits of playing volleyball. Include how much volleyball you would need to play each week to gain these benefits.

Reflection question

Do you think volleyball is an activity you would like to play as an adult? Why or why not? If you believe you'd like to play volleyball, would you rather play in an organized recreation league, in pick-up games at a park, or in your own backyard with friends and family?

Bonus question

Attend an adult recreation league volleyball game and write a brief paper on what you liked and didn't like about the way the game was played and add whether or not you'd like to participate in this league as an adult (include why or why not). Also add whether you'd rather play in a coed league.

From *Complete Physical Education Plans for Grades 7–12* by Isobel Kleinman, 2001, Champaign, IL: Human Kinetics.

Volleyball Teaching Tips

1. Allow noncompetitive practice time during each lesson so students can improve their skills without pressure.
2. Develop a short tournament.
3. If students are unable to participate fully in class activities, remember that they can be involved by coaching, officiating, keeping score, or conducting a research project.

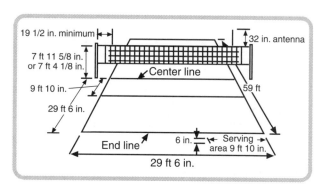

19 1/2 in. minimum
32 in. antenna
7 ft 11 5/8 in. or 7 ft 4 1/8 in.
Center line
9 ft 10 in.
59 ft
29 ft 6 in.
End line
6 in.
Serving area 9 ft 10 in.
29 ft 6 in.

Figure 16.1—Volleyball court dimensions.

Unit Setup

Facility

Overhead and wall obstructions should be removed.
Courts should be marked with sidelines and nets should be up and taut.

Equipment

A minimum of one ball for every four students. Leather-skinned balls are highly recommended, as plastic balls tend to burn students' skin.
Round-robin tournament schedules and charts (appendix A)

Unit Timeline

This unit is one of the best sports units to teach if you have large classes and are forced to stay indoors. It is also one of the longest in this text. With your guidance, the lesson plans will help students develop the skills they need to enjoy the games. And, have no fear, despite the length of the unit, student interest should be sustained.

There are three units in this chapter:

Four lessons to develop basic skills enough to enjoy a low-level game
Two lessons to work with new team groups in a cooperative learning environment
Ten to 12 lessons for a class double round-robin tournament
• Lessons 1-5 of the first round-robin tournament continue the development of skills
• Lessons 6-12 of the second round-robin tournament simulate match play
One lesson for a quiz and culminating activity

Unit Assessment

A student portfolio checklist is provided here for student use (table 16.1). Encourage students to track their progress as they master new skills. Quizzes at the

TABLE 16.1 Volleyball Student Portfolio Checklist

STUDENT NAME _____

- ☐ Knows how to and can perform the underhand volleyball serve
- ☐ Knows how to and can perform the bump pass
- ☐ Knows the rules of serve and how to rotate
- ☐ Can play a game while following the rules
- ☐ Knows how to and can perform the setup pass
- ☐ Has learned the tip-over
- ☐ Can direct the ball to different places on the court
- ☐ Knows and understands rules involving net play
- ☐ Has learned and can perform the overhead serve
- ☐ Has learned the spike
- ☐ Has learned the block
- ☐ Is able to play an offensive game
- ☐ Knows the official rules
- ☐ Has learned basic volleyball strategies
- ☐ Exhibits responsibility and good sporting behavior during competition
- ☐ Can, within the rules, interchange positions

From *Complete Physical Education Plans for Grades 7–12* by Isobel Kleinman, 2001, Champaign, IL: Human Kinetics

end of the chapter are available to test students' knowledge of the sport. Students' skills development can be assessed and graded using the appropriate-level performance assessment rubric. Further general assessment rubrics can be found in appendix B.

Additional Resources

American Sport Education Program. 1996. *Coaching Youth Volleyball.* Champaign, IL: Human Kinetics.

Asher, Kinda, editor. 1996. *Basic Elements of the Game.* Vol. 1 of *Best of Coaching Volleyball.* Indianapolis: Master Press.

Bertucci, Bob. 1995. *Volleyball Drill Book: Individual Skill.* Indianapolis: Master Press.

Neville, William. 1990. *Coaching Volleyball Successfully.* Champaign, IL: Human Kinetics.

Volleyball Lesson 1 — Beginner level

Lesson Setup

Facility

A wall with no obstructions
A large area of cleared floor space

Equipment

One ball for every four students

Performance Goal

Students will hit a bump pass.

Cognitive Goals

Students will learn

a brief history of volleyball and its evolution,
that to hit something up they need to hit from beneath it, and
the necessity of hitting the ball up.

Lesson Safety

Groups need their own space in which to practice—the minimum is 15 feet from any group near them.
Establish rules for how to deal with errant balls and teach students to follow them daily:
- Wait for the person closest to the ball to throw it back
- Throw it back on one bounce so that it doesn't cause more disturbance

Warm-Up

Students will

1. Jog around the playing area
2. Complete push-ups and sit-ups
3. Practice mimetics for the bump pass, practicing each component five times:
   - Proper hand and forearm position—practice it fast five times
   - Leg preparation—bending both knees and getting in a forward stride position while preparing the arms
   - Coordinate the arms and legs together, adding what is done on contact so it takes place in one smooth, flowing motion:
     Train students to keep their eyes on the imaginary ball as it touches the forearm
     Keep their legs bent
     Move their forearms in the direction they want the ball to go (forward and up)
   - Add getting to the "imaginary" ball, preparing for the hit, the contact, and follow-through

Motivation

Volleyball was developed in the United States and has become so popular that it is difficult to go to any resort, beachside community, or park without seeing nets set up and people playing. The game in its original form is played with six players. Six-on-six is the way it is played in the Olympics, in class, and in interscholastic activities.

Ask students if any of them have seen beach volleyball on TV or at the beach. If two people are opposite each other at a beach volleyball net, their only chance to get to each other's pass may be when they are able to hit the ball up in the air. In today's class, students will learn to do that: the bump pass.

Lesson Sequence

1. Teach and demonstrate the bump pass (figure 16.2).
2. Teach the following rules:
   - An open hand below the waist is illegal.
   - A ball that hits fixtures on the ceiling or the walls is out of bounds.
3. Set up progressive drills for the bump pass, providing as much repetition as possible:
   - A student takes a ball and practices bumping (blocking off the forearm) to himself.
   - He bumps to the wall, bumping back what the wall returns.
   - He receives a toss from somebody and bumps the ball back to the passer in the direction of the wall (figure 16.3).
   - A group circle is made, which tries to keep the ball alive by bumping it toward the middle.
4. Create some kind of contest to keep the enthusiasm high as students master the skill. Try the following questions:

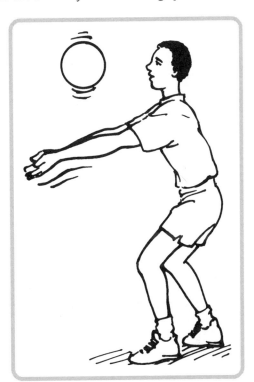

Figure 16.2—Bump pass to self.

- Who can keep the ball up 5 times, 10 times, or more before allowing it to get out of control?
- Which circle can keep it up, legally, the most times before it hits the floor?
- Can anyone beat the best team of the class, which got [however many] bumps?

Review

Ask students why they should use a bump pass for balls coming below their waists.

If they cannot control the height of the ball, review what rule might be broken.

If the ball is not going up and it's going straight ahead, discuss what adjustments should be made.

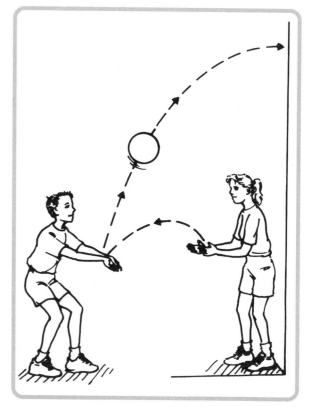

Figure 16.3—Working in pairs to practice the bump pass.

Volleyball Lesson 2   Beginner level

Lesson Setup

Facility

Nets up

Performance Goals

Students will

be able to serve underhand (or use other serves of their preference), and improve their bump passes.

Cognitive Goals

Students will learn

to make their arm a striking implement;

that to hit something forward, the point of contact is in the back; and basic service rules—boundaries, foot fault, and faultless flight.

Lesson Safety

Allowing students to hit every time they get a ball is great for practice, but it means that volleyballs will be coming at players who do not always expect them. Their safety is not a problem if all students remember that they are practicing a serve that should land within the court. Some will get excited and forget. They might try to serve as hard as they can, hitting the wall or even a classmate on the other side of the net. Unexpected hard-hit balls will not be welcomed if a person gets hit by one. Be aware of this problem and be vigilant to guard against it. If that is not possible, stop the progress of the serving and have all hitters on the same side of the net, round up the balls, and switch sides of the court.

Warm-Up

Students will

1. Run—side to side with crossover steps, backward and forward
2. Complete push-ups and sit-ups
3. Practice mimetics for the bump pass
4. Practice mimetics for an underarm serve:
   - The stance
   - The arm swing
   - The point of contact (using the other hand, aiming for the palm as the "middle of the ball")

Motivation

No game can start if players cannot put the ball into play. Tell students that in this lesson, everyone will learn how to serve the ball. Ask if someone can tell you which is most likely to fly from one end of the court to the other—something that is hit with a stick or something that is hit with a feather. Students will learn to make their arms like a stick.

Lesson Sequence

1. Teach and demonstrate the underhand serve.
2. Set up a short practice drill:
   - Start with hitting the ball underhand to a wall 10 feet away
   - Allow a few chances at a time, with quick rotation, and several repetitions per person
   - Move back gradually, each time encouraging a flight that hits the wall 12 feet high
3. Teach the following rules:
   - The net serve: this serve must pass over the net without touching anything.
   - The foot fault: the server must be off the court to serve.

4. Make a shooting gallery for the serve (figure 16.4):
   - Distribute every ball, having students behind either side of the court, allowing as much repetition as possible within the time parameters.
   - Some suggestions:

     After 10 successes, have students sit so that others can get the balls and get more repetition.

     Do not spend the whole period on this because arms will hurt and students will get bored.

     If a student or two is having a particular problem, let them know you will work with them on it during free play in the next class.

5. Put the groups in a circle and give them five minutes to practice their bump pass.

6. Afterward, ask them to count the number of legal taps they can control of the ball as a group. Remind them of the legally required rules:
   - No open hands.
   - No one player can tap it twice in a row.
   - If it touches the wall or ceiling, it is out.

7. Ask which team can keep the ball up the most in the class. See if anyone can beat the best team of the class, which got however many taps.

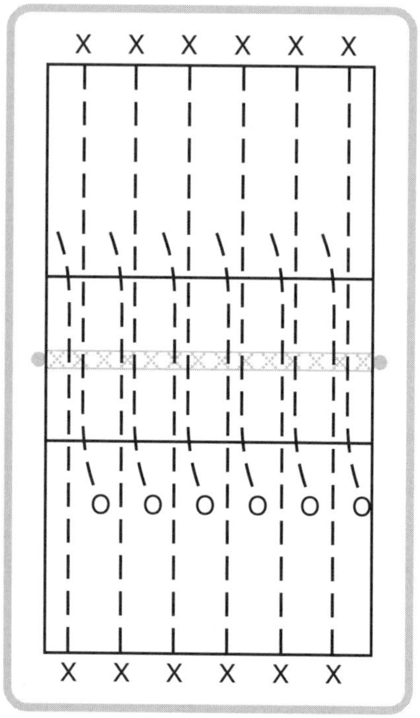

Figure 16.4—Practicing the serve.

Review

Ask the class what part of the body should meet the ball on a serve.

Ask students, if they think of the ball as having a face, what part of the face they would hit when they serve.

Review what constitutes a foot fault.

Ask if they still believe in "do-overs."

Volleyball Lesson 3 — Beginner level

Performance Goals

Students will

be able to legally hit balls with open upward setup passes, and improve their service and bump passes.

Cognitive Goals

Students will learn

to judge when to use a bump pass and when to use a set, when a pass is illegal and how to avoid illegal passes, and the importance of making passes go *up*.

Warm-Up

Students will

1. Participate in free play to practice before the class formally begins
2. Practice mimetics for the setup pass:
   - Have students begin with the hand position, the window over their eyes through which they spot the ball
   - Have them use the proper arm and hand motion.
   - Add the legs, one forward, one back, with a knee bend.
   - Add the footwork, moving to the knee bend, seeing the ball through the window, and following through up.
3. Practice the mimetic for the bump.
4. Practice the mimetic for the serve, having students use their free hand as the imaginary ball they have to look at and hit. Tell them to keep their target arm loose, so they don't hurt themselves when they hit it. (The target arm should swing away on contact with the serving arm.)

Motivation

Tell students that when a ball is dropping from above their head and they can get their eyes under it easily, it is better to use a setup pass. Eventually, this pass begins (sets up) the "attack," since this pass can be sent to someone or someplace specific. Tell the class that control takes time to develop, so it should be started now.

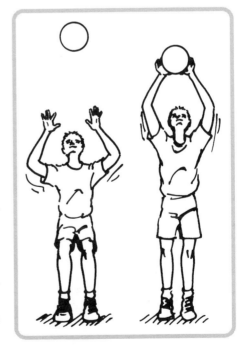

Figure 16.5—Set to self.

Lesson Sequence

1. Teach and demonstrate the set, half done in the progressive mimetic introductions in the warm-up.
2. Teach the rules:
   - Both hands have to contact the ball at one time.
   - The ball cannot appear as if it is resting in the hands.
3. Set up a progressive drill:
   - Start with a set to oneself for a few seconds to get under the ball and follow through up (figure 16.5)

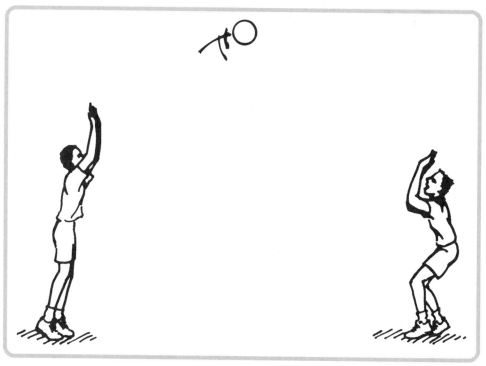

Figure 16.6—Practicing the set in partners.

- Set to the wall, aiming for height and continuous returns that are high
- Receive a toss from someone and return it high directly to that person (figure 16.6)
- Make a circle in a larger group and practice setting high balls and bumping any low-dropping ball or emergency save
4. If any time remains, devise a game or contest situation. Some examples:
    - The number of continuous legal taps a circle group can complete to control the ball
    - A short game

Review

Review what pass the class worked on in this lesson.
Ask why players would use this pass instead of the bump pass.
Discuss what pass they should use if the ball is dropping from a high arc.
Ask for a demonstration of how they would prepare to hit it.
Review what part of the hand touches the ball on a set.
Review what part of the arm touches the ball when hitting a bump pass.

Volleyball Lesson 4   Beginner level

Performance Goal

Students will use practiced skills in a game situation.

Cognitive Goals

Students will learn

how to rotate, and
game rules:
- Three taps per team
- Point scored only when serving
- Rotation after the opposing team loses serve
- The boundary lines

Warm-Up

Students will

1. Participate in free play to practice before the class formally begins
2. Practice mimetics for the setup, bump, and serve

Motivation

Ask if the class is ready to start. Announce that it's time to learn the rest of the game rules and to play.

Lesson Sequence

1. Teach the remaining game rules:
   - Rotation
   - Three taps per team
   - Staying on one's own side of the court
2. Assign groups of six to different courts.
3. Begin with a few minutes of volleying in a circle (figure 16.7).
4. Have students play games, while you move around to assist with rotation questions and any other questions.
5. After about eight minutes, change the teams that are playing each other.

Review

Review whether a player can serve twice before everyone on the team has served.
Ask the class if the team not scoring can ever win a point.
Review that the rotation is clockwise

Volleyball Lesson 5 — Beginner level

Performance Goals

Students will

react to a serve with a bump pass *up*, and
improve their skills in a game situation.

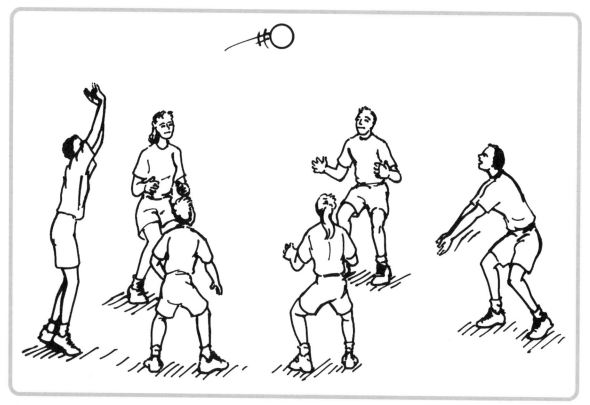

Figure 16.7—Circle volley.

Cognitive Goals

Students will learn

how important positioning is to success, and
the importance of using a controlled bump pass as the first tap.

Warm-Up

Students will

1. Participate in free play to practice before the class formally begins
2. Practice mimetics for the setup, bump, and serve

Motivation

Tell students that although they all can bump and set reasonably well in a circle, it becomes more difficult during a game. Hitting a served ball with a bump pass that stays on the court is difficult. The reason is because the serve is traveling farther and feels like it has been hit harder. It takes some practice to be able to convert a hard serve into a high pass that their teammates can work with. Suggest they take a little extra practice time before the games start to practice both their serve and how to control a bump pass off their opponent's serve.

Lesson Sequence

1. Demonstrate how you want partners to practice:
   - One serves and the other receives by bumping the ball up.
   - There should be a maximum of three couples per court.
   - Allow enough time so that each person gets to serve six times and receive six times.
2. For game time, allow students to get in their own group of six and assign the court.
3. Begin with a few minutes of volleying in a circle.
4. Have them play games, while you spend time at each court.

Review

Ask students if they noticed that when they bumped the serve, instead of it going up, it went into the net.
Ask if they want that and why it happened.
Discuss what things their body could do to prevent it.

Teacher Homework

Make up teams of equal gender and ability.

Volleyball Lesson 6 — Beginner level

Performance Goals

Students will

be able to use the skills already taught in a game situation,
meet and play with their tournament teams, and
choose their own captains and co-captains. (If the captain is a girl, the co-captain should be a boy and vice versa.)

Cognitive Goals

Students will

understand that everyone has different abilities and weaknesses;
identify the best server—someone who can get it over again and again; and
begin to think about building rotation order around strengths.

Warm-Up

Students will

1. Participate in free play to practice before the class formally begins
2. Move forward and back, side to side

3. Move to a spot on the gym floor and use the mimetics for the setup, then move back again—repeat five times
4. Repeat the same as above with the bump
5. Practice the mimetic for the serve

Motivation

Announce the permanent tournament teams. Tell students that it is important they get to know each other and how each will respond to a ball falling between them. Knowing one's teammates and how they play lets one know which players will go the extra yard, who needs a little more backup, and who is the best server. Discuss that the best server is someone who is able to get the ball over the net and onto the court over and over again. By the end of the class, students should agree on who their team's best server is.

Lesson Sequence

1. Announce the teams.
2. Assign teams to different courts.
3. Begin with a few minutes of volley practice in a circle.
4. Have students play games, while you move around to assist with rotation questions and any other questions.
5. Stop the games and ask the teams to decide their captains and co-captains. Have the captains report to you.

Review

Ask students who their best server is. Tell them that the next class will cover how to take advantage of a team's best server.

Teacher Homework

Complete the game schedule for the tournament, the team standings chart, and post them. Examples of these can be found in appendix A.

Volleyball Lesson 7 — Beginner level

Lesson Setup

Equipment

A blackboard or other visual aid
A posted game schedule (see appendix A)
A posted team standings chart

Performance Goals

Students will

set up their team with the best rotation they can think of,
encourage each other to hit the ball up, and
play round 1 of their tournament.

Cogntive Goals

Students will learn

more about rotation order:
  • Where the receiving team's first server will be at the beginning of the game
  • Where the last server is at the start of the game
  • Some thinking about setting up the team before the game starts
to adjust to the strengths and weaknesses of their team members, and
that the team that wins must lead by two points or a tie is recorded.

Warm-Up

Students will

1. Participate in free play to practice before the class formally begins
2. Move forward and back and side to side to practice setup and bump mimetics

Motivation

Discuss the identification of the best server on each team. Ask students, if they want to win a game, should they put their best server first or last. Talk about how to arrange their team to take advantage of its strengths so they are best positioned to win in the tournament games.

Lesson Sequence

1. Diagram and explain rotation order for serving and receiving teams.
2. Begin with a few minutes of volleying in a circle.
3. Have students play round 1 games, while you assist with questions and officiate.

Review

Ask students what their team should do if their best server is standing in the right
  back position when their captain announces that the other team serves first.
Ask the winning captains to please stand.
Review whether there are any ties. Ask the captains of the tying teams to
  please stand.

Volleyball Lesson 8   Beginner level

Lesson Setup

Equipment

A blackboard or other visual aid with the rotation order on display

Performance Goals

Students will

> try to save errant balls hit by teammates as long as their tap will not exceed the third tap, and
> play round 2 of their tournament.

Cognitive Goals

Students will

> start to deal with the excitement and pressure of wanting to win;
> be encouraged to hit the ball—even if it looks hopeless—as long as the team still has one tap left and the ball has not yet bounced on the ground, walls, or ceiling; and
> learn more about rotation order and the pairing of players.

Warm-Up

Students will

1. Participate in free play to practice before the class formally begins
2. Complete setup and bump mimetics that include moving forward and backward and side to side

Motivation

Announce to the class that the second round of the tournament is about to start. Mention what teams are in the lead after round 1 and with how many tournament points. The point system is as follows: If class is over before a game is finished, a team gets two points if they lead by two points. If no one was in the lead, both teams get one point for a tie. A loss means a team gets no points. Tell the students that, while they are playing their second round, you would like them to try to notice who on the team is able to make incredible saves. And if they already know, they should discuss where they would like to put them in the rotation order.

Lesson Sequence

1. Diagram and explain more about the rotation order:
   - The order should do more than just put good servers up earlier in the rotation.
   - The order must divide the team's talent:

     Some players are great at making saves. They should be next to the teammates who keep the ball from landing but can't seem to get it where they want it to go.

     Some players are great at judging whether the ball is going over the net and are able to give it that last bit of help. Such players are more valuable near the left front of the net. This way, even through rotations, they are near the net most of the game.
2. Begin with a few minutes of volleying in a circle.
3. Have students play games, while you move around to assist with rotation questions and any other questions.

Review

Find out if the teams know who their best server is.

Ask if their best server is serving first.

Review whether the best servers got to serve more than once during the game.

Ask the winning captains to please stand.

Also ask captains whose teams tied to please stand.

Volleyball Lesson 9   Beginner level

Performance Goals

Students will

be able to hit a ball backward over the net—a tip-over; and

play round 3 of the tournament.

Cognitive Goals

Students will

learn that the follow-through can make the ball go in a direction other than the direction they are facing,

accept their teammates' individual differences, and

learn the difference between backing up and taking over for those who cannot control the ball.

Warm-Up

Students will

1. Participate in free play time to practice before the class formally begins
2. Move forward and back and side to side to practice setup and bump mimetics.
3. Practice mimetics for the set and the bump pass following through backward.

Motivation

Tell your students that before they start, you would like to teach them all how to be a hero for their team so that they, too, can get the ball over the net even if they have their back to the net. They will take a little time before the games to do this.

Lesson Sequence

1. Demonstrate hitting a tip-over from a high set (figure 16.8).
2. Have teams toss high to a player with her back to the net—wait for three successes before rotating.
3. Demonstrate saves of low balls with a bump pass when the back is to the net (figure 16.9).
4. Have teams toss the ball below the waist to a player waiting with her back to the net. The hitter's turn is up once she has had three successes.
5. Announce the standings and court assignments, and have students play round 3.

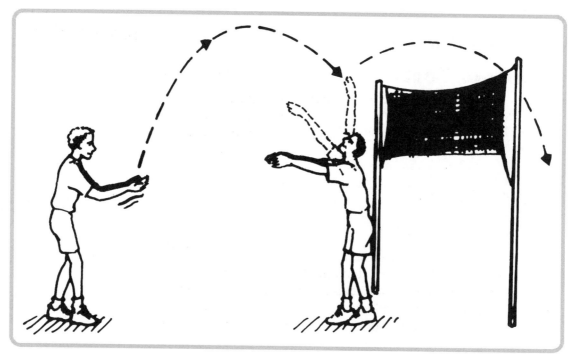

Figure 16.8—Tip-over from a high set.

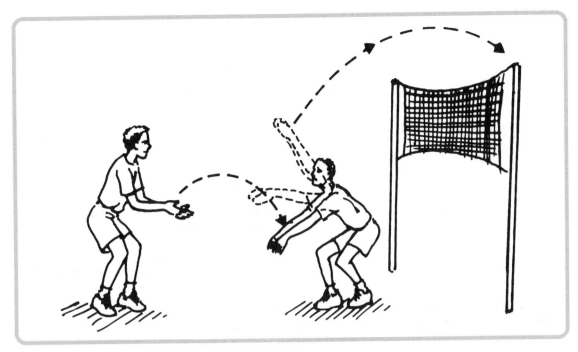

Figure 16.9—Tip-over from a low pass.

Review

Ask the class if anyone knows why it is more important to back up one's
   teammates than to allow the best player to always jump in and take over.
Review what backing up someone means.
Ask students if using the tip-over can be considered making a save.
Find some teachable moment that occurred on one of the courts and review it aloud.
Ask the winning captains to please stand.
Ask the captains whose teams tied to please stand.

Volleyball Lesson 10   Beginner level

Performance Goals

Students will

be able to hit the ball out of the net, and
play round 4 of the tournament

Cognitive Goals

Students will learn

that it is legal to recover a ball out of the net,
to identify how differently the ball rebounds from the net if it hits the net high
   and low, and

561

the rules involving the net:
- For the serve (serves cannot touch the net)
- During play (the ball is alive if it touches the net, people cannot touch the net)
- When the ball is dead (when it hits something outside the boundary line, not when it hits the net)

Warm-Up

Students will

1. Participate in free play to practice before the class formally begins
2. Practice mimetics of all skills, including the moving approach and directional follow-through

Motivation

Announce that round 4 of the tournament is about to start. The students have been introduced to just about everything a seventh- or eighth-grader needs to learn to be a good player, although they have not had the opportunity to really master it all. Explain that the trouble is, no matter how much they practice and get better, like all people, they will make mistakes and hit the ball into the net when they were planning on passing it up to the front-line players or hitting it over. Tell them that today they will learn how to save the balls hit into the net.

Lesson Sequence

1. Demonstrate hitting the ball out of the net (figure 16.10, a-b):
   - Show how the ball rolls down the net if it contacts the net at the top.
   - Show how the ball bounces back from the net if it hits in the middle.
   - Demonstrate getting under it, by squatting and using the bump pass to get it up.

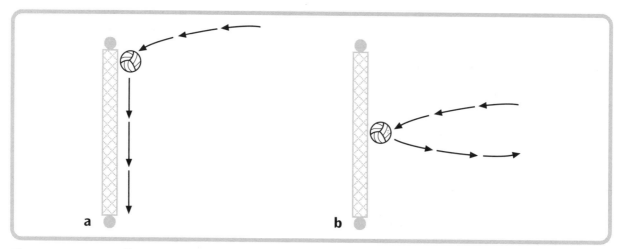

Figure 16.10—Reading the ball's rebound off the net: *(a)* hits the top and rolls down near the center line and *(b)* hits the center and bounces back several feet.

2. Have teams throw the ball into the net and practice recovering it. They should practice until each player has three successes.
3. Announce the standings, opponents, and court assignments.
4. Leave a few minutes for the circle volley.
5. Have students play round 4.

Review

Ask students if any net recovery occurred in their game.

Ask if there still are any teammates who think that when the ball hits the net it is dead.

Request the winning captains, and the captains whose teams tied, to stand.

Volleyball Lesson 11   Beginner level

Performance Goals

Students will

improve their teamwork, and
play round 5.

Cognitive Goal

Students will improve their sporting behavior by recognizing and appreciating the improvement of their teammates.

Warm-Up

Students will

1. Participate in free play to practice before the class formally begins
2. Practice mimetics for all skills with approach and directional follow-through

Motivation

Announce that round 5 of the tournament is about to start. If there are six teams, then after today, students will have played everyone in the class. Tell them that this makes today special. It is the last round of the round-robin tournament. During this first round robin, players only had time to play one game. If they're undefeated so far, the most tournament points their team could have gotten was eight points for winning all four games. Announce which teams are in what place and with how many points after four rounds.

Starting in the next class, they will begin their second round robin. Tell students that the games will begin as soon as they warm up. There will be no more instruction before the games. And, during the period, if they start right away, it will be possible to play more than one game. Should a team be able to play and win more than one game, they will get many more points than they've been able to get to date. For that reason, the standings can change dramatically. If a team can win a match (playing three games against the same team) in one class period, they could win up to six points that day, because they will earn two tournament points for each game their team wins.

Basically, tell the students, this is the last chance for their team to practice for half of the class time. After this day, they will warm up and start their games. Leave 10 minutes for open practice. As a team, on their own side of the net, they should practice what they think needs the most work: bumps, serves, sets, net recovery, or tip-overs. If they do any work on net recovery or tip-overs, they should remember they are sharing the net with the team on the other side of the court, so remind them not to interfere with that team.

Lesson Sequence

1. Announce court assignments.
2. Give the class a full 10 minutes to practice before the games begin.
3. Have students play round 5.

Review

Ask the winning captains, and the captains whose teams tied, to please stand.

Volleyball Lesson 12 — Beginner level

Performance Goals

Students will

improve their teamwork, and
play round 6 of the tournament.

Cognitive Goal

Students will learn about match play.

Warm-Up

Students will

1. Participate in free-play volleyball before the class formally begins
2. Perform a circle volley with the team

Motivation

Announce that round 6 of the tournament—the first round of the second round robin—is about to begin. This means that today, students will play the same team they played when the tournament first started. Announce the standings to date—what places the teams are in and with how many points.

What makes this tournament still wide open is that teams today will get two tournament points for each game they win in the match. Tell them that in interscholastic competition a match is the best of three or five games, depending on the school and level of play. There's not enough time for that, however, so you'll have them start as many games as they have time for, awarding two points for each one considered a win.

Lesson Sequence

1. Explain the procedure and scoring for match play:
   - A game is 15 points.
   - After one game is over, the rotation order for the second is the same as the start of the first.
   - Players should switch sides of the net for each game.
   - A partial win will count if the team can get a minimum of eight points. Partial games might occur if the class ends during the middle of a game:
     - If a team is ahead by two, it gets a win.
     - If not, it gets a tie.
2. Announce court assignments and the time for the practice period: allow three minutes.
3. Have students play round 6.

Review

Ask the winning captains, and the captains whose teams tied, to please stand.

Assessment

Post and start observing for performance standards based on one of the seventh- and eighth-grade volleyball performance assessment rubrics (on page 569).

Volleyball Lessons 13-16   Beginner level

Lesson Setup

Equipment

A posted performance rubric for the seventh and eighth grades
Regularly updated and posted tournament standings

Performance Goal

Students will improve their teamwork while they complete a 10-round tournament.

Cognitive Goals

Students will learn basic strategies to enhance team play:

Team organization of rotation
Keeping the ball high on the first and second taps
Thinking about winning the point instead of simply getting the ball over the net:
  • Changing direction
  • Hitting to the weak player
  • Hitting the ball deep
  • Hitting to where the person who is like to play the ball the most is not
  • If that person leaves his position right away, hitting to the position he vacated
  • Knowing that players who want to play every ball reduce team effectiveness

Warm-Up

Students will

1. Participate in free play to practice before the class formally begins
2. Perform a circle volley with the team

Motivation

Announce what round of the tournament the students are in, and the standings to date.

Lesson Sequence

1. Teach a strategy of the day, using the strategies listed in "Cognitive Goals." Choose the one that will do the most good for your class and work in descending order. If teams are still suffering with players who constantly want the ball, go for the strategy against those players first. If teams are losing out because their rotation order is leaving big weak zones or they are starting out with servers who cannot serve, start with that strategy.
2. Invite any team to request your services as its coach.
3. Post court assignments and team records.
4. Have students practice setting and bumping in a circle for at least three minutes.
5. Set up minimum performance goals, explain, and post.
6. Have students play the round.

Review

Ask the winning captains, and the captains whose teams tied, to please stand. Announce there will be a quiz during the next class.

Assessment

Throughout the last few rounds, observe for students' skills and effort for how they meet performance standards as defined in the performance assessment rubrics on page 569.

Give students a short quiz (page 607) at the conclusion of the unit.

Volleyball Lesson 17 | Beginner level

Lesson Setup

Equipment

Quizzes for each student
Pens and pencils

Performance Goals

Students will

take a volleyball quiz, and
have a culminating game after the quiz is over, either final playoffs or
- an all-star court
- boys versus girls, or
- making up new teams of the players' choice.

Cognitive Goal

Students will test their volleyball knowledge via a quiz.

Warm-Up

Students will

1. Complete push-ups
2. Jog in place
3. Complete a circle volley with a team

Motivation

Tell students that they played a great tournament. They should all feel like winners because the real winners are all the people who had fun learning, playing with new classmates, and making new friends. Announce the tournament winners and congratulate the following teams:

The one that made a great comeback
The one with the best teamwork
The one with the best sporting behavior

Although students may have been disappointed because their best friends were not on their team when the tournament teams were first announced, tell the class you're happy that they made some new friends and learned to appreciate people they did not know so well before. Ask them now if they want to stay with their teams and have play-off games or play their last day with different teams. Announce the current standings. If they would like different teams, they could choose an "all-star" game, a battle of the sexes, or picking any teams of their choice. Have the class take a quick vote.

Lesson Sequence

1. Distribute the quiz and pencils as students arrive so they can space out and begin.
2. Collect the quiz 10 minutes after it starts. If students are not finished, allow them to finish on the sidelines or after school or during their free period and let the rest of the class get underway.
3. After students vote on how they want to play the last game, send them to warm up on the court.
4. Begin the last volleyball game of the season.

Review

Ask students if they could change anything about this unit, what it would be. Ask if any questions stumped them.

Assessment

Students can be assessed using one of the two volleyball performance assessment rubrics in table 16.2, a-b. The first rubric focuses on specific volleyballs skills while the second rubric focuses on game skills. Further general assessment rubrics are available in appendix B.

Volleyball Lesson 1   Intermediate level

Lesson Setup

Facility

A volleyball court for every 12 players

Equipment

One ball for every three to four players

TABLE 16.2A Beginner Volleyball Performance Assessment Rubric

STUDENT NAME _____

	0	1	2	3
Serve	No effort	• Puts opposite foot forward • Uses correct arm motion • Contacts the ball in front	• Puts the ball in play	• Legally serves in the game
Bump pass	No effort	• Uses proper arm position • Keeps knees bent • Does a proper follow-through	• Is able to direct the ball upward	• Moves to the ball • Keeps the ball on the same side of the court
Setup pass	No effort	• Uses proper hand position • Keeps knees bent • Does a proper follow-through	• Directs the ball upward	• Moves eyes under the ball • Has high arch • Ball reaches its destination
Tip-over	No effort	• Maintains stance on contact with the ball • Does a proper follow-through	• Is able to direct the ball backward • Makes an effort to clear the ball over the net	• Ball passes over the net
Teamwork and sporting behavior	No effort	• Keeps eye on the ball during play • Gets to the court on time • Gets along with teammates	• Rotates properly • Covers the ball in own zone • Makes an effort to improve weaknesses	• Avoids touching the net • Plays within the rules • Covers balls inside the court

TABLE 16.2B Beginner Volleyball Performance Assessment Rubric

STUDENT NAME _____

	0	1	2	3	4	5
Offense	No effort	• Keeps eye on the ball • Uses proper body mechaniccs for the serve and the set	• Serves clear the net • Bumps go up • Sets go up	• Puts the ball in play during a game • Moves to the ball	• Is a reliable server • Saves errant taps by teammates and redirect them over the net	• Gets the third tap over the net • Uses strategy
Defense	No effort	• Contacts the ball in own zone • Uses correct bump-pass mechanics • Keeps eye on the ball	• Blocked ball goes up • Moves under the ball	• Bumps go up and forward • Blocks opponents' serves	• Directs a bump pass to teammate • Uses a bump to save a ball out of the net • Recovers wild teammate passes	• Backs up teammates • Is consistently able to block the ball up • Leaves and returns to the position for saves
Position, teamwork, and attitude	No effort	• Goes to court assignment promptly • Warms up with the team • Rotates properly	• Takes responsibility for position • Maintains concentration on the ball when in play	• Works well with teammates • Plays within the rules	• Recognizes good teammate effort and success • Never blames others • Has good sporting behavior	• Inspires the team • Backs up, not takes over, for teammates • Provides reliable, consistent leadership

Performance Goals

Students will

review a bump pass,
review a set, and
play a game.

Cognitive Goals

Students will

see the need for high passes until sending the ball to the other side, and
have to decide whether to use a set or a bump pass during a game.

Lesson Safety

Practice areas should be well spaced.
Reestablish rules for how to deal with errant balls:
- Players should not run across anyone's court to get their balls.
- Balls should be returned by throwing them back.
- Players should return the balls to their opponents by sending them under the net.

Warm-Up

Students will

1. Practice mimetics for the bump pass, setup pass, and overhead serve (see the beginner unit for more detail):
   - Practice each skill five times in the stationary position
   - Practice each skill five times with the proper footwork
2. Complete push-ups and sit-ups
3. Jump with arms straight up

Motivation

Ask your students how many enjoyed volleyball the previous year. This year, they will build on their skills so the games become even more exciting and they'll need even more teamwork than before. But tell them they must be able to control the ball on their own court and be able to hit the ball up to a specific place. For today's lesson, they will quickly review and warm up some rusty skills and then conclude with a short game.

Lesson Sequence

1. Review the bump pass: preparation, contact point, and follow-through.
2. Have students drill for the most repetition—for example, bumping to themselves at the wall, aiming for height and control.

3. Review the set: preparation, contact point, and follow-through.
4. Have students set to the wall.
5. Have students get in groups of six, as in figure 16.7. Then they should practice volleying in a circle on one side of the net:
   - Ask them to tell you when they have kept the ball up 10 times.
   - Then they should go for 15 times—and they're ready for a game.
6. Arrange the more successful groups to play each other the remainder of the period. Groups that are still aiming for 15 times should be allowed to continue practicing in a circle without going to a game.

Review

Review illegal tap rules and any rules that came up during the games.

Volleyball Lesson 2   Intermediate level

Performance Goals

Students will

learn an overhead serve, and
improve their set.

Cognitive Goals

Students will learn

strategy for sending an offensive serve onto the court, and
the value of accurate skills.

Warm-Up

Students will

1. Practice mimetics for the bump pass, setup pass, and overhead serve—with steps
2. Complete a wall volley in attendance lines

Motivation

Ask students if they watch highly competitive volleyball games. Now that they're older, they want to put the ball in play so that it is even more difficult for their opponents to return it. This lesson is about the overhead serve, or, in other words, the foundation for a spike. The overhead serve is the same motion with the feet on the ground. This serve is more difficult than the others because the ball is tossed. Hitting with two things moving—the arm and the ball—is more difficult than hitting with one thing moving.

Lesson Sequence

1. Teach and demonstrate the overhead serve.
2. Using every ball, with students on each side of court, have them practice the overhead serve, as shown in figure 16.4:
   - Interrupt the class to remind everyone of the boundary lines.
   - Interrupt to remind them of foot faults.
3. Have students get in teams and practice a circle volley on a half-court:
   - Ask them to tell you when they have kept the ball up 10 times.
   - Then they should go for 15 times—and they're ready for a game.
4. Have students play practice games, and encourage the following:
   - The use of the overhead serve
   - A high bump pass to the center of the court
   - Using a second pass—a set

Review

Review the motion and point of contact of the ball for the overhead serve.

Volleyball Lesson 3   Intermediate level

Lesson Setup

Facility

If possible, set up additional nets so that spiking practice can occur in groups of three.

Performance Goals

Students will

learn a spike,
improve their set, and
play a game.

Cognitive Goals

Students will learn

how angles affect spiking success and
the rules around the net:
   - No touching the net
   - No centerline violation
   - Simultaneous tap/block

Lesson Safety

Have groups that are practicing use one side of the court and keep the ball on their own side so they do not hinder the teams sharing the court with them.

Warm-Up

Students will

1. Practice mimetics for the bump pass, set, and overhead serve—with steps and a spike
2. Jump to spike

Motivation

Tell students that they have been working up to learning to spike for a long time now, and today is the day. If a player is small, her margin of error shrinks. Unless she times her jump just right and is behind the ball on the jump, she will not hit a successful spike. Tall players have a greater margin of error. For short players, poor timing or positioning can turn a spike into an offensive volley or a wild shot. Everyone should try anyway and then learn who will be the great spikers of the group.

Lesson Sequence

1. Teach and demonstrate the spike (figure 16.11).
2. Set up the smallest groups possible to guarantee the most repetition possible:
   • The player tosses, the spiker spikes, the retriever retrieves under the net.
   • Students rotate after two tries.
   • This practice continues until the lines have gone three or four times.

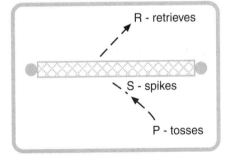

Figure 16.11—Drilling the volleyball spike.

3. After everyone gets a turn to be successful in their spiking efforts (this could be an offensive volley for shorter students), do the following:
   • Gather them together and go over the rules involved:
       No touching the net
       No centerline violation
   • Have them try to spike again, avoiding infractions of the rules.
4. Have students practice tapping in their circles—*the circle volley.*
5. Instruct them to play practice games, continuing to encourage
   • the use of the overhead serve;
   • a high bump pass to the center of the court;

- using a second pass—a set; and
- a third tap, either an offensive volley or a spike.

Review

Ask the class if anyone was able to spike during a game.
Ask students if they got a set from their teammate or if it was a friendly
mistake of their opponent that got the ball up there for a spike.

Assessment

Observe students, noting each one's strengths and weaknesses.
Use weaknesses for planning the next lesson.
Use strengths to help plan how to divide the class into teams.

Volleyball Lesson 4   Intermediate level

Performance Goals

Students will

practice setting to a target,
practice spiking, and
play a game.

Cognitive Goals

Students will learn

that they need good footwork and timing to have a successful spike,
that a team should try to set to its spikers during a game, and
that getting off their feet and meeting a ball above the net is a good offensive
strategy even if a hard spike is not the result.

Warm-Up

Students will

1. Practice mimetics for the bump pass, set, and overhead serve
2. Practice mimetics for the spike:
   - Doing the arm motions for the spike—practicing it five times
   - Taking a step to a spot on the ground, jumping, and, at the height of the
     jump, using the spiking motion (figure 16.2a)
   - Repeating several times until movement and motion are smooth
   - Checking the spot where they landed—is it the same one they took off
     from?
3. Jump to block (figure 16.12b)

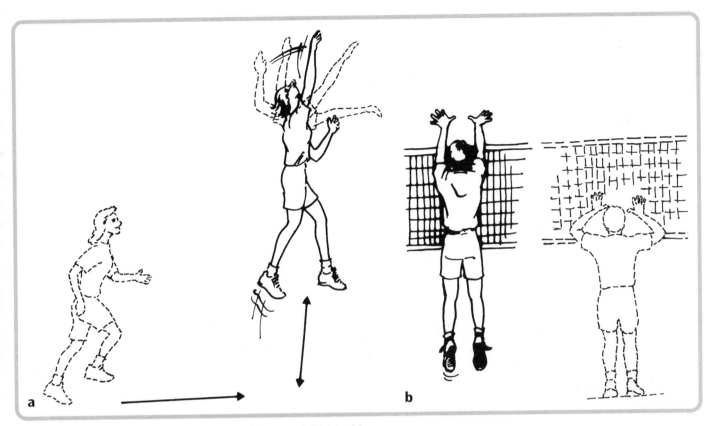

Figure 16.12—Nonball warm-ups: *(a)* spiking and *(b)* blocking.

Motivation

In this lesson, students will take part of the time to practice using the set so that the spikers on the team can move to the ball, jump, and spike. Tell the students it would be a shame if, once the tournament starts, their own team is unable to set to its spikers. Announce that you are going to present the tournament teams in the next class.

Lesson Sequence

1. Teach the point of aim for the setter.
2. Set up the smallest groups possible to guarantee the most repetition possible:
   - A player tosses to himself and sets to the spiker, with the retriever on the other side.
   - They rotate after two tries.
   - This practice continues until the lines have gone three or four times.
3. Have students play practice games, continuing to encourage
   - the use of the overhead serve;
   - a high bump pass to the center of the court;
   - using a second pass—a set; and
   - a third tap, either an offensive volley or a spike.

Review

Ask students how many sets were convertible to a spike in the class.
Ask if that number was more than in the last class.

Assessment

Observe each student for abilities and learning difficulties. Provide individual coaching help, making sure not to overlook the successful students.

Teacher Homework

Divide the students into tournament teams that are equal—boys to girls, spikers, setters, and good athletes.

Volleyball Lesson 5   Intermediate level

Performance Goals

Students will

meet and learn to work with new teams,
improve their skills, and
play a game.

Cognitive Goals

Students will learn

who their tournament team members are and assess their skills:
  • Who the spikers are
  • Who the strongest servers are
that turning before the ball arrives, rather than while trying to hit it, will yield
  better directional control.

Warm-Up

Students will

1. Practice mimetics for the bump pass and set, with footwork
2. Practice overhead service motion, taking care not to foot-fault
3. Practice mimetics for the spike—stepping to a spot, jumping, and swinging
   at the height of the jump ("jumping to spike"):

- Check the takeoff and landing spot
- Learn to "block" their momentum, so they land where they take off
- Learn why—to avoid net and centerline violations
4. Practice "jump to block" mimetics

Motivation

Announce the tournament teams right away. Mention to students that it will take a few days for them to get accustomed to everyone and figure out who is the best at what. Tell them that when their teams meet today, they should make a circle and practice their sets.

Lesson Sequence

1. Announce the teams and have students practice a circle volley.
2. Stop the practice and teach how to turn under the ball to direct the set in another direction:
   - Explain the purpose—to set to a specific person.
   - Suggest that to get to know their teammates, players set the ball and call the name of the person the pass is intended for.
   - Advise them that if they don't already know everyone's name, they should find out before they start.
3. Have students play practice games, continuing to encourage
   - the use of the overhead serve;
   - a high bump pass to the center of the court;
   - using a second pass—a set; and
   - a third tap, either an offensive volley or a spike.

Review

Call the teams together and ask them to elect a captain and co-captain. (If the captain is a girl, the co-captain should be a boy, and vice versa.)

Assessment

Observe each team to make sure there are no glaring inequities. If so, make adjustments during class.

Teacher Homework

Complete the tournament schedules and team standings charts and post them. Examples of these schedules and charts can be found in appendix A.

Volleyball Lesson 6   Intermediate level

Performance Goals

Students will

practice the timing and positioning of the block, and
play a game.

Cognitive Goals

Students will

review rotation order concerns—setters, spikers, and best servers; and
learn to identify spikers on their teams.

Lesson Safety

Now that tournament play is about to begin, and players have not yet adjusted
to all their teammates, be vigilant and active about correcting anything that can
be perceived as physical or emotional harassment.

Warm-Up

Students will

1. Practice mimetics as before, with a drill for the spiking mimetics. As you
   toss a ball in front of the class, have them do the following:
   • Jump as the ball starts to come down
   • Then, on the toss, take two running steps forward, jumping as the ball
     comes down
   • Same thing as above, adding the spiking motion at the height of the
     jump
   • Same thing as above, but do a foot check after landing—are students
     passing the spot on the ground they took off from?
2. Perform a circle volley

Motivation

Tell students that their practice days are ending. The sole purpose of this lesson is
to organize for round 1 of the tournament, which will begin in the next class.

Lesson Sequence

1. Diagram the court and possible team configurations according to skill. An
   example appears in figure 16.13.
2. Explain that in today's class, the following applies:

- Every time the opponents change, it is a new game, and the rotation order can be changed or returned to the starting lineup.

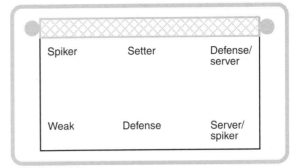

Figure 16.13—A strategic service lineup.

- A change of opponents and courts will be made every eight minutes. This will encourage teams to take time to make adjustments to their rotation order before beginning a new game.
- Players shouldn't bother keeping score today, they should just try to identify

  their best server,

  the spikers,

  the setters, and

  the best on defense.

3. Have students play practice games, rotating opponents every eight minutes.

Review

Ask if anyone has any questions.

Tell the class that round 1 will be played in the next lesson.

Instruct students that to get the most game time in the next class, they should meet on the court and begin a circle volley as soon as attendance is over. Teachers can speed up the process by taking attendance as students warm-up with their teams.

Assessment

Observe each group's ball control before play and students' interaction and dynamics during play. Disrupt any possible harassment to players viewed as not good enough.

Volleyball Lesson 7   Intermediate level

Lesson Setup

Equipment

A blackboard and chalk or other visual aid with the prior lesson left on

A tournament chart with individual team standings and game and court schedules (appendix A)

Performance Goals

Students will

make up their own rotation order and follow all rules associated with proper rotation, and

play round 1 of their tournament.

Cognitive Goals

Students will

learn how to read and follow the daily tournament schedule;

learn not to change their rotation order, beginning in the same positions each game;

understand that the receiving team rotates before it serves; and

understand that the receiving team's first server is in the right-front position when the game begins.

Lesson Safety

Be prepared to disrupt psychologically damaging comments to teammates or opponents.

Warm-Up

Students will

1. Participate in free play before the games start
2. Perform a circle volley before the games

Motivation

Announce round 1 and tell students not to start their games until both teams are ready. Suggest they include at least five minutes of warm-up volleying in a circle. Tell them they will each choose a teammate for the first serve, and they should assign serving order positions carefully because they will apply for the whole day.

Lesson Sequence

1. Post the tournament schedule and team lists, updating the standings after each game is completed.
2. Explain how to read the chart and follow the explanation up with an announcement of assignments.
3. Have students play round 1.

Review

Ask the captains of the teams that won a game by two points to please stand.
Ask the captains whose games were tied or there was only a one-point lead to please stand.
Tell the class that the winning teams will get two points per game won, while the tying teams get one.
Ask if there are any questions.

Volleyball Lesson 8   Intermediate level

Performance Goals

Students will

learn to block and practice it,
practice their offensive skills before the game begins, and
use offensive strategies during round 2 of their tournament.

Cognitive Goals

Students will

learn that practice improves their skills, and
learn the rules that affect the block:
- Touching the net
- The centerline violation
- What happens if there is a simultaneous tap or block
- What happens if the block leaves the ball on the team's own side of the net—can they tap it again? Yes, they can.

Warm-Up

Students will

1. Participate in free play before the games start
2. Complete a circle volley before the games

Motivation

Announce round 2. Tell students that their teams should set up spiking and blocking practice before they get into their circles today. If a player is not a designated spiker, there still will be occasions when he will have to hit the third tap over. Even if a student has given up on the idea of spiking, he should practice an offensive volley—hitting the ball deep and trying not to arch it easily over the net.

581

Lesson Sequence

1. Set up a drill as shown in figure 16.14, in which teams practice a set, spike, and block for five minutes.
2. Explain the rules that affect the success of a block:
   - Touching the net
   - The centerline violation
3. Explain what happens when the block is successful and how the rules apply:
   - If there is a simultaneous tap or block
   - If the blocked ball remains on the team's own side of the net—can they tap it again?
4. As each team member gets a sixth shot at spiking and blocking, have them begin volleying counterclockwise.
5. Have students play round 2.

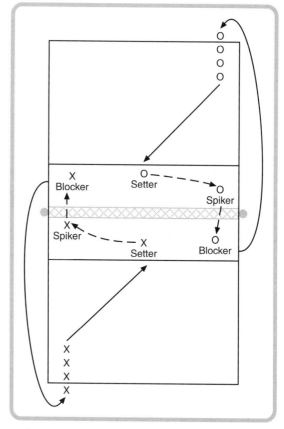

Figure 16.14—Spike and block drill.

Review

Ask the winning captains and the tying captains to please stand.
Any if there are any questions.
Share with the class some overall problems that could be seen by an outsider looking in:
- Rushing the game by not taking advantage of all three taps
- Setting the ball to the wrong place on the front line
- Taking for granted that the serve will go over
- Missing because the player wasn't paying attention
- Too eager to kill, forcing plays that result in netted balls

Volleyball Lesson 9   Intermediate level

Performance Goals

Students will

learn to practice their offensive skills before the game begins, and play round 3.

Cognitive Goals

Students will learn that sometimes strategy can make up for an outright skill:

> Keeping the ball on the court often makes up for razzle-dazzle, uncontrollable skills.
> Effective team play begins with defense—keeping the ball up.

Warm-Up

Students will

1. Participate in free play before the games start
2. Perform a circle volley before the games

Motivation

Announce round 3 and what the standings are after two rounds—who's in first place, second place, and third place, and with how many points in the tournament. Talk about a team being as strong as its weakest link, before students begin round 3.

Lesson Sequence

1. Have the teams practice tip-overs, as shown in figures 16.8 and 16.9.
2. Have teams practice volleying clockwise.
3. Call the class together before beginning the games and explain the following:
   - That keeping the ball on the court often makes up for razzle-dazzle, uncontrollable skills.
   - That effective team play begins with defense—keeping the ball up.
4. Have students play round 3.

Review

Ask the winning captains and the tying captains to please stand.
Any if there are any questions.
Share with the class some overall problem that could be seen by an outsider looking in:
- Rushing the game by not taking advantage of all three taps
- Setting the ball to the wrong place on the front line
- Taking for granted that the serve will go over
- Missing because the player wasn't paying attention
- Too eager to kill, forcing plays that result in netted balls

Assessment

Observe each student's progress toward moving up the performance assessment rubric (page 590).

For those lagging, help will come during free play and targeted warm-ups.

Volleyball Lesson 10   Intermediate level

Performance Goal

Students will play round 4.

Cognitive Goals

Students will learn

that back-line players should use their bump pass to direct the ball to the center of their court, and

that using three taps slows down the game and gives the team a chance to set up.

Warm-Up

Students will

1. Participate in free play before the tournament play starts
2. Complete a circle volley before the games

Motivation

Announce round 4 and what the standings are after three rounds—which teams are in what place and with how many points.

Lesson Sequence

1. Remind the back line of the following:
   • Not to send the ball over the net
   • To try to bump it to the center of the court
2. Have teams practice volleying counterclockwise.
3. Have students play round 4.

Review

Discuss problems, ideas, and positive situations that arose in the day's play.
Ask the winning captains and the tying captains to please stand.
Ask if there are any questions.

Volleyball Lesson 11 — Intermediate level

Lesson Setup

Equipment

A blackboard or magnetic board
Two balls for each team

Performance Goal

Students will play round 5.

Cognitive Goals

Students will review

what the difference is between backing up a teammate and taking over;
that the ball is not dead when it hits the net, but that recovery is possible; and
that anticipation is half the game:
  • How to anticipate a spike and what to do once a spike is anticipated
  • How to anticipate the angles a hitter can use and be ready to cover them

Warm-Up

Students will

1. Participate in free play before the games start
2. Complete a circle volley before the games

Motivation

Announce round 5, the last game of the first round robin (a six-team round robin). It is the last class in which there will be so much time set aside for practicing. Tell students that their team will be given two balls. They can practice anything they need to as long as it doesn't interfere with the other team sharing their court. Suggest that some students might want to practice serving, setting, or bumping, others the spike and block. They should use their team's time wisely. Tell them you will stop the practice with 15 minutes of class time left, so if they are organized, they can have the whole 15 minutes for the game.
Announce the class standings after four rounds.

Lesson Sequence

1. Have students on court for round 5, with the captains deciding what their teams need to practice and if they want to have work stations on the court for doing a variety of things.

2. Call the class together at the blackboard and review the following:
   - What the difference is between backing up a teammate and taking over
   - That the ball is not dead when it hits the net, that recovery is possible
   - That anticipation is half the game:

     If you can anticipate that a setup pass is coming down in front of a spiker, you can react to either block the pass at the net or drop back and defend it after it arrives on your court.

     If you can see the hitter and where the ball is coming from you can cover the possible angles of the hitter.
3. Have students play round 5.

Review

Ask the winning captains and the tying captains to please stand.
Ask if there are any questions.

Assessment

Observe students to assess their performance, using the intermediate performance assessment rubric on page 590.

Volleyball Lesson 12   Intermediate level

Lesson Setup

Equipment

A posted performance assessment rubric for intermediate-level volleyball players
Updated tournament standings charts

Performance Goals

Students will

play more than one game, and
play round 6.

Cognitive Goals

Students will

learn match play—both the official and the class modifications of official match play; and
learn how to use every minute wisely so they can accumulate the most tournament points.

Warm-Up

Students will

1. Participate in free play before the games start
2. Complete a circle volley before the games

Motivation

Announce round 6. Tell students that as they start their matches, it is important to remember the following:

The game ends at 15 points when one team is ahead by two.

Players should switch sides of the court, return to the starting lineup, and begin the next game immediately.

If the last game is incomplete, a win will be recorded for any team with eight points that is ahead by two points before the period ends. A tie will be awarded if there are at least as many as eight points and no team is leading by two points.

Announce the class standings after five rounds.

Lesson Sequence

1. Have students do warm-up practice on the court assigned for round 6.
2. Have them play round 6.

Review

Ask the captains to report their game scores.

Volleyball Lessons 13-16   Intermediate level

Performance Goal

Students will play more than one game a period, and complete the tournament, playing rounds 7, 8, 9, and 10.

Cognitive Goals

Students will

learn to value and maintain good sporting behavior, and
explore other strategies during their matches:
  • Doing the unexpected—look like spiking, but hit soft
  • Changing the direction of the hit

- Sending the ball deep
- Hitting to the weak player on the other side of the court

Warm-Up

Students will

1. Participate in free play before the games start
2. Complete a circle volley before the games

Motivation

Tell students that over the next few weeks, you will be evaluating their skills. Explain what you are looking for and tell them it will be on the board for them to look at in their leisure. Announce the class standings.

Lesson Sequence

1. Explain the strategy of the day.
2. Explain and post the grading standards.
3. Have students practice on their assigned court before the round begins.
4. Have them play their scheduled rounds.

Review

Call the students' attention to the posted performance assessment rubric, if they haven't already noticed it. Tell them you will be grading them on it. And remind them that when the tournament is over, there will be a quiz (see pages 608-609).
Ask the captains to report their game scores.
Discuss whether anyone exercised his right to look tough and hit soft.
Ask if anyone served to a lot of different spots on the court.

Assessment

Grades will be based on the level reached in the performance rubric.
A teacher, friend, teammate, or other student may evaluate by using the rubric.

Volleyball Lesson 17   Intermediate level

Lesson Setup

Equipment

Quizzes for each student
Pens and pencils

Performance Goals

Students will

take a quiz, and
play their last volleyball game of the class.

Cognitive Goals

Students will

evaluate their understanding of the game via feedback from the volleyball quiz, and
choose their final volleyball event:
- Playoffs if necessary
- Rearranged teams—a battle of the sexes or an all-star game

Warm-Up

Students will

1. Complete sit-ups and push-ups
2. Run in place
3. Complete a circle volley before the games

Motivation

Compliment the play of the tournament. Announce the winners and the standings after all the rounds of the tournament.

Lesson Sequence

1. Distribute the quiz, while inviting final questions.
2. After 10 minutes, collect the quizzes. Make arrangements with students who need more time to either complete the test while the class is playing or have them come during their study hall, lunch period, or after school.
3. Review the standings. Pay personal compliments for play, improvement, assists, spikes, sporting behavior, leadership, and so forth.
4. Assign any playoff teams to their court. Have the other players choose what they want to do:
   - Form their own teams
   - A battle of the sexes
   - A contest with friends
   - Sticking with their volleyball teams and having a rematch against opponents of their choice

Review

Ask if there are any questions about the quiz. Tell students you will try to have the quizzes back to them the next time they meet.

Assessment

Students can be assessed by using the intermediate performance assessment rubric in table 16.3. Appendix B also has general assessment rubrics that can be used. The quiz also provides a good means of assessing student's knowledge of the sport.

TABLE 16.3 Intermediate Volleyball Performance Assessment Rubric

STUDENT NAME _____

	0	1	2	3
Serve	No effort	• Uses proper mechanics • Inconsistent success • Serves behind the service line	• Consistently puts the ball in play • Has a legal serve	• Has good placement • Has good speed
Bump pass	No effort	• Uses proper mechanics • Directs in an upward arch • Has legal contact with the ball	• Moves under the ball • Is able to direct the ball upward after moving to it	• Ball stays on the same side • Directs the ball to a spot or player
Setup pass	No effort	• Uses proper mechanics • Has legal upward tap	• Moves eyes under the ball to tap legally	• Controls direction, height, and target • Sends over if the third tap
Strategy	No effort	• Tries to send the third tap over	• Uses speed and direction for taps going over the net • Makes an effort to set or to spike	• Spikes or uses the third tap offensively • Controls depth, speed, and direction
Teamwork and sporting behavior	No effort	• Avoids the rules • Blames others	• Tries to develop and improve • Works well with the team • Violations are unintentional	• Plays within the rules • Is a team leader • Helps others

Volleyball Lesson 1 {Advanced level}

Lesson Setup

Facility

A wall with no obstructions
A volleyball court with the net up

Equipment

One ball for every three students

Performance Goals

Students will review

a bump pass,
sets,
an overhead serve, and
a game.

Cognitive Goals

Students will review

the need for bumps that reach the middle of the court,
sets that drop on their own side of the net and are directed to a specific player,
the idea of defensive players and offensive players in volleyball, and
how to control the arch of each pass.

Lesson Safety

Space out practice so there is at least 15 feet between groups.
Reestablish rules for how to deal with errant balls.

Warm-Up

Students will

1. Practice mimetics for the bump pass, setup pass, and overhead serve—with steps
2. Complete push-ups and sit-ups
3. Jump with arms straight up

Motivation

Tell students that they all have the fundamental skills necessary to play volleyball. This year, you will teach them to play challenging volleyball. Since they all can hit the ball, this year's lesson is about hitting it the way they want to—in order to win. That strategy requires control, planning, and taking advantage of the individual strengths of each team member, because, as they should know by now, no one player can do it all. Mention that many sets that occurred last year happened by accident—they were too long, passed over the net, and became sets for the opposing team. This wasn't what the setter had in mind. Equally frustrating is seeing spikers underutilized because no one can set to them. To start off right, have them work on controlling those sets and bumps so that they go where they want them to.

Lesson Sequence

1. Review the bump pass: stress footwork and follow-through for control and placement.
2. Set up a drill, such as bumping from the low toss, and speeding up the toss for each new turn.
3. Review the set: stress footwork and follow-through for control.
4. Have students do a set-to-wall drill, as seen in figure 16.15: it uses a relay formation in which player 1 sets, then runs to the back of the line, the second player moves up, sets, and then moves to the back of the line, the third moves up to set, and so forth.

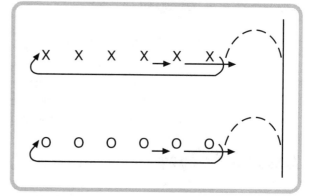

Figure 16.15—Relay wall volley.

5. Have them practice overhead serves—a minimum of 10 serves.
6. Allow games if practice seems too long and the students lose motivation.

Review

Review illegal tap rules and any rules that come up during games.

Assessment

Observe each student's ball control to determine
  whether to proceed to lesson 2, and
  the best way to break the class into teams.

Volleyball Lesson 2   Advanced level

Lesson Setup

Facility

A volleyball court for every 12 players in class
Additional practice areas with a net, if possible, and space for students to work in threes

Performance Goals

Students will

review the spike,
develop a spike or offensive volley, and
conclude the lesson with a short game if time remains.

Cognitive Goals

Students will review

the necessary mechanical features of the spike:
  • Timing the jump
  • The sequence and arm motion
  • Blocking their forward motion so on landing they don't break rules
the rules about what's not allowed around the net:
  • Reaching over the net to meet the ball
  • Touching the net during the play
  • Having any part of the body cross the centerline

Lesson Safety

There should be a minimum of 15 feet between each group for practice.
Reestablish classroom routines for dealing with errant balls.

Warm-Up

Students will

1. Practice mimetics for the bump pass, setup pass, overhead serve, and spike—with steps
2. Practice mimetics for getting under a ball and, before hitting, turning to a target, as seen in figure 16.16
3. Practice passing in a circle of one's choice—encouraging directional control by either
   • calling out a name, or
   • passing the ball to the person on the right or counterclockwise

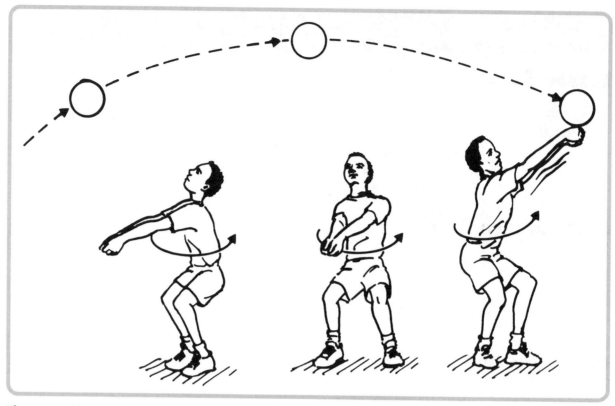

Figure 16.16—Turning under the ball to control pass in other direction.

Motivation

Tell your students that the only offensive skill you can teach them in volleyball is the spike. All other offensive efforts require thinking and outwitting their opponents. For today, since their tournament teams are not made up yet, they can practice the set and spike with their friends. Suggest they allow their friends to give them some coaching hints. With a little hint here or there, they might be able to make adjustments that will help them be more successful.

For instance, students might notice that a player jumps too late or runs under the path of the ball before she leaves the ground. Both of these would cause a problem with the spike. The first usually would make the ball go into the net. The second would lead to the spiking problem of the ball being hit out of bounds. If a player's friends see that she swings too hard and is finished before the ball arrives, or notice that she hasn't been able to adjust to an improperly placed set, they might help her adjust better. Tell students to use their friends' insights to help them. Mention that you'll always be there to offer advice. If they are having problems and you are on another court, tell them they should call you over.

Lesson Sequence

1. Demonstrate and review the spike. Try through demonstration to teach the results of

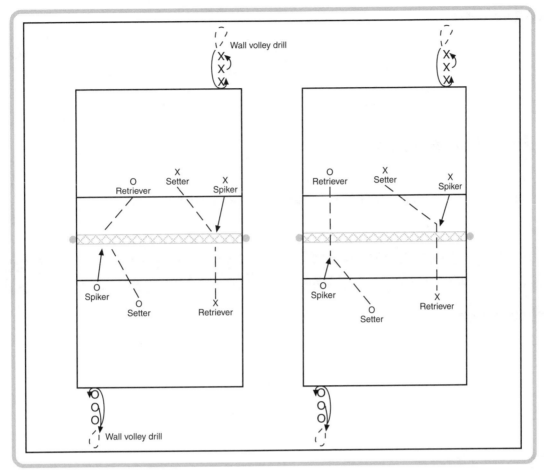

Figure 16.17—Using space wisely during team warm-ups.

- overrunning the ball,
- jumping too late,
- jumping too early, and
- swinging too late.
2. Have students drill in groups of three to practice setting and spiking:
   - Demonstrate to show rotation and positioning of setter, spiker, and retriever.
   - Rather than having students wait, set up other groups at the wall, as shown in figure 16. 17, in a three-person wall volley drill, rotating practice stations after everyone in a group has a certain number of successes.
3. Allow games if practice seems too long and the students lose motivation.

Review

Review all rules around the net:
Centerline violations
No touching the net
A second tap after a block

Assessment

This review moves along rather quickly. If the students are not up to it and if you have not been able to figure out who the good class spikers, setters, and defensive players are, it would be difficult to move on to lesson 3, which starts to teach students the specialization of jobs on the court.

Teacher Homework

Make up tournament teams, being certain to include an equal number of spikers, setters, and defensive players on each team whose skills make the teams as even as possible.

Volleyball Lesson 3   Advanced level

Performance Goals

Students will

meet their tournament teammates,
play practice games, and
choose their captains and co-captains.

Cognitive Goals

Students will

learn to identify how their own strengths fit in with that of their teammates; learn the concepts and rules that apply to interchanging positions; and define their roles on their new teams as either defense, offense, or setter.

Warm-Up

Students will

1. Practice mimetics for the approach-jump-swing for the spike and the approach-jump-block for the block
2. Complete push-ups and sit-ups

Motivation

Discuss spiking and blocking with the class and how some students may think that learning spiking, for them, is useless. There may be at least four people on the team who they think are better spikers than they are, and when they see a big opponent on the other side of the net ready to spike, all they really want to do is run away.

Unless students have been on competitive interscholastic teams or have seen their games, they probably don't realize that some people on the team never set and others never spike or block. They have positions, just like in all the other team sports in school. In this class, you'll explain how that works and how to do it legally, so students can begin to organize in their new teams.

Lesson Sequence

1. Announce the teams.
2. Demonstrate how to interchange positions legally.
3. Teach the applicable rules:
   - The players must be in the proper rotation order before and during the serve.
   - The players can go anywhere on the court to play the ball once the serve has been struck.
   - The back-line players may not spike if they are in front of the 10-foot line.
4. Show how the court usually is broken down—where the setter goes, where the spiker waits.
5. Have students play games.

Review

Identify if students think they should be the spikers, setters, or defenders. Have the captains and co-captains identify themselves to you.

Assessment

Observe to

confirm that new teams are well balanced, and
beware of conflict and intercede to get the group moving forward cooperatively.

Volleyball Lesson 4 — Advanced level

Performance Goals

Students will

continue to improve their skills;
begin experimenting with assuming specialized roles as defenders, setters, or spikers for their team; and
play games, interchanging positions.

Cognitive Goals

Students will

have the idea of interchanging positions reinforced, and learn to assume roles for their teams.

Warm-Up

Students will

1. Participate in free play
2. Practice mimetics for sets and bumps and
   - approach-jump-swing for the spike, and
   - approach-jump-block for the block

Motivation

Tell students that in today's game, you will spend the period reminding them to switch after every serve is hit, so that their teams have their defensive players in place to bump the serves and spikes to the center of their court. Explain that getting used to moving on the serve is going to take a while, but the challenge will be worth the effort in the end. Tell students that it is done in school games and on TV. So, before they start, they should establish their setter, and remind the setter to go to the center of the court to receive the bump pass. Otherwise their team will have mini-disasters. Also remind the spikers to shift to the nearest corner so the setter can set to them. And remind the whole class that on each serve, the players must go back to their original spots in the service order. That means that if a player is server 3, he must be between servers 2 and 4 during service.

Lesson Sequence

1. Announce the courts that students should go to.
2. Have them practice in a circle, volleying with the bump or set before the game begins. During this volley practice, change the direction, asking students to send the ball right, left, or across.
3. Have students play games.

Review

Ask if everyone is in agreement—if their team has identified its members who should be the spikers, setters, and defense.

Ask students what this master plan all hinges on: execution. If they cannot get the ball to the center of the court, the setter cannot set.

Discuss whether that means they should let the ball drop on the ground because the play did not work. Ask what they would do.

Assessment

Observe, looking for common problems to share with the class during the summary or in the next lesson.

Volleyball Lesson 5   Advanced level

Performance Goal

Students will play games, interchanging positions and rotating opponents.

Cognitive Goals

Students will

find the repetition reinforcing,
assume and understand the value of their roles during the game, and
learn and confirm the best rotation order for their teams.

Warm-Up

Students will

1. Participate in free play
2. Practice mimetics

Motivation

Announce that this is the last practice day before the tournament. Tell students it is important to review any questions they have about the notion of taking on a job for the team. Ask for questions. Also instruct them that before starting each game, they should work with rearranging their rotation order to take advantage of their team's assets. Ask in what position they should have their best net player, and why. Ask where they would like to put a defensive player who is a fine server. If one can change positions during play, ask if the other issues in service order are so important. And if a team has two people who play well at the net, discuss where they both should go.

Tell students that they should get used to interchanging positions but they also should pay attention to setting up their service order. You are going to stop the games every eight minutes so they can rearrange their players, switch courts, and get to see what other classmates are like to play against. Tell them not to worry about the score in this lesson.

Lesson Sequence

1. Announce the courts that students should go to.
2. Have them practice in a circle, volleying with the bump or set before the game begins. This time you might have everyone bump to the setter and the setter set to the person whose name is called.

3. Have students play games.
4. Rotate opponents every eight minutes.

Review

Ask if there are any questions.

Ask students if they are getting used to the interchanging of positions on the court and if they like it better.

Discuss whether players found themselves a little confused if they had to do something to save the ball that they had not anticipated doing because it wasn't their job.

Instruct the captains to write up their permanent team lineups before the next class.

Teacher Homework

Complete and post the tournament schedules and team standing charts. Examples of these are found in appendix A.

Volleyball Lesson 6   Advanced level

Lesson Setup

Equipment

Three balls for every team
Posted tournament charts (see appendix A) that are updated after each round

Performance Goal

Students will play round 1 of a double round-robin tournament.

Cognitive Goals

Students will learn

to take responsibility for their own performance,
to play competitively with good sporting behavior,
to anticipate their opponents' abilities, and
to enjoy their teammates' successes.

Lesson Safety

During warm-up, make sure that teams know to keep the balls on their own side of the court until everyone is allowed to take serving practice.

Now that the competition has started, be vigilant about bad sporting behavior, particularly if it threatens the physical or emotional health of the class. Students who lose control must be taught to make amends (apologize for hurting someone and/or hurting their feelings) and correct their behavior.

Warm-Up

Students will

1. Participate in free play
2. Practice mimetics

Motivation

Announce that the tournament is about to start. Tell students that they will only get credit for one game during this first round robin because they should take their team warm-up seriously. There are people on their team who need to practice, since timing and the feel for the ball are so important in the bump-set-spike strategy they are using. Tell them they will warm up their serves, sets, and bumps, and then their spikes, before the games start.

Inform the class that a game is won by scoring at least 15 points and being ahead by 2. Tell students that if their games are over early, they should not start a second game—they will not get credit for it. They should use the time to practice the things that need improvement.

Lesson Sequence

1. Alert students to the fact that their schedule and court assignments are posted. Announce the courts they should go to.
2. Have students practice three minutes for each skill—serving, passing, and spiking.
3. Have them play games.

Review

Ask if there are any questions.

Ask students what they think their team should do if the rotation order has not turned out to be as good as was thought. Discuss changing it.

Review how teams can legally change their service order: the positions and the rotation order must be designated in writing and be followed throughout the game.

Ask what, then, the captains can do if it needs to be in writing: they can change the rotation order that night.

Ask the winning captains to stand, and ask if there are any ties.

Suggest the captains review the service order before the next class.

Assessment

Observe to provide teams with specific coaching hints.

Volleyball Lessons 7-10 — Advanced level

Performance Goals

Students will

spend about 12 minutes of each lesson improving bumps, sets, spikes, and serves; and

complete the first round-robin tournament, playing rounds 2, 3, 4, and 5.

Cognitive Goals

Students will learn

to take responsibility for improving their performance,

to maintain their sense of sporting behavior and fair play no matter how heated the competition, and

to applaud their teammates' successes.

Warm-Up

Students will

1. Participate in free play
2. Practice mimetics

Motivation

After so many rounds, announce which team is leading with how many points. Also announce the teams in second and third place, and what their points are. Ask if anyone needs any help. Tell students you will remind them when to stop practice; they will start with three minutes for the serve, three minutes for the passes, and three minutes for spiking.

Lesson Sequence

1. Have the captains choose whose team gets first serve while the teams are practicing on their assigned courts.
2. Instruct the teams to practice, spending three minutes on each skill—the serve, bump, set, and spike.
3. Have them play the tournament game.

Review

Ask if there are any questions.
Ask the winning captains to stand, and find out if there are any ties.

Suggest that the captains review their service order before the next class and make it as efficient as possible.

Assessment

Observe while officiating. Use your observations about the play in the day's summary.

Volleyball Lessons 11-15 — Advanced level

Lesson Setup

Equipment

Continuously updated team standings
A posted performance assessment rubric for the advanced volleyball student

Performance Goal

Students will play a second round-robin tournament using match play.

Cognitive Goals

Students will learn to

focus on the future and let go of previous mistakes,
use their knowledge about their opponents to play offensive strategy,
reinforce each other, and
recognize and approve of individual accomplishment.

Lesson Safety

In the advent of matches, and the near completion of the tournament, highly competitive students will be very intense about the use of time and their scores. Guard against any difficulties that might arise if tempers get short.

Warm-Up

Students will

1. Participate in free play
2. Complete a circle volley

Motivation

After so many rounds, announce which team is leading with how many points. Also announce the teams in second and third place, and what their points are. Tell students that the only warm-up time they have is the circle volley. In the second round-robin tournament they will get credit for every game that is completed; suggest they don't waste any time. Winning more than one game in a period can dramatically change their standings. Inform them that from here on out, their games will be actively officiated either by you rotating from court to court or a student assigned to the job. Wish them luck.

Lesson Sequence

1. Start off the practice and games with some thought-out questions. Announce one idea a day. Some examples:
   - "Does everyone pat the player on the back who makes the kill shot?" Today students should acknowledge the great set that allows the spiker to do that.
   - "When is the last time you recognized the outstanding job your defenders do to keep the ball in play?" Suggest they start today if they have not already.
   - "What choices are there if a big blocker or spiker is facing you down on the other side of the net and you have the ball?"
   - "Have you recognized the personal accomplishment of the person on your team who is so into winning but does not explode or make you feel bad when you make a mistake?"
   - Tell students to think about their teammates and how they felt when the team was first organized. Ask them to think about whose personal effort made the biggest leap forward during the past few weeks. Suggest they let them know how much they appreciate their effort.
2. Have students practice for three minutes.
3. Have them play matches.

Review

Review strategies that might improve play in the next class.
Get the teams' scores.
On the last day of the tournament, remind students about the quiz coming up in the next lesson and invite any questions they still might have.

Assessment

Post assessment goals and answer any questions related to them.
Begin the evaluation process during match play.
Plan a short quiz (page 610) for the conclusion of the round-robin tournament.

Volleyball Lesson 16 — Advanced level

Lesson Setup

Equipment

One quiz for each student
Pens or pencils
A complete chart of the team records

Performance Goals

Students will

take a volleyball quiz, and
choose a culminating activity (new teams, separate genders, or a final play-off).

Cognitive Goals

Students will get

an objective measure of how much they understand about volleyball via their quiz, and
publicly recognized for their accomplishments.

Lesson Safety

Use the established rules.

Motivation

Instruct students to pick up a quiz and find a place to take it. When it is complete, they may turn it in and then go to the court for a warm-up. Tell them that when everyone is done, they will play their last day of the volleyball unit.

Lesson Sequence

1. Distribute the quiz and supervise.
2. Take a vote: Do the students want to make up new teams? Would they like to play games with all-girl teams and all-boy teams? Or are there any requests for rematches?
3. Have students play games after a brief warm-up.

Review

Congratulate the class on its accomplishments, being as specific as possible and crediting as many students and good plays as possible.

Announce the final standings of the tournament.

Tell students that the completed skills grades are available for discussion after class or after school.

Assessment

Grade students based on the posted performance assessment rubric (table 16.4). Further general assessment rubrics are available in appendix B. Grade the quizzes.

TABLE 16.4   Advanced Volleyball Performance Assessment Rubric

STUDENT NAME _____

	0	1	2	3	4	5
Skills	No effort	• Serves legally • Blocks most incoming balls up • Tries to send the third tap over the net	• Has consistent serve • Bump pass goes to the center of the court • Is developing a specialty	• Serves deep • Interchanges position to fit the team strategy • First and second taps remain on own side	• Varies speed, depth, and direction of serve • Either directs pass to setter or spiker, or spikes	• Attacks the serve • Defense or setters are offensive when necessary • As net person, varies touch or anticipates blocks • As setter, sets backward
Strategy	No effort	• Hits the ball over the net on the first or second tap • Uses correct body mechanics • Concentrates on play • Tries to take over	• Moves to prevent the ball from landing on own side • Sets up own attacker, avoids opponent's	• Plays a specialty in bump-set-spike strategy • Anticipates teammates • Varies depth, direction, and speed on the hit over	• Interchanges correctly • Backs up, not takes over • Anticipates the angles of opponent's attack	• Helps the team focus and adjust when losing • Detects deficiencies and redirects focus constructively
Position, teamwork, and attitude	No effort	• Blames others • Needs supervision to stay on task • Interferes with the other team	• Gets to the court on time • Warms up with the team • Plays within the rules	• Works well with teammates • Takes responsibility for position	• Consistently tries to play at personal best • Recognizes good teammate effort and success • Has good sporting behavior	• Inspires the team • Backs up, not takes over, for teammates • Provides reliable, consistent leadership • Assists individual team members to personally improve

Volleyball Quiz—Beginner level

NAME _____ TEACHER _____

DATE _____ CLASS PERIOD _____

True or False: Read each statement below carefully. If the statement is true, put a check under the True box in the column to the left of the statement. If the statement is false, put a check under the False box in the column to the left of the statement. If using a grid sheet, blacken in the appropriate column for each question, making sure to use the correctly numbered line for each question and its answer.

True **False**

☐ ☐ 1. If there are seven players on a volleyball team, only six may play at one time.

☐ ☐ 2. Rotation occurs after each point is won.

☐ ☐ 3. To follow a legal rotation order, a team must rotate in a clockwise direction.

☐ ☐ 4. A ball hitting the net during play always ends the point.

☐ ☐ 5. The left-back player is the server.

☐ ☐ 6. A bump pass is used when the ball looks like it is falling into a player's eyes.

☐ ☐ 7. If player A hits the first tap, and player B hits the second tap, then player A can hit the third tap.

☐ ☐ 8. A server who is off the court when serving is doing something illegal.

☐ ☐ 9. A player should open his hands and hit a setup pass when the ball falls below his waist.

☐ ☐ 10. It is good team strategy to hit the ball away from the strongest player on the other team.

☐ ☐ 11. Using a firm arm is bound to be more successful than a soft, feathery arm when you hit a serve.

☐ ☐ 12. Volleyball games are 15 points, but they must be played out to find a winner if the score is 14-15, because a team cannot win until it is in the lead by 2 points.

☐ ☐ 13. If player A hits the ball sending it to player B, who is only able to hit it so it goes straight up in the air, player B should hit it again to send it over the net.

☐ ☐ 14. The server should run onto the court as soon as he hits the ball because he is needed to cover the play on the court.

☐ ☐ 15. Neither the serve nor a person is allowed to touch the net.

From *Complete Physical Education Plans for Grades 7–12* by Isobel Kleinman, 2001, Champaign, IL: Human Kinetics.

Volleyball Quiz—Intermediate level

NAME _____ TEACHER _____

DATE _____ CLASS PERIOD _____

Diagram: It may help you to understand some of the questions by referring to the diagram. In some questions, you are to choose among the multiple-choice answers provided. In others, you must simply decide whether the statement is true or false. Place your answers on the line to the left of the question.

_____1. According to the diagram, which team will be serving first?
   a. purple
   b. gold

_____2. Player 3 on either team can legally spike a ball set up at the net.
   a. True
   b. False

_____3. Player 5 on the purple team may not spike in front of the 10-foot line.
   a. True
   b. False

_____4. Player 1 on the purple team will commit a service violation if she remains at this place on the court when she serves.
   a. True
   b. False

_____5. The team that serves first during the first game is the team that must serve first in the second game.
   a. True
   b. False

_____6. If playing time elapses when the score is 8 to 7, with the purple team in the lead, the game is a tie.
   a. True
   b. False

_____7. Volleyball players may not enter another team's court even if they go over the centerline an inch.
   a. True
   b. False

_____8. If the ball has been hit, players may contact the net on the follow-through.
   a. True
   b. False

_____9. Opposing blockers and spikers may hit the ball a second time if the ball was hit by both of them but didn't go anywhere.
   a. True
   b. False

_____10. The best first-tap strategy for the gold team is to bump the ball in the area marked by 4.
   a. True
   b. False

Matching Questions: Read one numbered item at a time. Then look at each of the possible choices in the column on the right. Decide which item in the right-hand column best matches up with that of the left-hand column. Put the corresponding letter on the blank space left of the number it best matches.

_____1. The legal limit of taps per team   **a.** A spike

_____2. The number of team players on a court   **b.** 15 points

_____3. A skill used by a teammate   **c.** 6

_____4. The back line cannot spike closer than   **d.** 2

_____5. A team serves twice, and the serve is not returned   **e.** 3

_____6. The number of points one player can get in a game   **f.** 10 feet

_____7. A kill shot   **g.** A set

_____8. A surprise   **h.** A reverse set

From *Complete Physical Education Plans for Grades 7–12* by Isobel Kleinman, 2001, Champaign, IL: Human Kinetics.

Volleyball Quiz—Advanced level

True or False: Read each statement below carefully. If the statement is true, put a check under the True box in the column to the left of the statement. If the statement is false, put a check under the False box in the column to the left of the statement. If using a grid sheet, blacken in the appropriate column for each question, making sure to use the correctly numbered line for each question and its answer.

True   False

☐   ☐   1. It is better to spike a ball dropping slightly in front of your face than to try and spike it when it drops behind your head.

☐   ☐   2. The setter should stay in rotation and wait for the set there.

☐   ☐   3. It is illegal to post a two-person block.

☐   ☐   4. If the ball bounces off your shoulder and goes over the net, the other team must play it.

☐   ☐   5. Neither spiker nor blocker can reach over the net.

☐   ☐   6. A server can legally step inside the court before contacting the serve.

☐   ☐   7. When the game seems to be getting too fast, the best way to slow it down is to use one hit and send the ball back over the net immediately.

☐   ☐   8. The right-back player will be the last server if the game starts with the opponents serving.

☐   ☐   9. The bump pass is the only skill that every person on the team must be able to execute.

☐   ☐   10. Going down the line is a placement strategy for serves and third taps.

From *Complete Physical Education Plans for Grades 7–12* by Isobel Kleinman, 2001, Champaign, IL: Human Kinetics.

Volleyball Answer Key—Beginner level

1. T. Only six are allowed on the court at one time; substitution provisions must be made for the extra team members.
2. F. Rotation occurs after the opposing team loses the serve.
3. T
4. F. A ball hitting the net is still in play.
5. F. The right-back player is the server.
6. F. The set is used when high passes descend.
7. T. A player can tap the ball twice as long as the taps are not consecutive.
8. F. The serve must be hit from off the court; once the serve is hit, the player should enter the court.
9. F. The bump pass should be used for balls below the waist. Hands should be closed.
10. T
11. T
12. T
13. F. Player B cannot hit the ball twice in a row.
14. T
15. T

Volleyball Answer Key—Intermediate level

Questions based on the diagram:

1. A. The purple team will be serving first—the first server is in the proper place in the rotation order.
2. T. Both are net players.
3. T. Player 5 is still a back-line player and may only spike from behind the 10-foot line.
4. T. The server must move off the court until the serve is hit.
5. F. Teams alternate who serves first at the beginning of each new game in a match.
6. T. Unless one team leads by two points, the game is a tie.
7. T. Crossing the centerline is a centerline violation.
8. F. Touching the net is illegal at any time.

Continued on next page ☞

Volleyball Answer Key—Intermediate level *(continued)*

9. T

10. F.   The best bump pass goes to the middle of the court.

Matching:

1. E
2. C
3. G
4. F
5. D
6. B
7. A
8. H

Volleyball Answer Key—Advanced level

1. T
2. F
3. F
4. T
5. T
6. F
7. F
8. T
9. T
10. T

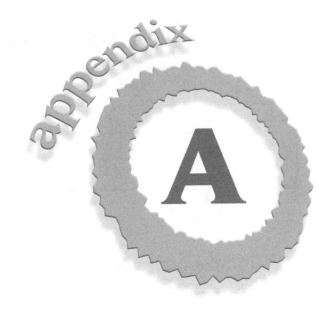

appendix

A

Tournament Charts

Round Robin Schedule for 3 courts, 3 days, 6 teams

	COURT 1	COURT 2	COURT 3
DAY 1	1 v 6	2 v 5	3 v 4
DAY 2	6 v 4	1 v 5	2 v 3
DAY 3	5 v 3	6 v 2	1 v 4

Sample Round-Robin Tournament Chart After Two Rounds

	1	2	3	4	5	6	7	8
1	X	2						
2	0	X	0					
3		2	X	2				
4			0	X	2			
5				0	X	1		
6					1	X		
7							X	
8								X

Win = 2 points

Tie = 1 point

Loss or default = 0

Team Tournament Record by Game and Class

CLASS	TEAM NUMBER	CAPTAINS AND CO-CAPTAINS	TOURNAMENT POINTS FOR EACH MATCH	TOTAL POINTS	CLASS PLACE
	1				
	2				
	3				
	4				
	5				
	6				

12 Team Round-Robin Tournament Schedule

	COURT 1	COURT 2	COURT 3	COURT 4	COURT 5	COURT 6	MATCHES	
Round 1	1 v 12	2 v 11	3 v 10	4 v 9	5 v 8	6 v 7	1-12 2-11 3-10	4-9 5-8 6-7
Round 2	5 v 6	1 v 11	12 v 10	2 v 9	3 v 8	4 v 7	1-11 2-9 4-7	12-10 3-8 5-6
Round 3	2 v 7	3 v 6	4 v 5	1 v 10	11 v 9	12 v 8	1-10 12-8 3-6	11-9 2-7 4-5
Round 4	3 v 4	2 v 3	12 v 6	11 v 7	10 v 8	1 v 9	1-9 11-7 2-5	10-8 12-6 3-4
Round 5	1 v 8	9 v 7	10 v 6	11 v 3	12 v 4	2 v 3	1-8 10-6 12-4	9-7 11-5 2-3
Round 6	8 v 6	1 v 7	9 v 5	10 v 4	11 v 3	12 v 2	1-7 9-5 11-3	8-6 10-4 12-2
Round 7	11 v 12	10 v 2	9 v 3	8 v 4	7 v 3	1 v 6	11-12 9-3 7-5	10-2 8-4 1 - 6
Round 8	1 v 3	9 v 12	7 v 3	6 v 4	8 v 2	10 v 11	10-11 8-2 6-4	9-12 7-3 1-5
Round 9	5 v 3	1 v 4	6 v 2	7 v 12	9 v 10	8 v 11	1-4 6-2 8 - 11	5-3 7-12 9-10
Round 10	4 v 2	8 v 9	1 v 3	6 v 11	5 v 12	7 v 10	1- 3 5-12 7-10	4-2 6-11 8-9
Round 11	6 v 9	7 v 8	5 v 10	4 v 11	3 v 12	1 v 2	7-8 5-10 3-12	6-9 4-11 1-2

Round-Robin Tournament Chart

TEAM NAME: _____

	1	2	3	4	5	6	7	8	9	10	11	12	13	14
1	X													
2		X												
3			X											
4				X										
5					X									
6						X								
7							X							
8								X						
9									X					
10										X				
11											X			
12												X		
13													X	
14														X

Racket Sports: Scheduling a Large Class

	COURT 1	COURT 2	COURT 3	COURT 4	COURT 5
Play period 1	1 v 2 3 officiates	4 v 5 6 officiates	7 v 8 9 officiates	10 v 11 12 officiates	13 v 14 15 officiates
Play period 2	2 v 3 1 officiates	6 v 4 5 officiates	9 v 7 8 officiates	12 v 10 11 officiates	15 v 13 14 officiates
Play period 3	1 v 3 2 officiates	6 v 5 4 officiates	9 v 8 7 officiates	11 v 12 10 officiates	14 v 15 13 officiates

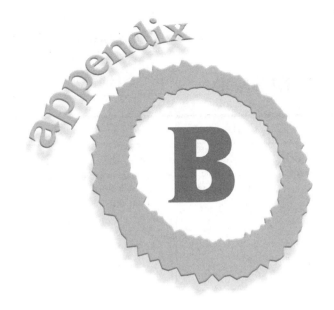

B

General Assessment Rubrics

Personality Attributes Assessment

STUDENT NAME _____

	0	1	2	3	4	5
Marking period	• Does not work with others • Does not participate	• Blames others • Does not assume responsibility for assignment • Needs outside supervision to stay on task • Interferes with others	• Is challenged • Is self-directed	• Is self-motivated to participate with others respectfully	• Cooperates with others and able to show care and concern for others	• Helps others achieve success • Has leadership • Has initiative • Has generosity of spirit
1						
2						
3						
4						

General Skills Assessment

STUDENT NAME _____

	0	1	2	3	4	5
	No effort	• Is awkward • Is unsuccessful • Is haphazard • Is unfocused	• Is intentional • Is focused • Is occasionally successful	• Is successful • Is automatic • Is consistent	• Combines skills • Reacts properly in predictable situations • Is accurate and controlled	• Performs in many changing conditions • Is able to modify own approach if situation demands it • Has complex performance
Catch						
Throw						
Body mechanics						
Footwork						
Defensive use of hands						
Defensive position						
Offensive position						

Team Play Assessment

STUDENT NAME _____

	0	1	2	3	4	5
	No effort	• Generally directs or controls an object	• Maintains possession in different ways and speeds • Is able to assist team • Combines two skills	• Plays the game within the context of the rules • Implements team strategies	• Successfully focuses on skills for an offensive or defensive game plan • Maintains team possession or effectively works to regain possession • Understands ones own space and responsibility and understands how it relates to the team	• Rarely violates rules while playing the game • Plays a flowing game • Uses specialized skills that integrate responsibilities with team members • Uses a variety of skills that can meet team objectives of maintaining possession or scoring
Football						
Basketball						
Volleyball						
Softball						
Soccer						
Badminton						
Tennis						

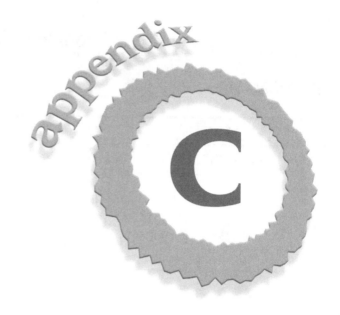

New York State Physical Fitness Norms

New York State Physical Fitness Norms: 7th Grade Fitness Conversion Table

BOYS

FITNESS LEVEL	PERCENTILE RANK	AGILITY (Side Step)	STRENGTH (Sit-ups)	SPEED (Shuttle Run)	ENDURANCE (Mile) 11 YRS	12 YRS	ACHIEVEMENT TOTAL	FITNESS LEVEL
10	99	25+	60+	18.5 or less	6.04-	5.4	33+	10
9	98	22-24	55-59	19	6.5	6.27	30-32	9
8	93	21	50-54	19.5-2.0	7.19	6.44	28-29	8
7	84	19-20	44-49	20.5-21	7.3	6.57	25-27	7
6	69	17-18	40-43	21.5-22	8.21	7.48	22-24	6
5	50	16	34-39	22.5	9.06	8.2	20-21	5
4	31	14-15	30-33	23	10.4	9.3	16-19	4
3	16	12-13	25-29	24-25	12.4	11.2	13-15	3
2	7	9-11	20-24	25.5-26.5	13.37	12.07	11-12	2
1	2	7-8	14-19	27-28	15.25	13.41	8-10	1
0	1	0-6	0-13	28.5			0-9	0

GIRLS

FITNESS LEVEL	PERCENTILE RANK	AGILITY (Side Step)	STRENGTH (Sit-ups)	SPEED (Shuttle Run)	ENDURANCE (Mile) 11 YRS	12 YRS	ACHIEVEMENT TOTAL	FITNESS LEVEL
10	99	23+	52+	16.5 or less	7.07	6.27	32+	10
9	98	21-22	46-51	17-18	7.46	7.26	30-31	9
8	93	19-20	41-45	18.5-20.5	8.1	7.44	27-29	8
7	84	18	36-40	21-22	8.36	8.05	25-26	7
6	69	16-17	32-35	22.5-23	9.44	9.08	22-24	6
5	50	15	28-31	23.5-24	10.27	9.47	19-21	5
4	31	13-14	23-37	24.5-25	11.51	11	16-18	4
3	16	11-12	18-22	25.5-26.5	13.16	12.35	13-15	3
2	7	9-10	12-17	27-28.5	14.41	13.34	10-12	2
1	2	7-8	11-14	30-31.5	16.56	14.46	8-9	1
0	1	0-6	0-10	32+			0-7	0

New York State Physical Fitness Norms: 8th Grade Fitness Conversion Tables

BOYS

FITNESS LEVEL	PERCENTILE RANK	AGILITY (Side Step)	STRENGTH (Sit-ups)	SPEED (Shuttle Run)	ENDURANCE (Mile) 13 YRS	ENDURANCE (Mile) 14 YRS	ACHIEVEMENT TOTAL	FITNESS LEVEL
10	99	26+	61+	18.5 or less	5.44	5.36	32+	10
9	98	24-25	56-60	19	6.11	5.51	30-31	9
8	93	22-23	51-55	19.5	6.22	6.05	28-29	8
7	84	20-21	46-50	20	6.33	6.13	25-27	7
6	69	18-19	42-45	20.5-21	7.06	6.48	22-24	6
5	50	17	37-41	21.5-22	7.27	7.1	19-21	5
4	31	15-16	32-36	22.5-23	8.24	7.54	16-18	4
3	16	13-14	27-31	23.5-24	9.09	8.43	13-15	3
2	7	10-12	21-26	24.5-25.5	9.39	9.3	10-12	2
1	2	7-9	15-20	26-27.5	10.23	10.32	7-9	1
0	1	0-6	0-14	28 or more			0-6	0

GIRLS

FITNESS LEVEL	PERCENTILE RANK	AGILITY (Side Step)	STRENGTH (Sit-ups)	SPEED (Shuttle Run)	ENDURANCE (Mile) 13 YRS	ENDURANCE (Mile) 14 YRS	ACHIEVEMENT TOTAL	FITNESS LEVEL
10	99	23+	56+	16 or less	6.2	6.44	32+	10
9	98	21-22	50-55	16.5-18	7.1	7.18	30-31	9
8	93	20	43-49	18.5-20.5	7.45	7.39	27-29	8
7	84	18-19	39-42	21-21.5	8.01	8.1	25-26	7
6	69	17	35-38	22-22.5	8.41	9.1	22-24	6
5	50	16	31-34	23-23.5	9.27	10.05	19-21	5
4	31	14-15	26-30	24-25	10.31	12.05	16-18	4
3	16	11-13	21-25	25.5-26.5	12.20	14.07	14-15	3
2	7	9-10	16-20	27-28	13.09	15.25	11-13	2
1	2	7-8	12-15	28.5-29.5	14.55	16.22	8-10	1
0	1	0-6	0-11	30 or longer			0-7	0

New York State Physical Fitness Norms: 9th Grade Fitness Conversion Tables

BOYS

FITNESS LEVEL	PERCENTILE RANK	AGILITY (Side Step)	STRENGTH (Sit-ups)	SPEED (Shuttle Run)	ENDURANCE (Mile) 14 YRS	15 YRS	ACHIEVEMENT TOTAL	FITNESS LEVEL
10	99	27+	62+	18.5	5.36	5.44	33+	10
9	98	26	58-61	19	5.51	6.01	31-32	9
8	93	22-25	53-57	19.5	6.05	6.08	29-30	8
7	84	21	48-52	20	6.13	6.18	25-27	7
6	69	19-20	44-47	20.5	6.48	6.56	22-24	6
5	50	18	40-43	21-21.5	7.1	7.14	19-21	5
4	31	16-17	35-39	22-23	7.54	7.52	16-18	4
3	16	14-15	31-34	23.5-24	8.43	8.48	13-15	3
2	7	10-13	24-30	24.5-25.5	9.3	9.25	11-12	2
1	2	9-9	20-23	26-27.5	10.32	10.37	9-10	1
0	1	0-7	0-19	28 or longer			0-7	0

GIRLS

FITNESS LEVEL	PERCENTILE RANK	AGILITY (Side Step)	STRENGTH (Sit-ups)	SPEED (Shuttle Run)	ENDURANCE (Mile) 14 YRS	15 YRS	ACHIEVEMENT TOTAL	FITNESS LEVEL
10	99	24+	54+	16 or shorter	6.44	6.36	32	10
9	98	23	48-53	16.5-18	7.18	7.39	30-31	9
8	93	21-22	43-47	18.5-20.5	7.39	8.01	28-29	8
7	84	19-20	39-42	21-21.5	7.54	8.1	25-27	7
6	69	18	34-38	22-22.5	8.37	9.1	22-24	6
5	50	16-17	29-33	23-23.5	9.35	10.05	19-21	5
4	31	14-15	24-28	24-25	11.11	12.05	16-18	4
3	16	12-13	20-23	25.5-26.5	13.56	14.07	13-15	3
2	7	10-11	14-19	27-28	15.20	15.25	10-12	2
1	2	8-9	10-13	28.5-29.5	16.59	16.22	9-9	1
0	1	0-7	0-9	30 or longer			0-7	0

New York State Physical Fitness Norms:
10th Grade Fitness Conversion Tables

BOYS

FITNESS LEVEL	PERCENTILE RANK	AGILITY (Side Step)	STRENGTH (Sit-ups)	SPEED (Shuttle Run)	ENDURANCE (Mile)		ACHIEVEMENT TOTAL	FITNESS LEVEL
					15 YRS	16 YRS		
10	99	27+	63+	18.5 or less	5.44	5.4	33+	10
9	98	25-26	59-62	19	6.01	5.48	31-32	9
8	93	24	53-58	19.5	6.08	6.02	29-30	8
7	84	22-23	50-52	20	6.18	6.12	26-27	7
6	69	20-21	44-49	20.5	6.56	6.47	22-25	6
5	50	18-19	40-43	21	7.14	7.11	19-21	5
4	31	16-17	35-39	21.5-22	7.52	7.51	16-18	4
3	16	14-15	31-34	22.5-23.5	8.48	9.1	13-14	3
2	7	11-13	26-30	24-25.5	9.25	9.52	10-12	2
1	2	9-10	22-25	26-27	10.37	10.40	7-9	1
0	1	0-8	0-21	27.5			0-6	0

GIRLS

FITNESS LEVEL	PERCENTILE RANK	AGILITY (Side Step)	STRENGTH (Sit-ups)	SPEED (Shuttle Run)	ENDURANCE (Mile)		ACHIEVEMENT TOTAL	FITNESS LEVEL
					15 YRS	16 YRS		
10	99	25+	58+	20.5 or less	6.36	6.33	34+	10
9	98	24	47-52	21	7.39	7.07	31-33	9
8	93	21-23	42-46	21.5	8.01	7.47	29-30	8
7	84	19-20	39-41	22	8.1	8.13	25-27	7
6	69	18	33-37	22.5-23.5	9.1	9.52	22-24	6
5	50	16-17	30-32	24-24.5	10.05	10.45	19-21	5
4	31	14-15	25-29	25-26	12.05	12.32	16-18	4
3	16	12-13	21-24	26.5-28	14.07	14.49	13-15	3
2	7	10-11	15-20	28.5-29.5	15.25	15.02	11-12	2
1	2	8-9	11-14	30-31.5	16.22	15.3	9-10	1
0	1	0-7	0-10	32			0-8	0

New York State Physical Fitness Norms:
11th Grade Fitness Conversion Tables

BOYS

FITNESS LEVEL	PERCENTILE RANK	AGILITY (Side Step)	STRENGTH (Sit-ups)	SPEED (Shuttle Run)	ENDURANCE (Mile) 16 YEARS OLD	ACHIEVEMENT TOTAL	FITNESS LEVEL
10	99	29+	66+	18 or less	5.4	33+	10
9	98	26-28	60-65	18.5	5.48	30-32	9
8	93	24-25	53-59	19	6.02	28-29	8
7	84	22-23	50-54	19.5	6.12	25-27	7
6	69	21	46-49	20	6.47	22-24	6
5	50	19-20	41-45	20.5-21	7.11	19-21	5
4	31	17-18	36-40	21.5-22	7.51	16-18	4
3	16	15-16	32-35	22.5-23	9.1	13-15	3
2	7	12-14	27-41	23.5-24.5	9.52	10-12	2
1	2	9-11	23-26	25-26.5	10.4	7-9	1
0	1	0-8	0-22	27+		0-6	

GIRLS

FITNESS LEVEL	PERCENTILE RANK	AGILITY (Side Step)	STRENGTH (Sit-ups)	SPEED (Shuttle Run)	ENDURANCE (Mile) 16 YEARS OLD	ACHIEVEMENT TOTAL	FITNESS LEVEL
10	99	25+	53+	19.5 or faster	6.33	34+	10
9	98	24	47-52	20-20.5	7.07	31-33	9
8	93	21-23	42-46	21-21.5	7.47	28-30	8
7	84	20	38-41	22	8.13	25-27	7
6	69	18-19	33-37	22.5-23	9.52	22-24	6
5	50	16-17	30-32	24-24.5	10.45	19-21	5
4	31	15	25-29	25-26	12.32	16-18	4
3	16	12-14	21-24	26.5-27.5	14.49	13-15	3
2	7	10-11	15-20	28-29.5	15.02	11-12	2
1	2	8-9	11-14	30-31	15.3	8-10	1
0	1	0-7	0-10	31.5+		0-7	0

New York State Physical Fitness Norms:
12th Grade Fitness Conversion Tables

BOYS

FITNESS LEVEL	PERCENTILE RANK	AGILITY (Side Step)	STRENGTH (Sit-ups)	SPEED (Shuttle Run)	ENDURANCE (Mile) 17 YRS.	ACHIEVEMENT TOTAL	FITNESS LEVEL
10	99	29+	70+	17.5 or less	5.42	35+	10
9	98	27-28	63-69	18	5.48	31-34	9
8	93	25-26	57-62	19.5	6.02	29-30	8
7	84	23-24	51-56	19-19.5	6.12	25-27	7
6	69	21-22	47-50	20	6.47	22-24	6
5	50	20	42-46	20.5	7.11	19-21	5
4	31	18-19	38-41	21-21.5	7.51	16-18	4
3	16	15-17	33-37	22-22.5	9.1	13-15	3
2	7	13-14	29-32	23-24	9.52	10-12	2
1	2	10-12	23-28	24.5-25.5	10.4	7-9	1
0	1	0-9	0-22	26 or longer		0-6	0

GIRLS

FITNESS LEVEL	PERCENTILE RANK	AGILITY (Side Step)	STRENGTH (Sit-ups)	SPEED (Shuttle Run)	ENDURANCE (Mile) 16 YEARS OLD	ACHIEVEMENT TOTAL	FITNESS LEVEL
10	99	26+	54+	19.0 or less	6.54	35+	10
9	98	24-25	49-53	19.5-20	7.26	32-34	9
8	93	22-23	44-48	20.5-21.5	8.08	29-31	8
7	84	20-21	39-43	22	8.28	25-27	7
6	69	18-19	34-38	22.5-23.5	9.41	22-24	6
5	50	16-17	30-33	24-24.5	9.47	19-21	5
4	31	15	25-29	25-26	10.5	16-18	4
3	16	13-14	21-24	26.5-27.5	12.5	13-15	3
2	7	10-12	16-20	28-29.5	13.05	10-12	2
1	2	8-9	12-15	30-31	15.24	8-9	1
0	1	0-7	0-11	31.5 or more		0-7	0

About the Author

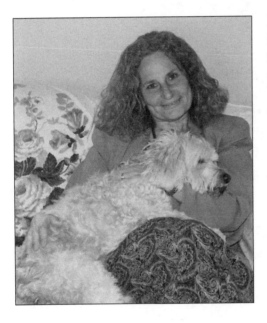

Isobel R. Kleinman has more than 30 years' experience teaching at the junior and senior high school levels, writing curricula, and supervising extracurricular activities. She has coached junior high soccer, field hockey, volleyball, basketball, tennis, gymnastics, archery, track and field, and softball, and she created and ran a performing arts dance group. She holds a BSE from the State University of New York College at Cortland, an MSE from New York City's Queens College, and an NYS Professional Certificate of School Psychology. She is a member of the American Alliance for Health, Physical Education, Recreation and Dance.

Throughout her teaching career, Kleinman has kept abreast of current trends and developed new programs in response to student interest. With the exception of team handball and wrestling, she has personally taught every unit presented in this text. Her well-rounded program provides depth and encourages multifaceted goals so that each student finds at least one place to shine.

Kleinman lives in Flushing, New York. In her leisure time, she enjoys playing tennis and a little golf, dancing socially, attending cultural performances, reading, and traveling around the world—sometimes on a bike.

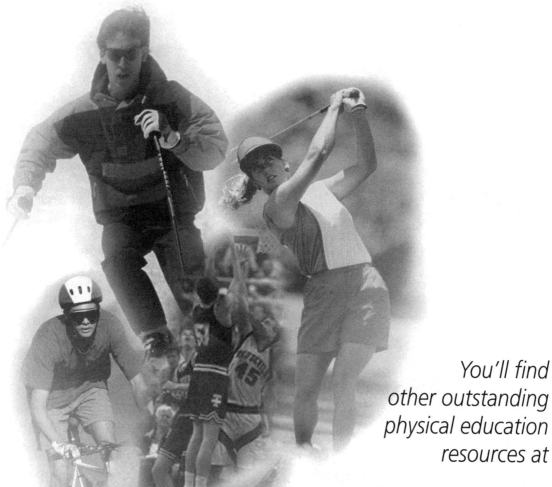